A·N·N·U·A·L EDI·T·I·O·N·S

Nutrition

06/07

Eighteenth Edition

D1514739

EDITOR
Dorothy Klimis-Zacas
University of Maine, Orono

Dorothy Klimis-Zacas is a Professor of Clinical Nutrition at the University of Maine and cooperating professor of nutrition and dietetics at Harokopio University, Athens, Greece. She teaches undergraduate and graduate classes in nutrition and its relation to health and disease for students of dietetics, nurses, and physicians.

Her current research interests relate to basic investigations in the area of trace mineral nutrition and its role in the development of atherosclerosis and to applied investigations that utilize nutritional interventions to reduce cardiovascular disease risk in adolescents both in the United States and in the Mediterranean region.

A Ph.D. and Fullbright Fellow, Dr. Klimis-Zacas is the author of numerous research articles and the editor of two books, *Manganese in Health and Disease* and the recently published second edition of *Nutritional Concerns for Women*. She is a member of Sigma Delta Epsilon, The American Society of Nutritional Sciences, The International Atherosclerosis Society, the American Dietetic Association, The Society for Nutrition Education, and The American Heart Association.

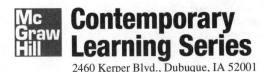
Contemporary Learning Series
2460 Kerper Blvd., Dubuque, IA 52001

Visit us on the Internet
http://www.mhcls.com

Credits

1. **Nutrition Trends**
   Unit photo—© Getty Images/PhotoLink/C. Sherburne
2. **Nutrients**
   Unit photo—The McGraw-Hill Companies, Inc./Tara McDermott
3. **Diet and Disease: Through the Life Span**
   Unit photo—© Getty Images/PhotoLink/S. Pearce
4. **Obesity and Weight Control**
   Unit photo—© Getty Images/Digital Vision
5. **Health Claims**
   Unit photo—© The McGraw-Hill Companies, Inc./Jill Braaten
6. **Food Safety/Technology**
   Unit photo—© Royalty Free/CORBIS
7. **World Hunger and Malnutrition**
   Unit photo—Photograph courtesy of USAID

Copyright

Cataloging in Publication Data
Main entry under title: Annual Editions: Nutrition. 2006/2007.
1. Nutrition—Periodicals. I. Klimis-Zacas, Dorothy, *comp*. II. Title: Nutrition.
ISBN-13: 978–0–07–351543–4   ISBN-10: 0–07–351543–4   658'.05   ISSN 1055–6990

Eighteenth Edition

Cover image © Photos.com and C. Sherburne/PhotoLink/Getty Images
Printed in the United States of America   1234567890QPDQPD9876   Printed on Recycled Paper

Editors/Advisory Board

Members of the Advisory Board are instrumental in the final selection of articles for each edition of ANNUAL EDITIONS. Their review of articles for content, level, currentness, and appropriateness provides critical direction to the editor and staff. We think that you will find their careful consideration well reflected in this volume.

Preface

In publishing ANNUAL EDITIONS we recognize the enormous role played by the magazines, newspapers, and journals of the public press in providing current, first-rate educational information in a broad spectrum of interest areas. Many of these articles are appropriate for students, researchers, and professionals seeking accurate, current material to help bridge the gap between principles and theories and the real world. These articles, however, become more useful for study when those of lasting value are carefully collected, organized, indexed, and reproduced in a low-cost format, which provides easy and permanent access when the material is needed. That is the role played by ANNUAL EDITIONS.

Since nutrition is an evolving science, it necessitates updating *Annual Editions: Nutrition* annually to keep up with the plethora of topics and controversies raised in the field. The main goal of this anthology is to provide the reader with up-to-date information by presenting current topics of information based on scientific evidence. *Annual Editions: Nutrition* also presents controversial topics in a balanced and unbiased manner. Where appropriate, international perspectives are presented in this book. We hope that the reader will develop critical thinking and be empowered to ask questions and to seek answers.

We are presently experiencing an obesity and diabetes epidemic with detrimental effects on the health of adults, of children, and teens. Globalization and the role a few mega-food companies play in providing consumers with products high in fat and added sugars along with the increased caloric intake from large portion sizes and reduction of activity have all contributed to the onset of the above degenerative diseases. In third world countries, obesity now coexists with hunger and malnutrition. Actually, the World Health Organization in its recent report on "Diet, Nutrition and the Prevention of Chronic Diseases" questions the role and contribution of global companies in the increasing incidence of obesity in developing countries.

The decoding of the genome has heralded the area of Nutrigenomics, which has enabled us to appreciate the interactions between genotype and nutrition and the effect of nutrients on gene expression. Thus the era of custom-made diets rather than "one diet fits all" was ushered to the forefront. This revolution will affect the way we diagnose and treat disease, design dietary interventions to reduce risk, and set nutrient requirements among many others. In fact the updated USDA Food Guide Pyramid uses the concept of personalization as its basis for making healthy and tasty choices for individuals.

"Nutrition experts" and "health advisors" seem to appear everywhere. We are at the parapet of a revolution in information technology and of nutritional research. Information is distributed at a very fast pace, across continents, and without consideration of country borders. Thus, informing the consumer regularly with reliable and current nutrition information is the duty of the professional.

Annual Editions: Nutrition 06/07 is to be used as a companion to a standard nutrition text so that it may update, expand, or emphasize certain topics that are covered in the text or present totally new topics not covered in a standard text.

To accomplish this, *Annual Editions: Nutrition 06/07* is composed of seven units that review current knowledge and controversies in the area of nutrition. The first unit describes current trends in the field of nutrition in the United States and the rest of the world, including the new dietary guidelines for the United States and the updated USDA Food Guide Pyramid. Units two, three, and four include topics that focus on nutrients and their relationship to health and disease, recent research finding on the role nutrients play in degenerative disease and the obesity epidemic. Unit five and six cover topics on health claims and focus on food safety, including subjects about which consumers are misinformed and are thus vulnerable to quackery. Finally, unit seven focuses on world hunger and malnutrition, including environmental sustainability and biotechnology. A topic guide will assist the reader in finding other articles on a given subject and World Wide Web sites will help in further exploring a particular topic.

Your input is most valuable to improve this anthology which we update yearly. We would appreciate your comments and suggestions as you review the current edition.

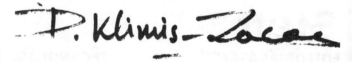

Dorothy Klimis-Zacas

Editor

Contents

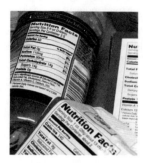

UNIT 1
Nutrition Trends

The concepts in bold italics are developed in the article. For further expansion, please refer to the Topic Guide and the Index.

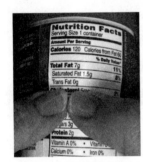

UNIT 2
Nutrients

The concepts in bold italics are developed in the article. For further expansion, please refer to the Topic Guide and the Index.

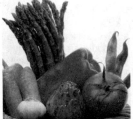

UNIT 3
Diet and Disease Through the Life Span

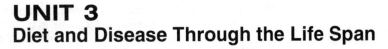

The concepts in bold italics are developed in the article. For further expansion, please refer to the Topic Guide and the Index.

UNIT 4
Obesity and Weight Control

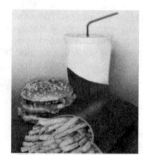

The concepts in bold italics are developed in the article. For further expansion, please refer to the Topic Guide and the Index.

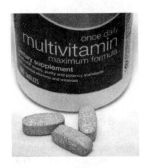

UNIT 5
Health Claims

The concepts in bold italics are developed in the article. For further expansion, please refer to the Topic Guide and the Index.

UNIT 6
Food Safety/Technology

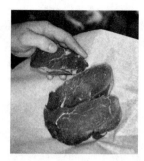

The concepts in bold italics are developed in the article. For further expansion, please refer to the Topic Guide and the Index.

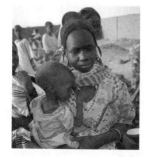

UNIT 7
World Hunger and Malnutrition

The concepts in bold italics are developed in the article. For further expansion, please refer to the Topic Guide and the Index.

The concepts in bold italics are developed in the article. For further expansion, please refer to the Topic Guide and the Index.

Topic Guide

This topic guide suggests how the selections in this book relate to the subjects covered in your course. You may want to use the topics listed on these pages to search the Web more easily.

On the following pages a number of Web sites have been gathered specifically for this book. They are arranged to reflect the units of this *Annual Edition.* You can link to these sites by going to the student online support site at *http://www.mhcls.com/online/.*

ALL THE ARTICLES THAT RELATE TO EACH TOPIC ARE LISTED BELOW THE BOLD-FACED TERM.

Adolescents
1. The Changing American Diet: A Report Card

Age related eye disorders
16. Feast For Your Eyes: Nutrients That May Help Save Your Sight

Allergies
23. Allergen Control
57. Assessment of Allergenic Potential of Genetically Modified Foods: An Agenda for Future Research

Attitudes and knowledge
1. The Changing American Diet: A Report Card
4. Healthier Eating
5. 10 Megatrends in the Supermarket
6. 51 Healthy Foods You Can Say "Yes" To
7. Getting Personal with Nutrition
8. The Slow Food Movement Picks Up Speed
9. Who's Filling Your Grocery Bag?
10. Moving Towards Healthful Sustainable Diets

Biotechnology
18. Fortifying with Fiber

Carbohydrates
14. Good Carbs, Bad Carbs

Children
24. Meeting Children's Nutritional Needs
26. The Role of the School Nutrition Environment for Promoting the Health of Young Adolescents

Controversies
28. Still Hungry? Fattening Revelations—and New Mysteries—About the Hunger Hormone
29. Eat More Weigh Less
36. Herbal Foods: Are They Efficacious and Safe?
37. Herbal Lottery
40. Are Your Supplements Safe?
41. Food Colorings: Pigments Make Fruits and Veggies Extra Healthful

Coronary heart disease
11. Omega-3 Choices: Fish or Flax?
13. Beyond Calcium: The Protective Attributes of Dairy Products and Their Constituents
20. Metabolic Syndrome: Time for Action
22. Coffee, Spices, Wine: New Dietary Ammo Against Diabetes?
35. Nutraceuticals & Functional Foods
38. The Latest Scoop on Soy
39. Multiple Choices: The Right Vitamins For You

Diabetes
14. Good Carbs, Bad Carbs
20. Metabolic Syndrome: Time for Action
21. The Magnesium-Diabetes Connection
22. Coffee, Spices, Wine: New Dietary Ammo Against Diabetes?

39. Multiple Choices: The Right Vitamins For You

Diet and disease
13. Beyond Calcium: The Protective Attributes of Dairy Products and Their Constituents
14. Good Carbs, Bad Carbs
15. Are You Getting Enough of This Vitamin?
16. Feast For Your Eyes: Nutrients That May Help Save Your Sight
17. Get the Lead Out, What You Don't Know *Can* Hurt You
19. Diet and Genes
20. Metabolic Syndrome: Time for Action
21. The Magnesium-Diabetes Connection
22. Coffee, Spices, Wine: New Dietary Ammo Against Diabetes?
23. Allergen Control
24. Meeting Children's Nutritional Needs
25. No One to Blame

Diet and genes
7. Getting Personal with Nutrition
19. Diet and Genes

Fats and substitutes
11. Omega-3 Choices: Fish or Flax?
12. Revealing Trans Fats
44. Hooked on Fish? There Might Be Some Catches

Fiber
18. Fortifying with Fiber

Food
1. The Changing American Diet: A Report Card
8. The Slow Food Movement Picks Up Speed
18. Fortifying with Fiber
34. Using Nutrition-Related Claims to Build a Healthful Diet
35. Nutraceuticals & Functional Foods
42. Certified Organic
43. Send in the Clones
44. Hooked on Fish? There Might Be Some Catches
46. Suspect Produce: How To Be Safe From Contaminated Fruits; Vegetables

Food labeling
43. Send in the Clones

Food safety and technology
40. Are Your Supplements Safe?
41. Food Colorings: Pigments Make Fruits and Veggies Extra Healthful
42. Certified Organic
43. Send in the Clones
44. Hooked on Fish? There Might Be Some Catches
45. Seafood Safety: Is Something Fishy Going On?
46. Suspect Produce: How To Be Safe From Contaminated Fruits; Vegetables
47. Ensuring the Safety of Dietary Supplements
57. Assessment of Allergenic Potential of Genetically Modified Foods: An Agenda for Future Research

Internet References

The following internet sites have been carefully researched and selected to support the articles found in this reader. The easiest way to access these selected sites is to go to our student online support site at *http://www.mhcls.com/online/*.

AE: Nutrition 06/07

The following sites were available at the time of publication. Visit our Web site—we update our student online support site regularly to reflect any changes.

General Sources

American Dietetic Association
http://www.eatright.org

This consumer link to nutrition and health includes resources, news, marketplace, search for a dietician, government information, and a gateway to related sites. The site includes a tip of the day and special features.

The Blonz Guide to Nutrition
http://www.blonz.com

The categories in this valuable site report news in the fields of nutrition, food science, foods, fitness, and health. There is also a selection of search engines and links.

CSPI: Center for Science in the Public Interest
http://www.cspinet.org

CSPI is a nonprofit education and advocacy organization that is committed to improving the safety and nutritional quality of our food supply. CSPI publishes the *Nutrition Action Healthletter,* which has monthly information about food.

Institute of Food Technologists
http://www.ift.org

This site of the Society for Food Science and Technology is full of important information and news about every aspect of the food products that come to market.

International Food Information Council Foundation (IFIC)
http://ific.org

IFIC's purpose is to be the link between science and communications by offering the latest scientific information on food safety, nutrition, and health in a form that is understandable and useful for opinion leaders and consumers to access.

U.S. National Institutes of Health (NIH)
http://www.nih.gov

Consult this site for links to extensive health information and scientific resources. Comprised of 24 separate institutes, centers, and divisions, the NIH is one of eight health agencies of the Public Health Service, which, in turn, is part of the U.S. Department of Health and Human Services.

UNIT 1: Nutrition Trends

Food Science and Human Nutrition Extension
http://www.fshn.uiuc.edu/

This extensive Iowa State University site links to latest news and reports, consumer publications, food safety information, and many other useful nutrition-related sites.

Food Guide Pyramid
http://www.foodguidepyramid.gov/

Visit this Web site and find out your daily needs for kilocalories and for protein intake.

Food Surveys Research Group
http://www.barc.usda.gov/bhnrc/foodsurvey/home.htm

Visit this site of the Beltsville Human Nutrition Research Center Food Surveys research group first, and then click on USDA to keep up with nutritional news and information.

UNIT 2: Nutrients

Dole 5 A Day: Nutrition, Fruits & Vegetables
http://www.dole5aday.com

The Dole Food Company, a founding member of the "National 5 A Day for Better Health Program," offers this site to entice children into taking an interest in proper nutrition.

Food and Nutrition Information Center
http://www.nal.usda.gov/fnic/

Use this site to find dietary and nutrition information provided by various USDA agencies and to find links to food and nutrition resources on the Internet.

Nutrient Data Laboratory
http://www.nal.usda.gov/fnic/foodcomp/

Information about the USDA Nutrient Database can be found on this site. Search here for answers to FAQs, a glossary of terms, facts about food composition, and useful links.

NutritionalSupplements.com
http://www.nutritionalsupplements.com

This source provides unbiased information about nutritional supplements and prescription drugs, submitted by consumers with no vested interest in the products.

U.S. National Library of Medicine
http://www.nlm.nih.gov

This site permits you to search databases and electronic information sources such as MEDLINE, learn about research projects, and keep up on nutrition-related news.

Fish Contamination Resource
www.epa.gov/waterscience/fishadvice/advice.html

This Environmental Protection Agency website gives the latest information on fish contamination issues.

UNIT 3: Diet and Disease Through the Life Span

American Cancer Society
http://www.cancer.org

Open this site and its various links to learn the concerns and lifestyle advice of the American Cancer Society. It provides information on alternative therapies, tobacco, other Web resources, and more.

American Heart Association (AHA)
http://www.americanheart.org

The AHA offers this site to provide the most comprehensive information on heart disease and stroke as well as late-breaking news. The site presents facts on warning signs, a reference guide, and explanations of diseases and treatments.

The Food Allergy and Anaphylaxis Network

http://www.foodallergy.org

The Food Allergy Network site, which welcomes consumers, health professionals, and reporters, includes product alerts and updates, information about food allergies, daily tips, and links to other sites.

Heinz Infant & Toddler Nutrition

http://www.heinzbaby.com

An educational section full of nutritional information and meal-planning guides for parents and caregivers as well as articles and reviews by leading pediatricians and nutritionists can be found on this page.

LaLeche League International

http://www.lalecheleague.org

Important information to mothers who are contemplating breast feeding can be accessed at this Web site. Links to other sites are also possible.

UNIT 4: Obesity and Weight Control

American Anorexia Bulimia Association/National Eating Disorders Association (AABA)

http://www.nationaleatingdisorders.org/

The AABA is a nonprofit organization of concerned people dedicated to the prevention and treatment of eating disorders. It offers many services, including help lines, referral networks, school outreach, support groups, and prevention programs.

American Society of Exercise Physiologists (ASEP)

http://www.asep.org/

The goal of the ASEP is to promote health and physical fitness. This extensive site provides links to publications related to exercise and career opportunities in exercise physiology.

Calorie Control Council

http://www.caloriecontrol.org

The Calorie Control Council's Web site offers information on cutting calories, achieving and maintaining healthy weight, and low-calorie, reduced-fat foods and beverages.

Eating Disorders: Body Image Betrayal

http://www.bibri.com/home/index.htm

This extensive collection of links leads to information on compulsive eating, bulimia, anorexia, and other disorders.

Shape Up America!

http://www.shapeup.org

At the Shape Up America! Web site you will find the latest information about safe weight management, healthy eating, and physical fitness. Links include Support Center, Cyberkitchen, Media Center, Fitness Center, and BMI Center.

UNIT 5: Health Claims

Federal Trade Commission (FTC): Diet, Health & Fitness

http://www.ftc.gov/bcp/menu-health.htm

This site of the FTC on the Web offers consumer education rules and acts that include a wide range of subjects, from buying exercise equipment to virtual health "treatments."

Food and Drug Administration (FDA)

http://www.fda.gov/default.htm

The FDA presents this site that addresses products they regulate, current news and hot topics, safety alerts, product approvals, reference data, and general information and directions.

National Council Against Health Fraud (NCAHF)

http://www.ncahf.org

The NCAHF does business as the National Council for Reliable Health Information. At its Web page it offers links to other related sites, including Dr. Terry Polevoy's "Healthwatcher Net."

QuackWatch

http://www.quackwatch.com

Quackwatch Inc., a nonprofit corporation, provides this guide to examine health fraud. Data for intelligent decision making on health topics are also presented.

UNIT 6: Food Safety/Technology

American Council on Science and Health (ACSH)

http://www.acsh.org/food/

The ACSH addresses issues that are related to food safety here. In addition, issues on nutrition and fitness, alcohol, diseases, environmental health, medical care, lifestyle, and tobacco may be accessed on this site.

Centers for Disease Control and Prevention (CDC)

http://www.cdc.gov

The CDC offers this home page, from which you can obtain information about travelers' health, data related to disease control and prevention, and general nutritional and health information, publications, and more.

FDA Center for Food Safety and Applied Nutrition

http://vm.cfsan.fda.gov

It is possible to access everything from this Web site that you might want to know about food safety and what government agencies are doing to ensure it.

Food Safety Project (FSP)

http://www.extension.iastate.edu/foodsafety/

This site from the Cooperative Extension Service at North Carolina State University has a database designed to promote food safety education via the Internet.

National Food Safety Programs

http://vm.cfsan.fda.gov/~dms/fs-toc.html

Data from the Food and Drug Administration, U.S. Department of Agriculutre, Environmental Protection Agency, and Centers for

Disease Control and Prevention expanding on the government policies and initiatives regarding food safety are presented on this site.

USDA Food Safety and Inspection Service (FSIS)
http://www.fsis.usda.gov

The FSIS, part of the U.S. Department of Agriculture, is the government agency "responsible for ensuring that the nation's commercial supply of meat, poultry, and egg products is safe, wholesome, and correctly labeled and packaged."

UNIT 7: World Hunger and Malnutrition

Population Reference Bureau
http://www.prb.org

A key source for global population information, this is a good place to pursue data on nutrition problems worldwide.

World Health Organization (WHO)
http://www.who.int/en/

This home page of the World Health Organization will provide you with links to a wealth of statistical and analytical information about health and nutrition around the world.

WWW Virtual Library: Demography & Population Studies
http://demography.anu.edu.au/VirtualLibrary/

A multitude of important links to information about global poverty and hunger can be found here.

We highly recommend that you review our Web site for expanded information and our other product lines. We are continually updating and adding links to our Web site in order to offer you the most usable and useful information that will support and expand the value of your Annual Editions. You can reach us at: *http://www.mhcls.com/annualeditions/*.

UNIT 1
Nutrition Trends

Unit Selections

Key Points to Consider

- Name some changes that have occurred in the American diet since the 1970s.

- How are you going to ensure that you are eating a healthful and sustainable diet?

- What are some of the ethical questions in the application of Nutrigenomics?

- What changes can you make in your diet, cooking, and life-style in general to be in agreement with the objectives of the Slow Food movement?

Student Website

www.mhcls.com/online

Internet References

Further information regarding these websites may be found in this book's preface or online.

Food Science and Human Nutrition Extension
http://www.fshn.uiuc.edu/

Food Guide Pyramid
http://www.foodguidepyramid.gov/

Food Surveys Research Group
http://www.barc.usda.gov/bhnrc/foodsurvey/home.htm

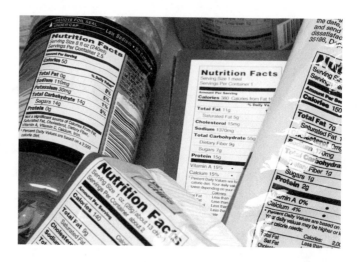

Consumers worldwide are bombarded daily with messages about nutrients and health. The first unit describes current trends and developments in the field of nutrition, the updated USDA Food Guide Pyramid and Dietary Guidelines for Americans, and offers practical advice for their application. Additionally, it presents the importance of personalizing nutrition based on the recent advances in the area of Nutrigenomics. Furthermore, it acquaints the reader with supermarket megatrends and explores the role that the food industry, agribusiness, and other special interest groups and institutions play in the increasing incidence of obesity.

The first article describes how Americans are doing with their eating. Compared to the decade of the 1970's, Americans are now eating more cheeses and breads, chicken and vegetables but have also increased their soda consumption dramatically. The good news is that they have decreased beef and whole milk consumption. This unit also addresses the challenges nutritionists face in educating consumers toward healthful sustainable diets that will not only improve quality of life but will also benefit the environment and support local agriculture.

Americans can refer to the updated USDA Food Guide Pyramid and the 2005 US Dietary Guidelines for guidance to construct a healthy diet. Personalizing your diet based on your age, gender and your activity is the focus of the 2005 Food Guide Pyramid. Physical activity and weight management, increasing consumption of fruits and vegetables to ensure adequate levels of antioxidant vitamins, minerals and fiber are the main focal points of the new Dietary Guidelines. Guidance on how to apply the Dietary Guidelines by controlling portion sizes, reading labels, and making lower fat choices among others are offered.

The decoding of the genome has revolutionized the way we think about the role of nutrition in health and disease and has influenced the focus of the updated USDA Food Guide Pyramid. The readiness and acceptability of Americans for personalized nutrition and the ethical issues that accompany nutrigenomics is discussed.

The monopoly large-food companies have on the kind of food we eat and our wallet is tremendous. Most snack foods are loaded with salt, sugar, and fat—and a big percent of Americans' food dollars goes there. So, not only personal behavior but also mega snack companies contribute to the obesity epidemic.

Thankfully, consumers are becoming aware of the relationship between nutrition and health and have started to demand healthier products. In response food companies quickly filled the supermarket shelves with whole-grain products, foods with less sugar and trans-fat and more functional fiber. Questions to ask before you buy these new products are raised in one of the articles.

Still, most Americans think that eating certain types of food while avoiding others is more critical to weight management than reducing their portion sizes and thus caloric intake. One of the articles discusses the role packaging, size, and shape of containers has in influencing consumers' buying decisions and their impression that they eat less than they actually do.

Fast food, convenience cuisine, and fast-life pace was the cause of the emergence of the Slow Food movement whose mission is based on buying fresh, local produce; slowing down to cook and enjoy the taste of food; and preserving traditional foods and ways of cooking. An article published in Today's Dietitian, describes how the Slow Food movement is being introduced to culinary arts and school wellness programs.

The importance and immediacy of nutritionists educating consumers toward a healthful diet that will benefit the environment, support local economy and agriculture, and prevent disease is discussed in the last article of this unit by Joan Gassow a professor of Nutrition at Columbia and a homesteader.

The Changing American Diet

A Report Card

BY BONNIE LIEBMAN

What are Americans eating? Are we turning towards vegetarian diets or indulging in more steak? Are we getting fat on fat-free ice cream, cake, and cookies or rewarding ourselves with fat-laden cheesecake, ice cream, and pastries? Are we eating more fruits and vegetables or more french fries?

Since the early 1900s, the U.S. Department of Agriculture has been tracking the amount of food available for Americans to eat. (The numbers over-estimate what we actually swallow, since some food never gets sold, some spoils, and some gets left on our plate. But they're valid for year-to-year comparisons.)

Every few years, we use that data to size up the American diet. The "grades" look not just at what we're eating, but whether we're moving in the right direction. Here's our latest report card.

Beverages: D

In 1977, soda became the most popular American beverage, and it never looked back. We now drink roughly 50 gallons of soda per person per year. And that doesn't include the eight gallons of uncarbonated soda that masquerades as "fruit" drinks. Of the healthier beverages—milk, fruit *juice*, and bottled water—only water is clearly climbing. The bottom line: The soft-drink industry keeps filling our ever-larger cups with its high-calorie sugar water, and we keep drinking as though there were no (bathroom scale to get on) tomorrow.

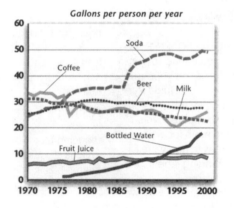

Gallons per person per year

Dairy Products: D

We're eating only slightly less ice cream than we did in 1970. And most of it is as fatty as it was 30 years ago (except for Ben & Jerry's and Häagen-Dazs, which are even fattier).

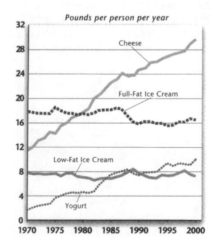

Pounds per person per year

As for cheese: The sky's the limit. We eat more than twice as much as we did in 1970. Cheese has now passed beef as our number-one source of saturated fat. Pizza and cheeseburgers started the trend back in the 1960s. But now cheese is everywhere: in your tacos and nachos, your soups and salads, your rice and potatoes, your chicken and fish… and your arteries.

Flour & Cereal: B

We're eating more flour than we did in the 1970s (in the U.S., flour means wheat). Some goes into breads, bagels, pasta, and pancakes; some ends up in cakes, cookies, Cinnabons, doughnuts, and other sweets.

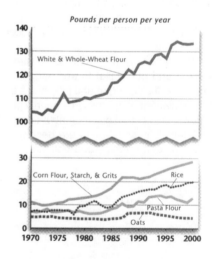

Pounds per person per year

Are all those carbs making us fat? You bet they are … along with all the fat, protein, and alcohol we scarf down. And only a tiny fraction of the wheat flour is whole-grain, the kind that may help lower the risk of heart disease and diabetes.

Added Fats & Oils: B

The big trends in fats and oils are clear: Since 1970, we've been eating slightly less butter and margarine, more shortening, and (much) more oil.

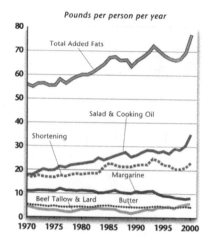

Pounds per person per year

Shortening, butter, and some margarines have saturated or trans fat, which clogs arteries. Oils don't. But all fats have calories...and that's one thing we don't need more of. Some people blame America's obesity epidemic on a low-fat diet (see "Big Fat Lies," November 2002). Can you find the low-fat diet on this graph?

Sweeteners: F

We now produce 152 pounds of added sugars each year for every man, woman, and child in America. That's 25 percent more than in 1970. Soft drinks account for a third of our intake. So-called "fruit" drinks supply another ten percent, while cookies, cakes, and other sweet baked goods contribute 14 percent (thank you, Mrs. Fields and Cinnabon). Candy, breakfast cereals, and ice cream each chip in about five percent. Does the tiny dip in 2000 signal the end of our runaway sweet tooth? Stay tuned.

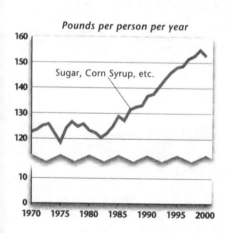

Pounds per person per year

Meat, Poultry, & Seafood: B

Beef and pork were neck-and-neck for the first half of the 20th century. But in the 1950s, beef started a steep climb that finally peaked in the mid-1970s. Chicken's growth keeps clucking along. But we still eat far more red meat (111 pounds per person) than poultry and seafood (83 pounds) each year.

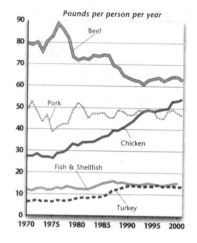

Pounds per person per year

Fruits & Vegetables: A

We're eating more fruits and vegetables than we did 30 years ago. On the upswing are bell peppers, broccoli, carrots, cucumbers, mushrooms, onions, spinach, squash, and tomatoes (but not brussels sprouts, cabbage, celery, or sweet potatoes). Also rising are bananas, grapes, mangos, melons, papayas, pears, pineapples and strawberries (but not apples, apricots, cherries, grapefruit, oranges, peaches, or plums). We still don't eat enough fruits and vegetables, but at least we're moving in the right direction.

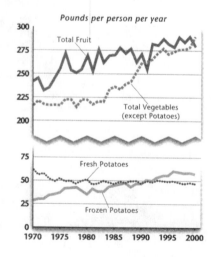

Pounds per person per year

Milk: C

Whole milk is down (that's good). So is reduced-fat (2 percent) milk (also good). But low-fat (1 percent) and skim (fat-free) aren't replacing the fattier milks. And we still drink more than twice as much of the two fattier milks than their two low-fat cousins.

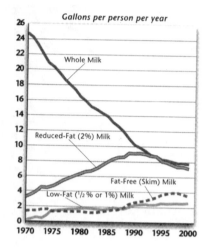

Gallons per person per year

Heather Jones DeMino helped compile the information for this article. Source: Economic Research Service, U.S. Department of Agriculture. (To access the U.S.D.A.'s per capita food consumption database on-line, go to www.ers.usda.gov/data/foodconsumption.)

---

pyramid power

THE FOOD GUIDE PYRAMID HAS A NEW LOOK. HERE'S HOW TO USE IT TO HELP YOU.

Libby Tucker

Each school day you face the same lunch dilemma: Soda or milk? Mystery meat or pizza? Choices abound, but how do you decide what to spend your money on? If only food came with directions.

Look no further than the new Food Guide Pyramid. Last spring, nutritionists at the U.S. Department of Agriculture (USDA) updated the old food pyramid with a new design that can help people make healthful—and tasty—choices.

"The message we have in the new pyramid is any positive change in the diet is wonderful," Jackie Haven, a nutritionist with the USDA, tells Choices. "Small steps over time is a way to build a healthy diet."

My Pyramid, as it's called, can be found on the Web site www.mypyramid.gov. The pyramid has a rainbow of vertical stripes instead of horizontal boxes, and it shows a figure running up the side. (See it at right.) The idea is to emphasize the importance of eating a variety of foods along with exercising.

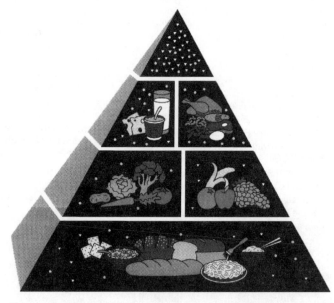

This is what the Food Guide Pyramid used to look like.

serving sizes	1-OUNCE SERVINGS OF GRAIN	1/2 CUP SERVING OF VEGGETABLES	1/2 CUP SERVING OF FRUIT	1 SERVING OF MILK
What's a serving size? For instance, if you're supposed to eat 7 ounces of grains a day, how much bread, pasta, or cereal equals 7 ounces? The list, shown at right, can help.	= 1 slice of bread	= 1 cup of raw leafy vegetables	= 1 medium apple	= 1 cup of fat-free or low-fat milk
	= 1 cup of breakfast cereal		= 1/4 cup of dried fruit	= 1 ounce of low-fat or fat-free cheese
	= 1/2 cup of cooked rice or pasta	= 1/2 cup of cut-up raw or cooked vegetables	= 1/2 cup of fresh, frozen, or canned fruit	= 1 cup of fat-free or low-fat yogurt

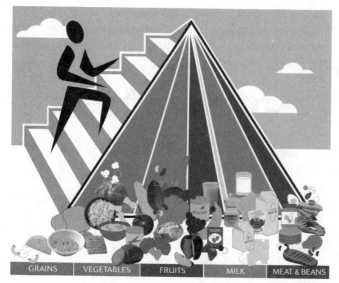

GRAINS | VEGETABLES | FRUITS | MILK | MEAT & BEANS

The new Food Guide Pyramid, shown above includes an exercise component. Each section in the pyramid represents one of the five basic food groups. (The smallest section is for oils and fats.) The bars on the left side are wider than those on the right side. A healthful meal includes more foods from the larger bars on the left, and fewer servings from the bars on the right.

"It's not just about what we choose to eat, it's also about what we do to be healthy," says Keith Ayoob, assistant professor of nutrition at Albert Einstein College of Medicine in New York.

Do you ever feel as if you're eating the same things over and over again? Well, you may be. Bread, pasta, meat, and cereal are staples of the American diet and they're all the same bland colors. Fruit and vegetables don't often make it to the dinner table.

your turn

My Pyramid is available online at www.mypyramid.gov. Log on and in the "My Pyramid Plan" box personalize the pyramid for yourself by typing in your age, gender, and the mount of exercise you get on most days. When you're done, ask yourself how you could improve your eating habits and exercise routine.

The different colored bars in the new pyramid give eaters one basic rule: "Make sure your plate has a lot of color on it, and that comes from fruits and vegetables," says Susan Moores, a nutritionist and spokesperson for the American Dietetic Association.

Each section in the pyramid represents one of the five basic food groups. For a healthful diet, you should eat foods from each group at every meal. You should also limit the amount of fats and oils in the foods you choose.

Some food groups, should take up a bigger portion on your plate. That's why the bars on the pyramid come in different sizes. The bars on the left side are wider than those on the right side. A healthful meal includes more foods from the larger bars on the left, and fewer servings of foods from those on the right.

Think of your plate as a pie cut into four pieces. Three of those pieces should come from grains, fruits, and vegetables; the fourth piece is the protein. "Visualize your plate coming from those kinds of foods for every meal," Moores says.

more serving size tips

■ A cup of food is about the size of a human fist.

□ Three ounces of meat or poultry or fish are about the size of a deck of cards.

■ Three ounces of meat are equal to two raw eggs.

□ One ounce of cheese is about the size of your thumb.

A big part of the pyramid is its exercise component. Teenagers should be physically active at least 60 minutes every day, according to the USDA. The more you exercise, the more calories your body needs to fuel that activity. That also means you can eat more. "If you're active, there's more wiggle room for things such as fats," Moores says.

Combining a healthful diet with exercise can have a powerful effect. Doctors have linked a healthful diet to brain power. Kids who eat well do better in school. Getting the proper nutrients also helps the body's immune system fight infection. Healthful eaters get ill less often and recover more quickly when they do get sick. And a good diet leads to shinier hair, brighter teeth, and healthier skin. "What you eat affects all cells in your body," Moores says.

A typical lunch for Rachel Davidson, 15, is a turkey sandwich, Goldfish crackers, and chocolate milk. It's a healthy lunch, but she knows she can do better. "I don't eat enough veggies and fruit," says Rachel, a ninth-grader at Roosevelt High School in Seattle, Washington. For many teens, evaluating their diets is a good first step toward better eating.

It's not hard to make changes to your diet, if you do it gradually. Drink milk instead of a soda for lunch one day. Have a salad instead of a hamburger. Eventually, you'll have a colorful plate again. "If people are eating mountains of french fries, I think they can swallow three broccoli florets," Ayoob says.

Dietary Guidelines for Americans 2005

Executive Summary

The *Dietary Guidelines for Americans [Dietary Guidelines]* provides science-based advice to promote health and to reduce risk for major chronic diseases through diet and physical activity. Major causes of morbidity and mortality in the United States are related to poor diet and a sedentary lifestyle. Some specific diseases linked to poor diet and physical inactivity include cardiovascular disease, type 2 diabetes, hypertension, osteoporosis, and certain cancers. Furthermore, poor diet and physical inactivity, resulting in an energy imbalance (more calories consumed than expended), are the most important factors contributing to the increase in overweight and obesity in this country. Combined with physical activity, following a diet that does not provide excess calories according to the recommendations in this document should enhance the health of most individuals.

An important component of each 5-year revision of the *Dietary Guidelines* is the analysis of new scientific information by the Dietary Guidelines Advisory Committee (DGAC) appointed by the Secretaries of the U.S. Department of Health and Human Services (HHS) and the U.S. Department of Agriculture (USDA). This analysis, published in the DGAC Report (http://www.health.gov/dietary guidelines/dga2005 /report/), is the primary resource for development of the report on the Guidelines by the Departments. The *Dietary Guidelines* and the report of the DGAC differ in scope and purpose compared to reports for previous versions of the *Guidelines*. The 2005 DGAC report is a detailed scientific analysis. The scientific report was used to develop the *Dietary Guidelines* jointly between the two Departments and forms the basis of recommendations that will be used by USDA and HHS for program and policy development. Thus it is a publication oriented toward policymakers, nutrition educators, nutritionists, and healthcare providers rather than to the general public, as with previous versions of the *Dietary Guidelines,* and contains more technical information.

The intent of the *Dietary Guidelines* is to summarize and synthesize knowledge regarding individual nutrients and food components into recommendations for a pattern of eating that can be adopted by the public. In this publication, Key Recommendations are grouped under nine inter-related focus areas. The recommendations are based on the preponderance of scientific evidence for lowering risk of chronic disease and promoting health. It is important to remember that these are integrated messages that should be implemented as a whole. Taken together, they encourage most Americans to eat fewer calories, be more active, and make wiser food choices.

A basic premise of the *Dietary Guidelines* is that nutrient needs should be met primarily through consuming foods. Foods provide an array of nutrients and other compounds that may have beneficial effects on health. In certain cases, fortified foods and dietary supplements may be useful sources of one or more nutrients that otherwise might be consumed in less than recommended amounts. However, dietary supplements, while recommended in some cases, cannot replace a healthful diet.

Two examples of eating patterns that exemplify the *Dietary Guidelines* are the USDA Food Guide (http://www.usda. gov/cnpp/pyramid.html) and the DASH (Dietary Approaches to Stop Hypertension) Eating Plan.[1] Both of these eating patterns are designed to integrate dietary recommendations into a healthy way to eat for most individuals. These eating patterns are not weight loss diets, but rather illustrative examples of how to eat in accordance with the *Dietary Guidelines*. Both eating patterns are constructed across a range of calorie levels to meet the needs of various age and gender groups. For the USDA Food Guide, nutrient content estimates for each food group and subgroup are based on population-weighted food intakes. Nutrient content estimates for the DASH Eating Plan are based on selected foods chosen for a sample 7-day menu. While originally developed to study the effects of an eating pattern on the prevention and treatment of hypertension, DASH is one example of a balanced eating plan consistent with the 2005 *Dietary Guidelines*.

Throughout most of this publication, examples use a 2,000-calorie level as a reference for consistency with the Nutrition Facts Panel. Although this level is used as a reference, recommended calorie intake will differ for individuals based on age, gender, and activity level. At each calorie level, individuals who eat nutrient-dense foods may be able to meet their recommended nutrient intake without consuming their full calorie allotment. The remaining calories—the *discretionary calorie allowance*—allow individuals flexibility to consume some foods and beverages that may contain added fats, added sugars, and alcohol.

The recommendations in the *Dietary Guidelines* are for Americans over 2 years of age. It is important to incorporate the food preferences of different racial/ethnic groups, vegetarians, and other groups when planning diets and developing educational programs and materials. The USDA Food Guide and the DASH Eating Plan are flexible enough to accommodate a range of food preferences and cuisines.

Taken together, [the *Dietary Guidelines*] encourage most Americans to eat fewer calories, be more active, and make wiser food choices.

The *Dietary Guidelines* is intended primarily for use by policymakers, healthcare providers, nutritionists, and nutrition educators. The information in the *Dietary Guidelines* is useful for the development of educational materials and aids policymakers in designing and implementing nutrition-related programs, including federal food, nutrition education, and information programs. In addition, this publication has the potential to provide authoritative statements as provided for in the Food and Drug Administration Modernization Act (FDAMA). Because the *Dietary Guidelines* contains discussions where the science is emerging, only statements included in the Executive Summary and the sections titled "Key Recommendations," which reflect the preponderance of scientific evidence, can be used for identification of authoritative statements. The recommendations are interrelated and mutually dependent; thus the statements in this document should be used together in the context of planning an overall healthful diet. However, even following just some of the recommendations can have health benefits.

The following is a listing of the *Dietary Guidelines* by chapter.

ADEQUATE NUTRIENTS WITHIN CALORIE NEEDS

Key Recommendations

- Consume a variety of nutrient-dense foods and beverages within and among the basic food groups while choosing foods that limit the in-

take of saturated and *trans* fats, cholesterol, added sugars, salt, and alcohol.
- Meet recommended intakes within energy needs by adopting a balanced eating pattern, such as the USDA Food Guide or the DASH Eating Plan.

Key Recommendations for Specific Population Groups

- *People over age 50.* Consume vitamin B12 in its crystalline form (i.e., fortified foods or supplements).
- *Women of childbearing age who may become pregnant.* Eat foods high in heme-iron and/or consume iron-rich plant foods or iron-fortified foods with an enhancer of iron absorption, such as vitamin C-rich foods.
- *Women of childbearing age who may become pregnant and those in the first trimester of pregnancy.* Consume adequate synthetic folic acid daily (from fortified foods or supplements) in addition to food forms of folate from a varied diet.
- *Older adults, people with dark skin, and people exposed to insufficient ultraviolet band radiation (i.e., sunlight).* Consume extra vitamin D from vitamin D-fortified foods and/or supplements.

WEIGHT MANAGEMENT

Key Recommendations

- To maintain body weight in a healthy range, balance calories from foods and beverages with calories expended.
- To prevent gradual weight gain over time, make small decreases in food and beverage calories and increase physical activity.

Key Recommendations for Specific Population Groups

- *Those who need to lose weight.* Aim for a slow, steady weight loss by decreasing calorie intake while maintaining an adequate nutrient intake and increasing physical activity.
- *Overweight children.* Reduce the rate of body weight gain while allowing growth and development. Consult a healthcare provider before placing a child on a weight-reduction diet.
- *Pregnant women.* Ensure appropriate weight gain as specified by a healthcare provider.
- *Breastfeeding women.* Moderate weight reduction is safe and does not compromise weight gain of the nursing infant.
- *Overweight adults and overweight children with chronic diseases and/or on medication.* Consult a healthcare provider about weight loss strategies prior to starting a weight-reduction program to ensure appropriate management of other health conditions.

PHYSICAL ACTIVITY

Key Recommendations

- Engage in regular physical activity and reduce sedentary activities to promote health, psychological well-being, and a healthy body weight.
    - To reduce the risk of chronic disease in adulthood: Engage in at least 30 minutes of moderate-intensity physical activity, above usual activity, at work or home on most days of the week.
    - For most people, greater health benefits can be obtained by engaging in physical activity of more vigorous intensity or longer duration.
    - To help manage body weight and prevent gradual, unhealthy body weight gain in adulthood: Engage in approximately 60 minutes of moderate- to vigorous-intensity activity on most days of the week while not exceeding caloric intake requirements.
    - To sustain weight loss in adulthood: Participate in at least 60 to 90 minutes of daily moderate-intensity physical activity while not exceeding caloric intake requirements. Some people may need to consult with a healthcare provider before participating in this level of activity.
- Achieve physical fitness by including cardiovascular conditioning, stretching exercises for flexibility, and resistance exercises or calisthenics for muscle strength and endurance.

Key Recommendations for Specific Population Groups

- *Children and adolescents.* Engage in at least 60 minutes of physical activity on most, preferably all, days of the week.
- *Pregnant women.* In the absence of medical or obstetric complications, incorporate 30 minutes or more of moderate-intensity physical activity on most, if not all, days of the week. Avoid activities with a high risk of falling or abdominal trauma.
- *Breastfeeding women.* Be aware that neither acute nor regular exercise adversely affects the mother's ability to successfully breastfeed.
- *Older adults.* Participate in regular physical activity to reduce functional declines associated with aging and to achieve the other benefits of physical activity identified for all adults.

FOOD GROUPS TO ENCOURAGE

Key Recommendations

- Consume a sufficient amount of fruits and vegetables while staying within energy needs. Two cups of fruit and 2 ½ cups of vegetables per day are recommended for a reference 2,000-calorie intake, with higher or lower amounts depending on the calorie level.
- Choose a variety of fruits and vegetables each day. In particular, select from all five vegetable subgroups (dark green, orange, legumes, starchy vegetables, and other vegetables) several times a week.
- Consume 3 or more ounce-equivalents of whole-grain products per day, with the rest of the recommended grains coming from enriched or whole-grain products. In general, at least half the grains should come from whole grains.
- Consume 3 cups per day of fat-free or low-fat milk or equivalent milk products.

Key Recommendations for Specific Population Groups

- *Children and adolescents.* Consume whole-grain products often; at least half the grains should be whole grains. Children 2 to 8 years should consume 2 cups per day of fat-free or low-fat milk or equivalent milk products. Children 9 years of age and older should consume 3 cups per day of fat-free or low-fat milk or equivalent milk products.

FATS

Key Recommendations

- Consume less than 10 percent of calories from saturated fatty acids and less than 300 mg/day of cholesterol, and keep *trans* fatty acid consumption as low as possible.
- Keep total fat intake between 20 to 35 percent of calories, with most fats coming from sources of polyunsaturated and monounsaturated fatty acids, such as fish, nuts, and vegetable oils.
- When selecting and preparing meat, poultry, dry beans, and milk or milk products, make choices that are lean, low-fat, or fat-free.
- Limit intake of fats and oils high in saturated and/or *trans* fatty acids, and choose products low in such fats and oils.

Key Recommendations for Specific Population Groups

- *Children and adolescents.* Keep total fat intake between 30 to 35 percent of calories for children 2 to 3 years of age and between 25 to 35 percent of calories for children and adolescents 4 to 18 years of age, with most fats coming from sources of polyunsaturated and monounsaturated fatty acids, such as fish, nuts, and vegetable oils.

CARBOHYDRATES

Key Recommendations

- Choose fiber-rich fruits, vegetables, and whole grains often.
- Choose and prepare foods and beverages with little added sugars or caloric sweeteners, such as amounts suggested by the USDA Food Guide and the DASH Eating Plan.
- Reduce the incidence of dental caries by practicing good oral hygiene and consuming sugar- and starch-containing foods and beverages less frequently.

SODIUM AND POTASSIUM

Key Recommendations

- Consume less than 2,300 mg (approximately 1 tsp of salt) of sodium per day.
- Choose and prepare foods with little salt. At the same time, consume potassium-rich foods, such as fruits and vegetables.

Key Recommendations for Specific Population Groups

- *Individuals with hypertension, blacks, and middle-aged and older adults.* Aim to consume no more than 1,500 mg of sodium per day, and meet the potassium recommendation (4,700 mg/day) with food.

ALCOHOLIC BEVERAGES

Key Recommendations

- Those who choose to drink alcoholic beverages should do so sensibly and in moderation— defined as the consumption of up to one drink per day for women and up to two drinks per day for men.
- Alcoholic beverages should not be consumed by some individuals, including those who cannot restrict their alcohol intake, women of child-bearing age who may become pregnant, pregnant and lactating women, children and adolescents, individuals taking medications that can interact with alcohol, and those with specific medical conditions.

- Alcoholic beverages should be avoided by individuals engaging in activities that require attention, skill, or coordination, such as driving or operating machinery.

FOOD SAFETY

Key Recommendations

- To avoid microbial food borne illness:
  - Clean hands, food contact surfaces, and fruits and vegetables. Meat and poultry should *not* be washed or rinsed.
  - Separate raw, cooked, and ready-to-eat foods while shopping, preparing, or storing foods.
  - Cook foods to a safe temperature to kill microorganisms.
  - Chill (refrigerate) perishable food promptly and defrost foods properly.
  - Avoid raw (unpasteurized) milk or any products made from unpasteurized milk, raw or partially cooked eggs or foods containing raw eggs, raw or undercooked meat and poultry, unpasteurized juices, and raw sprouts.

Key Recommendations for Specific Population Groups

- *Infants and young children, pregnant women, older adults, and those who are immunocompromised.* Do not eat or drink raw (unpasteurized) milk or any products made from unpasteurized milk, raw or partially cooked eggs or foods containing raw eggs, raw or undercooked meat and poultry, raw or undercooked fish or shellfish, unpasteurized juices, and raw sprouts.
- *Pregnant women, older adults, and those who are immunocompromised:* Only eat certain deli meats and frankfurters that have been reheated to steaming hot.

Note

1. N/H Publication No. 03-4082, Facts about the DASH Eating Plan, United States Department of Health and Human Services, National Institutes of Health, National Heart, Lung, and Blood Institute, Karanja NM et al. *Journal of the American Dietetic Association (JADA)* 8:S19-27, 1999. http://www.nhlbi.nih.gov/health/public/heart/hbp/dash/.

United States Department of Health and Human Services, 2005.

Healthier Eating

Michelle Meadows

*M*ost Americans consume too many calories and not enough nutrients, according to the latest revision to the Dietary Guidelines for Americans. In January 2005, two federal agencies—the Department of Health and Human Services and the Department of Agriculture (USDA)—released the guidelines to help adults and children ages 2 and up live healthier lives.

Currently, the typical American diet is low in fruits, vegetables, and whole grains, and high in saturated fat, salt, and sugar. As a result, more Americans than ever are overweight, obese, and at increased risk for chronic diseases such as heart disease, high blood pressure, diabetes, and certain cancers.

Of course old habits are hard to break, and the notion of change can seem overwhelming. But it can be done with planning and a gradual approach, says Dee Sandquist, a spokeswoman for the American Dietetic Association (ADA) and manager of nutrition and diabetes at the Southwest Washington Medical Center in Vancouver, Wash.

"Some people can improve eating habits on their own, while others need a registered dietitian to guide them through the process," Sandquist says. You may need a dietitian if you are trying to lose weight or if you have a health condition such as osteoporosis, high blood pressure, high cholesterol, or diabetes.

Sandquist says that many people she counsels have been used to eating a certain way and never thought about what they were actually putting into their bodies. "Someone may tell me they drink six cans of regular soda every day," she says. "When they find out there are about nine teaspoons of sugar in one can, it puts things in perspective. Then I work with the person to cut back to three cans a day, then to two and so on, and to start replacing some of the soda with healthier options."

Others are eating a lot of food between mid-day and bedtime because they skip breakfast, Sandquist says. Another common scenario is when someone has grown up thinking that meat should be the focus of every meal. "We may start by having the person try eating two-thirds of the meat they would normally eat, and then decreasing the portion little by little," Sandquist says. Cutting portion size limits calories. So does eating lean cuts of meat and using lower-fat methods of preparation such as broiling.

Sandquist says that when people strive for more balance in their diets, they tend to enjoy mixing up their food choices. "A lot of times, they've been eating the same things over and over. So when they start trying new foods, they find out what they've been missing."

Barbara Schneeman, Ph.D., an FDA nutrition expert, says the latest revision of the *Dietary Guidelines for Americans* emphasizes calorie control, nutrient-rich foods, and physical activity.

Barbara Schneeman, Ph.D., director of the Food and Drug Administration's Office of Nutritional Products, Labeling, and Dietary Supplements, encourages consumers to make smart food choices from every food group, "The Nutrition Facts label is an important tool that gives guidance for making these choices," she says. The label shows how high or low a food is in various nutrients.

Experts say that once you start using the label to compare products, you'll find there is flexibility in creating a balanced diet and enjoying a variety of foods in moderation. For example, you could eat a favorite food that's higher in fat for breakfast and have lower-fat foods for lunch and dinner. You could have a full-fat dip on a low-fat cracker, "What matters is how all the food works together," Sandquist says.

Older people are most likely to improve their eating habits, but nutrition is important for people of all ages, says Walter Willet, M.D., chairman of the nutrition department at the Harvard School of Public Health, "We know that when people have health problems or their friends become ill, these are strong motivators of change," says Willet. "The more serious the health condition, the more serious the change. We'd rather people made changes early and prevent health problems in the first place."

So what if you're feeling trapped by a diet full of fast food burgers and cookies? You can work your way out slowly but surely. Here are tips to move your eating habits in the right direction.

Look at What You Eat Now

Write down what you eat for a few days to get a good picture of what you're taking in, suggests Cindy Moore, direc-

Differences in Saturated Fat and Calorie Content of Commonly Consumed Foods

Food Category	Portion	Saturated Fat Content (grams)	Calories
Cheese			
• Regular cheddar cheese	1 oz.	6.0	114
• Low-fat cheddar cheese	1 oz.	1.2	49
Ground beef			
• Regular ground beef (25% fat)	3 oz. (cooked)	6.1	236
• Extra-lean ground beef (5% fat)	3 oz. (cooked)	2.6	148
Milk			
• Whole milk (3.24%)	1 cup	4.6	146
• Low-fat (1%) milk	1 cup	1.5	102
Breads			
• Croissant (medium)	1 medium	6.6	231
• Bagel, oat bran (4")	1 medium	0.2	227
Frozen desserts			
• Regular ice cream	1/2 cup	4.9	145
• Frozen yogurt, low-fat	1/2 cup	2.0	110
Table spreads			
• Butter	1 teaspoon	2.4	34
• Soft margarine with zero *trans* fat	1 teaspoon	0.7	25
Chicken			
• Fried chicken (leg with skin)	3 oz. (cooked)	3.3	212
• Roasted chicken (breast no skin)	3 oz. (cooked)	0.9	140
Fish			
• Fried fish	3 oz.	2.8	195
• Baked fish	3 oz.	1.5	129

ARS Nutrient Database for Standard Reference, Release 17

tor of nutrition therapy at the Cleveland Clinic Foundation. "By looking at what you eat and how much you're eating, you can figure out what adjustments you need to make," she says.

Sometimes she asks patients to write down what they are feeling. Were you nervous, happy, or sad when you ate five slices of pizza in one sitting? "The very nature of writing things down in a food diary can help patients make changes," Moore says. "Someone will tell me, 'I didn't want to have to write that I ate nine cookies, so I ate two instead.'"

Start With Small Changes

You don't have to go cold turkey. In the end, you want to achieve a long-term healthy lifestyle. Small changes over time are the most likely to stick. "If you want to eat more vegetables, then try to add one more serving by sneaking it in," Moore says. "Add bits of broccoli to something you already eat like pizza or soup. If you need more whole grains, add barley, whole wheat pasta, or brown rice to your soup."

To make smart food choices quickly and easily, compare the Nutrition Facts labels on products.

When you think about what you need to get more of, the other things tend to fall into place, Moore says. "If you have some baby carrots with lunch or add a banana to your cereal in the morning, you're going to feel full longer." You won't need a food that's high in sugar or fat an hour later, she adds.

Also, look for healthier versions of what you like to eat. If you like luncheon meat sandwiches, try a reduced fat version. If you like the convenience of frozen dinners, look for ones with lower sodium. If you love fast-food meals, try a salad as your side dish instead of french fries.

"Pick one or two changes to start with," Moore says. "Once the changes have become habits, which usually happens in about two to four weeks, then try adding one or two more. In six to 12 months, you'll find that you've made substantial changes."

Use the Nutrition Facts Label

To make smart food choices quickly and easily, compare the Nutrition Facts labels on products. Look at the percent Daily Value (%DV) column. The general rule of thumb is that 5 percent or less

Nutrition Facts

Serving Size 1 cup (228g)
Servings Per Container 2

Amount Per Serving

Calories 260	Calories from Fat 120

	% Daily Value*
Total Fat 13g	**20%**
Saturated Fat 5g	**25%**
Trans Fat 2g	
Cholesterol 30mg	**10%**
Sodium 660mg	**28%**
Total Carbohydrate 31g	**10%**
Dietary Fiber 0g	**0%**
Sugars 5g	
Protein 5g	

Vitamin A 4%	•	Vitamin C 2%
Calcium 15%	•	Iron 4%

* Percent Daily Values are based on a 2,000 calorie diet. Your Daily Values may be higher or lower depending on your calorie needs:

	Calories:	2,000	2,500
Total Fat	Less than	65g	80g
Sat Fat	Less than	20g	25g
Cholesterol	Less than	300mg	300mg
Sodium	Less than	2,400mg	2,400mg
Total Carbohydrate		300g	375g
Dietary Fiber		25g	30g

Calories per gram:
Fat 9 • Carbohydrate 4 • Protein 4

of the Daily Value is considered low and 20 percent or more is high.

Keep saturated fat, *trans* fat, cholesterol, and sodium low, while keeping fiber, potassium, iron, calcium, and vitamins A and C high. Be sure to look at the serving size and the number of servings per package. The serving size affects calories, amounts of each nutrient, and the percentage of Daily Value.

The %DV is based on a 2,000-calorie diet, but recommended calorie intake differs for individuals based on age, gender, and activity level. Some people need less than 2,000 calories a day. You can use the %DV as a frame of reference whether or not you consume more or less than 2,000 calories. The %DV makes it easy to compare the nutrients in each food product to see which ones are higher or lower. When comparing products, just make sure the serving sizes are similar, especially the weight (grams, milligrams, or ounces) of each product.

Control Portion Sizes

Understanding the serving size on the Nutrition Facts label is important for controlling portions, Moore says. "Someone may have a large bottled drink, assuming it's one serving," she says. "But if you look at the label, it's actually two servings. And if you consume two servings of a product, you have to multiply all the numbers by two." When the servings go up, so do the calories, fat, sugar, and salt.

Moore also suggests dishing out a smaller amount on your plate or using smaller plates. "If you put more food in front of you, you'll eat it because it's there," she says. According to the ADA, an average serving size of meat looks like a deck of cards. An average serving size of pasta or rice is about the size of a tennis ball. Here are some other ways to limit portions: Split a meal or dessert with a friend at a restaurant, get a doggie bag for half of your meal, get in the habit of having one helping, and ask for salad dressing, butter, and sauces on the side so you can control how much you use.

Control Calories and Get the Most Nutrients

You want to stay within your daily calorie needs, especially if you're trying to lose weight, says Eric Hentges, Ph.D., director of the USDA Center for Nutrition Policy and Promotion. "But you also want to get the most nutrients out of the calories, which means picking nutritionally rich foods," he says. Children and adults should pay particular attention to getting adequate calcium, potassium, fiber, magnesium, and vitamins A, C, and E.

According to the *Dietary Guidelines*, there is room for what's known as a discretionary calorie allowance. This is for when people meet their recommended nutrient intake without using all their calories. Hentges compares the idea to a household budget. "You know you have to pay all the bills and then you can use the leftover money for other things," he says. "The discretionary calorie allowance gives you some flexibility to have foods and beverages with added fats and sugars, but you still

want to make sure you're getting the nutrients you need."

For example, a 2,000-calorie diet has about 250 discretionary calories, according to the *Dietary Guidelines*.

Smart Snacks

- Unsalted pretzels
- Applesauce
- Low-fat yogurt with fruit
- Unbuttered and unsalted popcorn
- Broccoli, carrots, or cherry tomatoes with dip or low fat yogurt
- Grapes
- Apple slices with peanut butter
- Raisins
- Nuts
- Graham crackers
- Gingersnap cookies
- Low- or reduced fat string cheese
- Baked whole-grain tortilla chips with salsa
- Whole-grain cereal with low-fat milk

Know Your Fats

Fat provides flavor and makes you feel full. It also provides energy, and essential fatty acids for healthy skin, and helps the body absorb the fat-soluble vitamins A, D, E, and K. But fat also has nine calories per gram, compared to four calories per gram in carbohydrates and protein. If you eat too much fat every day, you may get more calories than your body needs, and too many calories can contribute to weight gain.

Too much saturated fat, *trans* fat, and cholesterol in the diet increases the risk of unhealthy blood cholesterol levels, which may increase the risk of heart disease. "Consumers should lower all three, not just one or the other," says Schneeman. Saturated fat is found mainly in foods from animals. Major sources of saturated fats are cheese, beef, and milk. *Trans* fat results when manufacturers add hydrogen to vegetable oil to increase the food's shelf life and flavor. *Trans* fat can be found in vegetable shortenings, some margarines, crackers, cookies, and other snack

Some Nutrient Content Claims

fat-free	less than 0.5 grams of fat per serving
low-fat	3 grams or less per serving (if the serving size is 30 grams or less or 2 tablespoons or less, no more than 3 grams of fat per 50 grams of the food)
light	one-third fewer calories or half the fat of the "regular" version
low-sodium	140 milligrams or less per serving (if the serving size is 30 grams or less or 2 tablespoons or less, no more than 140 milligrams of sodium per 50 grams of the food)
lightly-salted	at least 50 percent less sodium per serving than the "regular" version
reduced	when describing fat, sodium, or calorie content, the food must have at least 25 percent less of these nutrients than the "regular" version

USDA

foods. Cholesterol is a fat-like substance in foods from animal sources such as meat, poultry, egg yolks, milk, and milk products.

Most of your fats should come from polyunsaturated and monounsaturated fatty acids, such as those that occur in fish, nuts, soybean, corn, canola, olive, and other vegetable oils. This type of fat does not raise the risk of heart disease and may be beneficial when consumed in moderation.

Make Choices That Are Lean, Low-fat, or Fat-free

When buying meat, poultry, milk, or milk products, choose versions that are lean, low-fat, or fat-free. Choose lean meats like chicken without the skin and lean beef or pork with the fat trimmed off.

If you frequently drink whole milk, switch to 1 percent milk or skim milk. Many people don't taste a difference. Some mix whole milk with lower-fat milk for a while so the taste buds can adjust. This doesn't mean you can never eat or drink the full-fat versions, Schneeman says. "That's where the discretionary calories come in."

Other tips to reduce saturated fat include cooking with non-stick sprays and using olive, safflower, or canola oils instead of lard or butter. Eat more fish, which is usually lower in saturated fat than meat. Bake, grill, and broil food instead of frying it because more fat is absorbed into the food when frying. You could also try more meatless entrees like veggie burgers and

add flavor to food with low-fat beans instead of butter.

Focus on Fruit

The *Dietary Guidelines* recommend two cups of fruit per day at the 2,000-calorie reference diet. Fruit intake and recommended amounts of other food groups vary at different calorie levels. An example of two cups of fruit includes: one small banana, one large orange, and one-fourth cup of dried apricots or peaches.

Eat a variety of fruits—whether fresh, frozen, canned, or dried—rather than fruit juice for most of your fruit choices. "The whole fruit has more fiber, it's more filling, and it's naturally sweet," says Marilyn Tanner, a pediatric dietitian at the Washington University School of Medicine in St. Louis. Still, some juices, such as orange and prune, are a good source of potassium.

Ways to incorporate fruit in your diet include adding it to your cereal, eating it as a snack with low-fat yogurt or a low-fat dip, or making a fruit smoothie for dessert by mixing low-fat milk with fresh or frozen fruit such as strawberries or peaches. Also, your family is more likely to eat fruit if you put it out on the kitchen table.

Eat Your Veggies

The *Dietary Guidelines* recommend two and one-half cups of vegetables per day if you eat 2,000 calories each day.

Tanner suggests adding vegetables to foods such as meatloaf, lasagna, om-

elettes, stir-fry dishes, and casseroles. Frozen chopped greens such as spinach, and peas, carrots, and corn are easy to add. Also, add dark leafy green lettuce to sandwiches. "Involve kids by letting them help pick vegetables in different colors when you're shopping," Tanner suggests. Get a variety of dark green vegetables such as broccoli, spinach, and greens; orange and deep yellow vegetables such as carrots, winter squash, and sweet potatoes; starchy vegetables like corn; legumes, such as dry beans, peas, chickpeas, pinto beans, kidney beans, and tofu; and other vegetables, such as tomatoes and onions.

'You can buy salad in a bag. Or buy a vegetable tray from the grocery store and put it in the refrigerator.'

"Look for ways to make it convenient," Tanner says. "You can buy salad in a bag. Or buy a vegetable tray from the grocery store and put it in the refrigerator. Everything's already cut up and you can just reach in and eat it throughout the week."

Make Half Your Grains Whole

Like fruits and vegetables, whole grains are a good source of vitamins, minerals, and fiber. The *Dietary Guidelines* recommend at least three ounces of whole grains per day. One slice of bread, one cup of breakfast cereal, or one-half cup of cooked rice or pasta are each equivalent to about one ounce. Tanner

Exercise Made Easy

The 2005 *Dietary Guidelines* recommend finding your balance between food and physical activity. Consuming more calories than you expend leads to weight gain. More than half of all Americans don't get the recommended amount of physical activity. To reduce the risk of chronic disease in adulthood, engage in at least 30 minutes of moderate activity a day on most days of the week. Children and adolescents should engage in at least 60 minutes a day on most, and preferably all, days of the week.

To manage body weight and prevent gradual weight gain, people should exercise about 60 minutes at a moderate to vigorous intensity on most days of the week, while not exceeding recommendations for caloric intake. Sixty to 90 minutes may be needed to maintain weight loss.

The more vigorous the activity and the longer the duration, the more health benefits you'll get. But every little bit counts. Here are some examples of easy ways to work exercise into your day:

- Take a 10-minute walk after breakfast, lunch, and dinner to reach the goal of 30 minutes per day.
- Park your car in the farthest spot when you run errands.
- Take a family walk after dinner.
- Walk your dog.
- Do yard work.
- Wash your car by hand.
- Pace the sidelines at kids' athletic games.
- Ask a friend to exercise with you.
- Run around and play with your children for 30 minutes a day.
- Walk briskly at the mall.
- Take the stairs instead of the elevator.

HHS Small Steps program, www.smallstep.gov

suggests baked whole-grain corn tortilla chips or whole-grain cereal with low-fat milk as good snacks.

In general, at least half the grains you consume should come from whole grains. For many, but not all, whole grain products, the words "whole" or "whole grain" will appear before the grain ingredient's name. The whole grain must be the first ingredient listed in the ingredients list on the food package. The following are some whole grains: whole wheat, whole oats or oatmeal, whole-grain corn, popcorn, wild rice, brown rice, buckwheat, whole rye, bulgur or cracked wheat, whole-grain barley, and millet. Whole-grain foods cannot necessarily be identified by their color or by names such as brown bread, nine-grain bread, hearty grains bread, or mixed grain bread.

Lower Sodium and Increase Potassium

Higher salt intake is linked to higher blood pressure, which can raise the risk of stroke, heart disease, and kidney dis-

ease. The *Dietary Guidelines* recommend that people consume less than 2,300 milligrams of sodium per day (approximately one teaspoon of salt). There are other recommendations for certain populations that tend to be more sensitive to salt. For example, people with high blood pressure, blacks, and middle-aged and older adults should consume no more than 1,500 milligrams of sodium each day.

Most of the sodium people eat comes from processed foods. Use the Nutrition Facts label on food products: 5%DV or less for sodium means the food is low in sodium and 20%DV or more means it's high. Compare similar products and choose the option with a lower amount of sodium. Most people won't notice a taste difference. Consistently consuming lower-salt products will help taste buds adapt, and you will enjoy these foods as much or more than higher-salt options.

Prepare foods with little salt. The DASH (Dietary Approaches to Stop Hypertension) eating plan from the

National Heart, Lung, and Blood Institute recommends giving flavor to food with herbs, spices, lemon, lime, vinegar, and salt-free seasoning blends. Consult with your physician before using salt substitutes because their main ingredient, potassium chloride, can be harmful to some people with certain medical conditions.

Also, increase potassium-rich foods such as sweet potatoes, orange juice, bananas, spinach, winter squash, cantaloupe, and tomato puree. Potassium counteracts some of sodium's effect on blood pressure.

Limit Added Sugars

The *Dietary Guidelines* recommend choosing and preparing food and beverages with little added sugars. Added sugars are sugars and syrups added to foods and beverages in processing or preparation, not the naturally occurring sugars in fruits or milk. Major sources of added sugars in the American diet include regular soft drinks, candy, cake, cookies, pies, and fruit drinks. In the ingredients list on food products, sugar may be listed as brown sugar, corn syrup, glucose, sucrose, honey, or molasses. Be sure to check the sugar in low-fat and fat-free products, which sometimes contain a lot of sugar, Tanner says.

Instead of drinking regular soda and sugary fruit drinks, try diet soda, low-fat or fat-free milk, water, flavored water, or 100 percent fruit juice.

For snacks and desserts, try fruit. "People are often pleasantly surprised that fruit is great for satisfying a sweet tooth," Tanner says. "And if ice cream is calling your name, don't have it in the freezer. Make it harder to get by having to go out for it. Then it can be an occasional treat."

From *FDA Consumer,* May/June 2005, pp. 10, 12-17. Published 2005 by U.S. Food and Drug Administration. www.fda.gov

10 MEGA-TRENDS
IN THE SUPERMARKET

Bonnie Liebman

If it's not Sugar Free Milanos, it's whole-grain Cocoa Puffs. If it's not calcium-enriched Goldfish Crackers, it's Pringles in 100-calorie packs. You can get cereal, oatmeal, and orange juice with antioxidants. Yogurt comes with added fiber or cholesterol-lowering phytosterols. Pasta, eggs, and bread have added omega-3 fats.

Why the sudden flood of healthy-sounding foods? It's a perfect storm—a confluence of forces striking the food industry:

■ **The pressure to sell health.** Food marketers must be feeling the heat. With an obesity epidemic that's left two out of three adults and one out of six children overweight, companies know that they're vulnerable to lawsuits or regulations.

Obesity isn't the only issue. By January 1, 2006, all Nutrition Facts labels on food packages will have to disclose trans fat, so some companies are trying to eliminate it by then.

And it's not just fear that's motivating the industry. When companies like General Mills boost the whole grains in their foods, they must see a marketing opportunity. Ditto for companies that are adding antioxidants, calcium, and other nutrients.

■ **Leftovers from the low-carb craze.** Last year, companies tripped over themselves trying to churn out foods to please low-carb dieters. The craze launched a rush to replace the usual carbs (sugars and white flour) with whole grains or "good" carbs (like artificial sweeteners, fiber, and sugar alcohols) that purportedly don't raise blood sugar levels.

When the craze petered out—not surprisingly, since many lower-carb foods were no lower in calories—companies still had plenty of reformulated products

in the pipeline, especially low-sugar foods made with Splenda (sucralose). It's the first artificial sweetener that hasn't been dogged by safety questions. And unlike NutraSweet (aspartame), Splenda works in cooked foods. Now it's showing up everywhere.

■ **Looser claims.** Lawsuits, the business-friendly Bush Administration, and pressure from the food industry have led the Food and Drug Administration to allow more health claims on foods.

The FDA used to require "significant scientific agreement" before a company could claim that a food could reduce the risk of heart disease, cancer, or other illness. Now it allows those claims when the evidence is skimpier, as long as the label says something like "scientific evidence suggests but does not prove...."

Mix these three forces together, sprinkle in the need to get an edge over your competitors, and you've got a revolution in the supermarket. Or do you? Are we talking healthier foods or just trans-free Oreos in smaller packages? Here's how to spot the difference in 10 trends that have invaded the grocery store.

1 MORE WHOLE GRAINS

"All General Mills Cereals Are Made With WHOLE GRAIN!" scream the boxes. GM made a big splash with its announcement last September, but the change isn't quite as dramatic as it sounds.

General Mills replaced some, but not all, of the refined flour in some of its cereals like Trix, Golden Grahams, Lucky Charms, and Rice Chex with whole grain. (Whole-grain cereals like Wheaties weren't touched.)

But few of the reformulated cereals have more than 1 gram of fiber per serving. Fiber isn't the only reason to eat whole grains, but it can be a good indicator of how much whole grain a food contains.

"Made with whole grain" often means made with both whole and refined grains.

What's more, even if a cereal had *no* white flour, that alone wouldn't make it a health food. Cereals like Boo Berry, Lucky Charms, Count Chocula, and Cocoa Puffs are nearly half sugar. With or without whole grains, they're nothing more than breakfast candy.

General Mills aside, whole grains are showing up throughout the supermarket. Boboli makes a 100% Whole Wheat pizza crust. Thomas' and Pepperidge Farm make 100% Whole Wheat English Muffins. Lean Cuisine's line of Spa Cuisine entrées uses only 100% whole-wheat pasta or brown rice. San Giorgio and Ronzoni make Healthy Harvest pasta that's part whole-grain (the companies won't say how much).

Keep in mind

Claims may sound alike, but they don't all mean the same thing:

■ **"100% whole grain"** means no refined flour.

■ **"Made with whole grain"** means the food may be made with either a lot or a little.

■ **"Whole grain"** may mean that only 51 percent of the flour is whole-grain. (That's the minimum a food needs to carry a health claim like "whole grains may reduce the risk of heart disease.")

■ **"Good source of whole grain"** means there may be as little as 8 grams of whole grains per serving. An **"excellent source"** means as little as 16 grams per serving. (That's what General Mills has asked the FDA to require. Several companies are using those minimums while waiting for the feds to set official levels.)

So a breakfast cereal—which usually weighs 30 to 55 grams per serving—could be "a good source of whole grain" if only 15 to 25 percent of its grain is whole (and 75 to 85 percent is refined).

■ **"Multigrain"** means a mixture of grains, so it could be mostly refined grain plus a sprinkling of whole grains.

You save a quarter of the calories by switching from regular to sugar-free Pillsbury Chocolate Chip cookies, but only 6 percent of the calories (3 calories per cookie) by switching from regular to sugar-free Milanos.

2 LESS SUGAR

"Not for weight control," says the tiny type on the label of Pepperidge Farm Sugar Free Milanos. That's for sure. Each cookie has only 3 fewer calories than a regular Milano, even though the regular's 4 grams of sugar are gone.

The same "not for weight control" (required by the FDA for "sugar-free" foods that aren't low-calorie) appears on SnackWell's Sugar Free Fudge Brownie or Oatmeal Cookies. No kidding. At 90 calories a cookie, it's no diet food.

The low-carb craze has left its legacy. Fewer consumers have blind faith that any food with a carb claim will restore their college physique. But they do seem to recognize that excess sugar is no friend to anyone's fanny.

Also fueling the sugar-free boom: companies can sweeten their foods with Splenda (sucralose), which the Atkins and South Beach diet books recommend. At this point, Splenda's manufacturers can't keep up with demand.

Keep in mind

■ **Is it lower in calories?** Sometimes. Expect half the calories in lower-sugar drinks like Minute Maid Light and Tropicana Light 'n Healthy orange juice, which replace half the juice with artificially sweetened water. Ditto for Pepsi Edge and Coca Cola's C2, which also have half the sugar.

But beyond beverages, you can't assume that cutting sugar means saving calories. Each Sugar Free Entenmann's Chewy Chocolate Chip Cookie, for example, has only 3 fewer calories than its regular counterpart. And General Mills Reduced Sugar Cinnamon Toast Crunch cereal has only 10 fewer calories per ¾-cup serving than the regular.

In contrast, you save about a quarter of the calories by switching from regular to Pillsbury Sugar-Free Chocolate Chip Cookie Dough. Hershey's Sugar Free Chocolate Candy, Chocolate Candy with Almonds, and Dark Chocolate Candy and Reese's Peanut Butter Cups also save you about a quarter of the calories versus a similar serving of the regular versions.

Why not more? Most companies replace the sugar not just with artificial sweeteners, but with sugar alcohols (like maltitol), polydextrose, inulin, maltodextrin, and other carbohydrates. They're safe—though the sugar alcohols can have what the labels delicately call "a laxative effect." And while most of the sugar substitutes have fewer calories than sugar, they're not calorie-free.

■ **Has the serving size changed?** If you calculate the calorie savings, make sure you're comparing equal servings. For example, both Kellogg's ¾ Less Sugar Frosted Flakes and regular Frosted Flakes have 120 calories, according to the labels. But if you eat ¾ cup of each, the regular still has 120 calories but the ⅓ Less Sugar has only 90 calories.

And once you adjust to a similar serving size (⅛ cake), Entenmann's Sugar Free Butter Loaf has about as many calories as its regular All Butter Loaf Cake.

■ **Does it use only Splenda?** Minute Maid Light orange juice, Breyer's Carb-Smart ice cream, and many other foods use both Splenda and acesulfame potas-

sium, a sweetener that may not be safe. Always check the ingredients list.

■ **Is it junk anyway?** If you're talking about healthful foods—like orange juice, yogurt, and whole-grain cereals—it's worth looking for less sugar. But cookies, chocolate candy, and refined-grain cereals are junk foods with or without sugar. The last thing you need is an excuse to pop an extra Milano in your mouth.

3 NO TRANS

"New! 0 grams Trans Fat" boasts the label of York Dark Chocolate Dipped Cookies. Hershey slaps the same claim on its three Milk Chocolate Dipped Cookies (with Almonds, Almond Joy, and Reese's).

"Trans-free" is showing up on more and more labels (whether or not the food ever had trans fat). And manufacturers of some foods that contain trans seem to be overhauling their recipes to get rid of it by the January 2006 deadline, when all Nutrition Facts labels must disclose trans.

Less trans is good news, since the fat—which comes largely from partially hydrogenated oil—promotes heart disease at least as much as saturated fat does. But don't assume that all trans-free foods are a gift for your heart.

Warning: Hershey's new trans-free cookies are high in saturated fat.

Hershey's new Chocolate Dipped cookies have about 5 grams of saturated fat per serving (that's two cookies at 80 calories each). Who needs a quarter of a day's sat fat in a couple of bites? And the company's sat-fat-laden Chocolate Dipped York cookies may trip up fans of York Peppermint Patties, which are one of the few chocolate candies that are fairly low in sat fat (1½ grams per patty).

Keep in mind

■ **Did it ever have any?** It's easy to eliminate trans fat from breads, chips, oils, salad dressings, and cereals, since most never had much to begin with. It's tougher to get trans out of crackers, margarine, cookies, pastries, and cakes. Hardest of all is replacing the more-solid, trans-heavy fats in foods like chocolate coatings, cake icings, and pie crusts.

■**Is it high in saturated fat?** So far, it looks like most companies are replacing trans fat with an equal amount of saturated fat, mostly from palm and palm kernel oil. But too much of either fat is bad news for arteries.

A food's saturated and trans fat shouldn't add up to more than 4 grams (more is considered "high") and should preferably be 1 gram or less (that's "low"). One gram doesn't sound like much, but with a sat-plus-trans limit of 20 grams a day, it adds up.

■**Is it really trans-free?** "Trans-free" or "0 grams trans fat" means less than 0.5 grams of trans per serving. But if a serving of, say, three cookies has 0.49 grams of trans and you eat, say, six cookies, you're getting close to one gram of trans. That's not trivial.

An advisory panel to the FDA recommended earlier this year that the agency set a limit of 2 grams of trans fat a day (for people who eat a typical 2,000-calorie diet). So watch out for foods—even "trans-free" foods—that have partially hydrogenated oil in the ingredients list, especially if you think you'll eat more than the serving size.

■**Is it junk anyway?** Just because your cookies, chips, or doughnuts are trans-free, that's no excuse to sink your teeth in.

4 MORE FUNCTIONAL FIBER

How does Dannon get fiber into its new Light 'n Fit Yogurt with Fiber? Many people will assume that it's from the apple, peach, or strawberries pictured on the labels.

In fact, it's not the yogurt's fruit, but its maltodextrin, that adds 3 grams of fiber to each ½-cup serving. Maltodextrin is what scientists call a *functional* fiber—a non-digestible carbohydrate that's isolated from foods, rather than the *dietary* fiber that occurs naturally in foods. (In theory, functional fibers should have some benefit, but it's too early to say whether they all do.)

Maltodextrin is just one of many functional fibers that are popping up in dozens of foods, thanks, in part, to the low-carb craze. (Manufacturers don't count fiber in their "net carb" totals, and some fibers can replace the bulk that sugars add to foods.)

Other functional fibers: Breyer's CarbSmart ice cream has 3 grams of fiber per serving from polydextrose, a chemical combination of dextrose (corn sugar) and sorbitol (a sugar alcohol) that's poorly digested (which is what makes it count as fiber). Quaker boosts the fiber in its Take Heart Oatmeal with inulin, an extract of chicory root.

And dozens of breads now contain cellulose, a functional fiber supplied by ingredients like oat hull fiber, wheat fiber, pea fiber, soy fiber, and cottonseed fiber. ("Light" breads used to get their cellulose from wood pulp.)

Functional fibers are safe, but they may not confer all the benefits of fruits, vegetables, and wheat bran, which is the fiber-rich outer layer of the wheat kernel.

"My guess is that these isolated fibers are low in the phytochemicals, antioxidants, and other constituents of wheat bran," says Joanne Slavin, a fiber expert at the University of Minnesota. "When you isolate fiber, you get rid of as much of its phytochemicals as you can."

Keep in mind

■**How much fiber?** Women need 25 grams of fiber a day (21 grams if they're over 50). Men need 38 grams a day (30 grams if they're over 50). The typical American gets half that much.

■**Is it naturally occurring fiber?** The evidence that fiber can lower the risk of heart disease, diabetes, or cancer comes almost exclusively from studies of people who ate *dietary*, not *functional*, fiber. So your best bet is to get most of your fiber from wheat bran, whole grains, beans, vegetables, and fruit.

■**Is it functional fiber?** It's not clear what isolated fibers can do, but so far, it looks like cellulose *does*, maltodextrin *doesn't*, and polydextrose and inulin *may* help prevent constipation (though cellulose doesn't work as well as bran does).

■**Could it cause cramps or diarrhea?** The FDA requires foods with high levels of some sugar alcohols to warn consumers that "excess consumption may have a laxative effect."

Dannon's new yogurt gets its fiber from maltodextrin, not fruit.

5 WEAKER CLAIMS

"Scientific evidence suggests but does not prove that eating 1.5 ounces per day of most nuts … may reduce the risk of coronary heart disease," says the label of Planters NUT-rition Heart-Healthy Mix.

"Suggests but does not prove"? Are consumers supposed to rush to the library to evaluate the evidence themselves?

Until the early 1980s, food labels couldn't mention high blood pressure or a disease like cancer or heart disease. Then Congress passed a law that allowed claims about disease (called "health claims"), but only if the FDA determined that the claim was backed by "significant scientific agreement."

No longer. The FDA now also allows claims based on weaker evidence (so-called "qualified health claims"), as long as the claim contains a phrase like "suggests but does not prove" or "the evidence is limited and not conclusive."

So far, the FDA has permitted only a few "qualified" claims for foods—nuts, EPA and DHA omega-3 fats, and olive oil. All promise to lower the risk of heart disease.

How can consumers judge claims like "evidence suggests but does not prove" that nuts may reduce the risk of heart disease.

But many companies take the easy way out and use claims like "supports healthy arteries" or "promotes a healthy immune system." Because they don't mention a disease, these so-called "structure or function" claims require no approval.

It's no wonder shoppers are befuddled. According to a new food-industry study, consumers have difficulty distinguishing between solid claims—ones supported by "significant scientific agreement"—and claims based on far weaker evidence.

Keep in Mind

■**Structure or function claims.** Words like "supports," "maintains," or "promotes" a healthy heart, immune system, blood pressure, cholesterol, bones, etc., are usually part of a structure or function claim. They require little or no evidence. And they can appear on any food, no matter how junky or high in saturated fat, trans fat, sodium, or cholesterol.

■**Qualified health claims.** These claims say that a food "may help reduce the risk" of a disease, but caution that "the evidence suggests but does not prove," "the evidence is limited and not conclusive," or something similarly vague.

At least the FDA prohibits qualified health claims on foods that are junky or too high in saturated fat, trans fat, cholesterol, or sodium.

■**Health claims.** If the label says a food "may help reduce the risk" of a disease but says nothing else about iffy evidence, the claim is backed by reasonably good science and the food is decent.

6 MORE OMEGA-3 FAT

"Rich in Heart Healthy Omega-3," crow the Barilla Plus pasta labels. "The ground flaxseeds in Barilla Plus are the highest plant source of Omega-3, an essential fatty acid that promotes heart health."

What's more, the labels compare the amount of omega-3s in the pasta (360 milligrams per ¼ box) to the amount in shrimp (375 mg in 3 ounces) and salmon (1,725 mg in 3 ounces), even though a typical restaurant serves 8 ounces of salmon. "Enjoying Barilla Plus several times per week provides as much Omega-3 as a serving of fish," says the small print.

Well, sort of. Barilla Plus's omega-3s come from ground flaxseed, which is rich in alpha-linolenic acid (ALA). It's not clear if ALA can lower the risk of sudden death heart attacks as well as the longer-chain omega-3 fats in fish oil, eicosapentaenoic acid (EPA) and docosahexaenoic acid (DHA).

So even if you have "several servings" of Barilla Plus each week, it may not protect your heart as much as a serving of salmon.

Barilla can still make the "heart healthy" claim because of a loophole: as long as the claim doesn't mention heart *disease*, it's a "structure or function" claim that needs no approval by the FDA.

Barilla is also sneaky with its serving size. The Nutrition Facts panel says that a serving is ⅛ box (about 1 cup cooked), but elsewhere on the package Barilla uses ¼ box as one serving. That's probably more realistic, but a harried shopper might inadvertently compare the protein, fiber, and other nutrients in ¼ box of Barilla to ⅛ box of other pasta.

Omega-3s are also showing up in spreads (like Smart Balance), breads (like Healthy Life Flaxseed), eggs (like Eggland's Best), and bars (like Odwalla Go-Mega). In several years, Kellogg's plans to roll out cereals fortified with DHA.

Keep in Mind

■**Which omega-3 does it have?** Check the ingredients list to see if the omega-3s come from fish oil or flaxseed. The ALA in flaxseed may lower the risk of cardiac arrest as well as fish oil, but it's too early to say.

And be careful. The front of the Smart Balance Light Buttery Spread package says "now with flax oil," while the front of Smart Balance Omega Plus Buttery Spread says "with...organic menhaden oil." (Menhaden is a fatty fish.)

But only 150 mg of every 550 mg of omega-3s in each tablespoon of Omega Plus is from fish oil. The rest is from "plant sources" (the ALA in canola and soy oil). And there's no way for shoppers to tell that from the confusing label, unless they know that "long-chain" omega-3s come from fish oil and "short-chain" omega-3s come from plant sources.

■**How much will you get per day?** The American Heart Association recommends about 1 gram of EPA plus DHA per day (preferably from fatty fish) for people with heart disease. That's because fish oil cut the risk of a second heart attack in some studies.

It's not clear if omega-3 fats from flax, canola, or soy oil protect the heart as well as omega-3 fats from fish oil.

Everyone else should eat a variety of (preferably fatty) fish at least twice a week, says the Heart Association. It also recommends ALA-rich foods like flaxseed, canola and soy oils, and walnuts, but doesn't say how much to shoot for.

However, the National Academy of Sciences recommends at least 1.1 grams of ALA a day for women and 1.6 grams for men. Most people can reach those levels by eating foods that contain canola oil (1.3 grams per tablespoon) or soy oil (0.9 grams). The list includes most salad dressings, mayonnaise, and anything sautéed in either canola or soy oil.

7 SELF-STYLED SYMBOLS

Quaker, Frito Lay, Aunt Jemima, Tropicana, Gatorade, Dole, SoBe, and other Pepsi-owned brands have a "Smart Choices Made Easy" logo on selected products.

Minute Rice, DiGiorno, Tombstone, Boca, Breakstone's, Kool-Aid, VeryFine, Crystal Light, Nabisco, Stella D'Oro, Jell-O, Miracle Whip, Louis Rich, Oscar Mayer, Planters, and other brands owned by Kraft have a "Sensible Solution" flag on the labels.

Kellogg's has a "Healthy Beginnings" program that slaps one of five logos—Heart Health, Fiber, Shape Management, Well-Being & Energy, or Pregnancy—on some of its cereals. General Mills puts symbols like "whole grain" or "low saturated fat" on the "Goodness Corner" of its boxes.

What's going on?

Stung by criticism that they're feeding the obesity epidemic by selling high-calorie junk, several food giants are trying to highlight their healthier products.

And it may help consumers to see logos on Tropicana juice, Quaker Oatmeal, and Boca Burgers, or on Light (but not regular) Oscar Mayer Wieners, Sugar Free (but not regular) Jell-O, Baked or Light (but not regular) Doritos, Fat Free or Light Done Right (but not regular) Kraft salad dressing, and Lite or Low Calorie (but not regular) Aunt Jemima syrup. If the logos catch on, they may even spur companies to develop more of those foods.

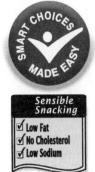

Symbols like these point you to a company's healthier products. But don't confuse a "healthier" food (like Baked Cheetos) with a "healthy" food (like fresh fruit).

But by coming up with their own criteria for logos, companies are taking the easy way out. They've ignored the FDA's criteria for "healthy" foods, which exclude a food that's, say, low in fat but high in salt. Nor can "healthy" appear on empty-calorie junk foods, like sugar-free Kool-Aid or Diet Coke, even if the company has tossed in some vitamin C.

Instead, companies make up their own criteria for their symbols, complete with plenty of weasel room. For example, Pepsi products can use a "Smart Choices Made Easy" logo if they're "fortified and contain other wholesome ingredients." Kraft products get a "Sensible Solution" flag if they have 25 percent less calories, fat, saturated fat, sugar, or sodium than an "appropriate reference product."

Translation: "Smart Choices" goes on decent foods like oatmeal and orange juice, but also on Quaker Quakes Sour Cream & Onion Potato Stix, Baked Cheetos, and Cap'n Crunch Peanut Butter Crunch cereal. And "Sensible Solution" appears on Premium Fat Free Saltines, Fat Free Fig Newtons, and Sugar Free Jell-O. None would qualify as a "healthy" food because they don't have enough naturally occurring nutrients.

Keep in mind

■ **Look for "healthy" foods.** But since only a few companies—like Healthy Choice—make "healthy" claims, it's also worth scanning the shelves for foods with company symbols. Just remember that they may appear on slightly-better-but-still-flawed products.

■ **Watch out for vague promises.** If the symbol makes a straightforward promise (like a "Fiber" symbol on Kellogg's cereals), it's probably trustworthy. Watch out for fuzzier, more-grandiose promises, like Kellogg's "Well-Being & Energy" symbol. The company puts it on cereals that are high in carbs (like any cereal) and are fortified with extra B-vitamins, even though there's no good evidence that those nutrients make people more energetic.

■ **Hit the produce aisle.** Concentrate on eating more fruits and vegetables (not "fruit" snacks or drinks or fruit-and-cereal bars).

8 MORE PHYTOSTEROLS

"Helps Lower Cholesterol," announces the label of Yoplait Healthy Heart (the "lowfat yogurt with plant sterols"). How?

Phytosterols are safe plant compounds that occur naturally in small amounts in fruits, vegetables, nuts, and beans. At higher levels, they can lower LDL ("bad") cholesterol by about 10 percent by keeping the cholesterol in your gut from being absorbed into the bloodstream.

Phytosterols are not in the same ballpark as prescription statin drugs, which can cut LDL cholesterol by 20 to 50 percent. But if you can lose a little cholesterol just by choosing one orange juice over another, why not?

When the FDA approved a health claim for phytosterols in 2000, only two spreads—Benecol and Take Control—could carry it. Now you can get phytosterols in Minute Maid Heart Wise orange juice, Yoplait Heart Healthy yogurt, Rice Dream Heartwise Rice Drink, and Lifetime Low Fat cheese. And the list is likely to grow.

You can now get cholesterol-lowering phytosterols in yogurt, orange juice, and spreads.

Keep in mind

■ **How much is enough?** The FDA allows a health claim on foods with at least 0.4 grams of sterols per serving. The label must explain how much plant sterols each serving contains and how much you need per day to lower the risk of heart disease (at least 0.8 grams).

■ **Twice a day.** Phytosterols work by trapping cholesterol in the gut, so it's better to eat them at least twice a day with meals, according to the FDA.

■ **More isn't better.** Once you exceed about 3 grams of plant sterols a day, cholesterol doesn't drop further.

9 ADDED VITAMINS & MINERALS

Forget regular oatmeal. Quaker now sells "Advanced Nutrition for your Heart." Its new Take Heart oatmeal is low in sodium and has added potassium "to maintain healthy blood pressure" and "antioxidant vitamins E & C plus B vitamins to help support healthy arteries."

Never mind that there isn't much evidence that extra C and E protect your heart. Never mind that anyone could get the same day's worth of B-vitamins (B-6, B-12, and folic acid) from an ordinary multivitamin (though the multi would supply many more nutrients). When it comes to marketing, none of that matters.

Kellogg's uses a similar strategy to sell its Smart Start Antioxidants. The cereal has antioxidants "to support a healthy immune system," says the label. And that "could help slow age damage to the body and help prevent disease," says the company Web site.

A multivitamin on top of Smart Start Antioxidants and other foods could give you too much iron and zinc.

Again, you're better off taking a multi than getting a handful of vitamins and minerals from your cereal. The extra vitamins won't hurt you, but the extra iron and zinc may.

Each cup of Smart Start Antioxidants has 18 mg of iron and 15 mg of zinc. Take a typical multi and you get the same amount of each.

So even without what you get from other foods, that's 36 mg of iron—far more than the 18 mg recommended for premenopausal women or the 8 mg recommended for other adults. And it's not too far from 45 mg—the maximum you can take without risking gastrointestinal distress.

Similarly, 30 mg of zinc is well over the 11 mg recommended for men and the 8 mg recommended for women. And it's not too far from the 40 mg maximum. More than that interferes with the absorption of copper and may impair immunity. So much for Smart Start Antioxidants' claims about "supporting a healthy immune system."

The latest nutrient-of-the-month may be potassium. Quaker adds potassium gluconate to Take Heart and Kellogg's adds potassium chloride to Smart Start Healthy Heart. Both kinds of potassium can help lower blood pressure, but only gluconate (and citrate) can also protect against kidney stones and osteoporosis (see Dec. 2004, p. 8).

Keep in Mind

■**Is it junk anyway?** Who cares if Hershey adds calcium to its chocolate syrup or Pepperidge Farm adds calcium to its Goldfish Crackers? Fortified junk food is still junk.

■**Do you need it?** If you take a multivitamin, odds are that you don't need the added vitamins and minerals in fortified foods, which are often less than a day's worth.

Exceptions: a multi rarely has a day's worth of calcium and has less than a day's worth of vitamin D for people over 70.

■**Are you getting too much?** If you take a multivitamin and eat fortified foods, you might get too much of nutrients like iron and zinc. That's no reason to drop the multi, though. It's more complete than the fortified food.

10 RE-PACKAGING

"Counting calories? Count with Pringles!" suggests the cheery label on Pringles Original 100 Calorie Packs.

Portion control can help dieters, but Procter & Gamble deserves the American Landfill Association's 2005 Overpackaging Award for stuffing six (overpriced) plastic tubs into each box. Smaller portions don't make snacks good for you. Pringles are mostly dried potatoes and oil—not exactly foods that Americans need to eat more of.

Nabisco's 100 Calorie Packs—Thin Crisps (wafers flavored like Chips Ahoy, Kraft Cheese Nips, Honey Maid Cinnamon, or Oreos), Ritz Snack Mix, Wheat Thins Minis, and Fruit Snacks—are mostly white flour, except for the Fruit Snacks, which are mostly sugar.

Yes, they're all low in fat, and the Thin Crisps are less fatty than original Chips Ahoys or Oreos. But they're not exactly baby carrots, peaches, and cantaloupe chunks.

Keep in Mind

■**Snack on fruits & vegetables.** Experts now recommend 8 to 10 servings—that's 4 to 5 cups—of fruits and vegetables a day. It's not easy to hit that target if your snacks are cookies and candy.

■**Make your own snack packs.** If you want portion control, fill some small (reusable) plastic containers with berries, grape tomatoes, pineapple or melon chunks, or any other fruit or vegetable. An apple, a pear, an orange, or a banana is nature's own 100-calorie "snack pack."

■**Go for whole grains.** For something more substantial than fruit or veggies, try a handful of nuts or some whole-grain crackers. All nine Triscuit varieties are 100 percent whole-grain, and all but the Cheddar are trans-free.

■**Keep the dairy light.** If you want small portions, grab a light yogurt or an individually wrapped light string cheese.

51 Healthy Foods You Can Say "YES" To

Tired of being told what not to eat? Here's a sampling of the many choices you can feel good about including as part of a balanced diet.

HARDLY A DAY GOES BY, it seems, without the news media reporting some food that's been found to be bad for you. One day it's processed meats; the next, it's baked goods made with trans-fatty acids. Faced with this litany of "don'ts," you can start to wonder whether *any* food is OK to eat.

In fact, scientists know of a whole cornucopia of healthy foods you can choose from. Not only are there plenty of food choices that are OK—many foods can actually give your body a boost. Your daily diet can supply everything from essential nutrients to compounds that have been positively associated with preventing diseases and minimizing the toll of aging. These are foods you can enthusiastically say "yes!" to as part of a well-rounded diet. Many of them have been covered in depth in previous issues of this newsletter.

But we're not talking about so-called "superfoods." Foods aren't magic pills; eating spinach won't cure what ails you any more than it will make you as strong as Popeye.

And even healthful foods like those mentioned in this Special Supplement are good for you only in the overall context of a balanced diet. Gorging on any one type of food, no matter how "healthy," won't give you the nutrients you need—regardless of what some fad diets would have you believe. Nor will simply adding healthful foods "fix" your diet: "Sprinkling nuts on top of a hot-fudge sundae, although nuts are 'good for you,' does not negate the saturated fat and calories in the sundae," cautions Alice H.

Lichtenstein, DSc, Stanley N. Gershoff Professor of Nutrition in Tufts' Friedman School of Nutrition Science and Policy.

Keep in mind, too, that even good food choices have calories. Robin B. Kanarek, PhD, a professor of nutrition and behavior at the Friedman School, cites the example of a friend who wanted to lose weight, and couldn't understand why it wasn't happening—she was eating only fruit. "The answer to why she wasn't losing weight was quite simple: Fruit has calories, and seven cantaloupes, six apples, six oranges, etc., had as many calories as what she regularly consumed before."

Some of the foods for which researchers have found positive health effects are particularly packed with calories; you should say "yes" to these only when saying "no" to other foods. Substitute nuts, for example, for candy bars when you need a snack—but if you just add nuts to your diet, you're upping your calorie intake. Similarly, vegetable oils can be a healthy choice instead of animal-derived fats such as butter or lard. That doesn't mean drinking a cupful of canola oil every day is a good idea, though.

The 51 healthy foods to say "yes" to listed on these pages represent merely a sampling of the variety of foods you can choose in a nutritious diet. (We could pretty much list all fruits and vegetables, for instance, but that would make this list either long or boring or both.) This sampling is designed to give you ideas for meals and even snacks that point your eating plan in the right

direction. Any one food on the list isn't necessarily "better" for you than other choices, cautions Jeanne P. Goldberg, PhD, RD, professor of nutrition and director of the Center on Nutrition Communication at the Friedman School. Take salmon, for example. "While salmon does have omega 3s, other fish are quite low in fat," Goldberg notes. So salmon isn't "better" than, say, flounder—the key is to include more fish of all kinds in your diet than most Americans now do. (And remember to bake or broil your fish, not fry it—preparation matters, too!)

If this list simply gives you some new foods to try, that's a big step in the right direction. Studies have shown the importance of eating a variety of healthy foods. But most Americans aren't doing a very good job at diversifying their diets: Potatoes and head lettuce account for nearly half our vegetables, and only six fruit choices (orange juice, bananas, apples, watermelon, apple juice, grapes) total half of our fruit consumption. Check out our list for some fresh ideas.

It's even OK—occasionally—to indulge, in moderation, in some of those foods you've been told to say "no" to. Don't feel guilty, says Kanarek, about having a small piece of chocolate or a little ice cream.

But we think you'll find some of these healthful choices—and the related options that they suggest—appealing enough that you might not even be tempted.

1 Acorn Squash—A source of lycopene, folate and vitamins A and C, winter squash of all sorts also gives you dietary fiber. Plus acorn squash, for example, is rich in potassium—almost 900 milligrams per cup.

2 Almonds—A good source of potassium, almonds, like other nuts, are low in saturated fat and high in unsaturated fats. But they're also high in calories, so substitute almonds for a snack that's high in trans- or saturated fat; otherwise the added calories offset any heart-healthy benefits. Recent research from the Antioxidants Research Laboratory at Tufts' Jean Mayer USDA Human Nutrition Research Center on Aging has demonstrated an antioxidant synergy between flavonoids and vitamin E in whole almonds. Almonds are also a source of riboflavin, magnesium and zinc.

3 Apples—You know what they say about keeping the doctor away? An apple a day may not be quite *that* powerful, but apples are a good source of fiber, and a medium-sized apple has only 80 calories. Red apples are among the fruits highest in quercetin, which researchers are studying for possible antioxidant benefits. But the antioxidants are concentrated in the skin, so don't peel before eating.

4 Apricots—A good source of vitamins A and C, apricots also are a way to get lycopene, which has been associated with cancer prevention in men (see tomatoes, below).

5 Asparagus—With just 25 calories in eight medium-sized asparagus spears, you get 25 percent of your daily vitamin A and 15 percent of vitamin C, plus essential folic acid.

6 Bananas—A good source of magnesium, which protects against bone loss and is associated with heart health, bananas are also packed with potassium. With 422 milligrams of potassium in one medium banana, you're getting almost 10 percent of the 4,700 milligrams the Institute of Medicine says you need. Potassium helps lower blood pressure and reduces the risk of kidney stones and bone loss.

7 Barley—Looking for ways to get the whole-grain servings recommended in the new federal dietary guidelines? (Six to 13 servings of grains depending on your caloric intake, of which at least half should come from whole grains.) Try cooking up some barley—also a good source of iron and minerals—in place of white rice. But make sure you're buying whole-grain barley, not the "pearl" variety with the healthful outer husk removed. Whole grains have been associated with protection against heart disease and cancer, and may help control diabetes. Other good whole-grain choices of this type include bulgur, buckwheat groats (also known as kasha), millet and quinoa (see below).

8 Beef eye of round—While studies continue to suggest it's smart to limit your red-meat consumption, when you've gotta have beef, eye of round is the leanest cut. A three-ounce serving has nearly half your daily protein and just 160 calories. Beef is a good source of zinc and vitamin B6.

9 Blueberries—Tufts researchers are studying blueberries for their antioxidant benefits, including the possibility that they may boost brain functions that weaken as we age. Other scientists have found in animal testing that blueberries may lower cholesterol levels. Blueberries are also a good source of vitamin K, which Tufts researchers suggest may play a role in preventing osteoporosis and hardening of the arteries. Berries of all sorts are good choices, too: Blackberries, for example, also deliver vitamin K, along with a quarter of your daily vitamin C in just a half-cup. If berries are out of season, try frozen berries blended into a smoothie.

10 Bran flakes—Research shows that breakfast really is "the most important meal of the day," and bran flakes can get you off to a good start. You'll get lots of fiber and magnesium—plus many other nutrients if you pick a moderately fortified cereal. Remember to use skim or low-fat milk and to go easy on the sugar. Need a touch of sweetness? Top your bran flakes with some berries (see above) or other fruit.

11 Broccoli—You probably don't need any convincing that broccoli, the classic "good for you" vegetable, is a healthy choice. But one of the biggest changes in the government's new food pyramid is an increased emphasis on dark green vegetables—like broccoli and leafy greens such as spinach and kale. Most Americans need to double or triple their intake of dark green veggies, according to the experts.

12 Brown rice—Part of the push to replace processed foods with whole grains means eating more brown rice instead of the white stuff you probably grew up on. Whole grains like brown rice include the bran and germ of the natural grain that are lost in processing to make white rice, which contains only the inner endosperm. A lot of good stuff gets lost in the bargain: Brown rice has almost 10 times as much phosphorus and potassium as white rice, for instance.

13 Brussels sprouts—Another no-surprise inclusion, brussels sprouts may do your body even more good than you'd guess. A half-cup of brussels sprouts—only about four sprouts—delivers 235 micrograms of vitamin K, which is almost double what the average American gets in a whole day.

14 Canola oil—Here's where substitution is really the key: Replacing butter, lard or other saturated fats with vegetable oils that contain monounsaturated and polyunsaturated fats can pay dividends for your heart. Canola oil is the very lowest in saturated fat, with other choices such as safflower and soybean oil close behind; the differences are small enough that you should pick whichever polyunsaturated oil you prefer. Olive oil has the highest proportion of monounsaturated fat and has earned heart-healthy labeling from the FDA, but it's not necessarily best. Let taste drive your choice: When you want flavor-free oil, go with polyunsaturated; when you want flavor, pick olive or peanut oils. Whichever you choose, remember that all fat contains 120 calories a tablespoon—so go easy, and don't *add* fat to your diet just to get more vegetable oil.

15 **Cantaloupe**—That orange color inside should clue you in that cantaloupe is a great source of beta-carotene—100 percent of your daily value in a single cup. Cantaloupe is no slouch in the vitamin C count, either, with 113 percent of daily needs per cup. Other melons such as honeydew are also good choices, though lower in both beta-carotene and vitamin C.

16 **Carrots**—You knew carrots were good for you, but did you know *how* good? Carrots are a prime example of why it's important to eat a "rainbow" of different fruits and vegetables representing the whole spectrum of colors. This orange option delivers 150 percent of your daily vitamin A in just half a cup, plus lesser percentages of a variety of other vitamins and minerals.

17 **Cauliflower**—Don't let the pasty white color fool you. Cauliflower is a cruciferous vegetable (meaning it's from the mustard family), just like broccoli and brussels sprouts. Compounds in cruciferous vegetables have been suggested as possible cancer protectors. In any case, cauliflower packs a nutritional punch, with 45 percent of your daily vitamin C in just half a cup.

18 **Chicken breasts**—Boneless, skinless chicken breasts offer great convenience and a good way to get protein (half your daily value in a three-ounce serving) without a lot of fat (three grams total, including just one gram of saturated fat) or calories (140, only 18 percent of them from fat). Broil, bake or grill—don't fry—to keep chicken a smart choice.

19 **Collard green**—Another option in the dark-green vegetable category, collard greens are packed with vitamin A. You'll get 150 percent of your daily value of A in just a half-cup of cooked collard greens, plus 30 percent of your vitamin C and 15 percent of calcium.

20 **Cranberry juice**—Studies suggest cranberry juice can help ward off urinary-tract infections and might even prevent periodontitis and gingivitis by keeping bacteria from adhering to your teeth and gums. It's also loaded with vitamin C. Look for juice that's artificially sweetened to avoid added sugar. (Note that cranberry juice can interact with the blood-thinning medication warfarin to cause bleeding.)

21 **Kale**—Here's another vitamin-A powerhouse as well as a way to up your intake of dark green vegetables. Like most leafy greens, kale is a source of lutein. A mere half-cup of cooked kale also rewards you with almost seven times the recommended daily amount of vitamin K.

22 **Kidney Beans**—Rich in fiber, iron and protein, beans of all sorts can be a key ingredient in an occasional meatless meal. They're also a source of potassium and magnesium, as well as folate, which some researchers are studying for potential benefits to the brain. Beans of all types—besides kidney, for instance, black, pinto and navy—are good choices and nutritionally similar. Kidney beans give you marginally the most protein and fiber with the fewest calories, but pintos are tops in folate. Cook your own using dried beans, to avoid added salt in canned beans.

23 **Mackerel**—Less familiar than other cold-water fish, mackerel is worth adding to your seafood repertoire because it also contains heart-healthy omega-3 fatty acids. It's also a good dietary source of vitamin D, as well as of selenium, which has antioxidant benefits. (Small children and pregnant women should eat mackerel sparingly, however, because of the risk that some fish may have high levels of mercury.)

24 **Milk (non- or low-fat)**—That ad campaign urging you to get milk is on-target—as long as you stick to skim or low-fat milk. Drinking milk makes it easy to meet the new dietary guidelines' recommendation to get the equivalent of three cups of dairy products daily. In addition to delivering calcium, fortified milk is among the best ways to get vitamin D, which your body needs in tandem with calcium to build bone strength to prevent osteoporosis.

25 **Oatmeal**—Besides the benefits of starting your day with a healthful breakfast, and besides the fact that oatmeal helps you get whole grains, oatmeal has been shown to lower cholesterol. You can also lower blood cholesterol with oat bran and with cold cereal made from oatmeal or oat bran. (Watch out for instant oatmeal packages, though, which typically contain lots of extra sugar.)

26 **Okra**—A food better known in southern states, okra is a good source of folate and also gives you 20 percent of your vitamin C needs in just half a cup. A recent study suggests that okra, along with eggplant and whole grains, among other foods, can be part of a cholesterol-lowering diet. (Breading and frying okra, southern-style, adds so many calories that it offsets any health benefits, however!)

27 **Oranges**—Of course, you already know about the benefits of eating from the "sunshine tree"—notably, getting more than a day's dose of vitamin C in just one navel orange. Oranges also are a pretty good source of potassium.

28 **Peaches**—Peaches and similar fruit such as nectarines deliver modest amounts of vitamins (especially A and C), niacin and minerals (particularly potassium), while satisfying your craving for something sweet—all at a tiny price in calories (only 40 in a medium-sized peach).

29 **Peanut butter**—Most of the fat in peanut butter remains monounsaturated, making "PB" an option as a sandwich substitute for meats high in saturated fat. A two-tablespoon serving has eight grams of protein and 25 percent of your daily niacin. There's no nutritional difference between creamy and crunchy peanut butter—just texture.

30 **Popcorn**—Air-popped popcorn (easy on the salt and butter!)

makes a filling whole-grain snack. A cup of plain air-popped popcorn has just 30 calories.

31 **Pork loin**—This is the leanest cut of "the other white meat" (actually a red meat). A three-ounce serving delivers 32 percent of daily protein needs with just 2.5 grams of saturated fat and 120 calories. Because it's so lean, be careful to cook pork loin to the safe internal temperature of 160 degrees but not beyond. Use a meat thermometer, and remove from the heat 5-10 degrees before it's done, as the pork will keep cooking while "resting." Even if still pink in the center, pork is safe to eat at 160 degrees.

32 **Prunes**—Prunes aren't just your mom's constipation cure. A half-cup of dried prunes does provide a quarter of your daily fiber, sure, but you're also getting potassium and vitamin A, plus vitamin B6 and powerful antioxidants.

33 **Quinoa**—Another whole-grain option (see the listing for barley for more), quinoa is catching on as an alternative to refined grains and other mealtime "starch" choices. Remember to rinse it well before cooking.

34 **Romaine lettuce**—This salad staple counts toward your daily goal of eating more leafy greens, and delivers vitamin A and C along with a tasty crunch. Boston, Bibb and red or green leaf lettuces are other good salad choices (easy on the fatty dressings!), though not as vitamin-packed. Iceberg lettuce has only a fraction of the nutritional value of its greener, darker kin.

35 **Salmon**—The classic example of fish with heart-healthy omega-3 fatty acids, salmon can be broiled, baked or grilled to make a main dish. Keep in mind, however, that even fat that's good for you comes with a caloric price tag—160 in a three-ounce serving of farmed salmon, 120 for the same portion of wild Atlantic salmon. If you occasionally opt for canned salmon with the bones, you'll also get calcium in the bargain.

36 **Sardines**—another fatty fish that's rich in omega-3s, sardines are also a good source of vitamin D and (eaten with the bones) calcium.

37 **Shredded-wheat cereal**—In addition to the benefits of a healthy breakfast, shredded-wheat cereal gives you a good start on your daily goal of 400 milligrams of magnesium, which has been associated with reduced risk of diabetes. Just two regular-sized biscuits have 80 milligrams of magnesium.

38 **Spinach**—Popeye was onto something here. Besides being the quintessential dark leafy green and rich in vitamins A and K (plus some folate), spinach is also packed with lutein. Researchers have found that lutein consumption is associated with a reduced risk of macular degeneration, the leading cause of vision loss and blindness in people age 65 and older.

39 **Strawberries**—Like most berries (see blueberries, above), grapes and prunes, strawberries contain anthocyanins, powerful antioxidants that improve circulation and may have other health benefits. Strawberries are also a good choice for folate and vitamin C.

40 **Sweet potatoes**—Try sweet potatoes instead of regular potatoes. They have more beta-carotene (a whopping 25,000 IU in one baked sweet potato with skin), vitamin C, folate, calcium and manganese than white spuds.

41 **Tea**—What to drink with all this? Try a nice cup of freshly brewed tea instead of a sugary soft drink. Research has suggested many possible benefits from the phytonutrient antioxidants in tea, called catechins; the strongest scientific evidence is for reducing heart disease. There's not a significant difference in antioxidants between caffeinated and decaffeinated tea, but we're not talking about herbal teas here. Iced tea contains only low concentrations of catechins, however. Premixed iced-teas and ready-to-drink teas are likewise low in antioxidants—but laden with sugar.

42 **Tofu**—The range of benefits hoped for from tofu and other soy products has been called into question, but tofu can still be a smart substitute for meat in your meal planning. It's a good source of protein and calcium if it's been prepared with calcium carbonate.

43 **Tomatoes**—Men have been gobbling tomatoes ever since research suggested that the lycopene therein may be protective against prostate cancer; a recent study points to a similar effect for pancreatic cancer in men. Tomatoes are also a good choice for lutein, and a single medium tomato contains half your daily value of vitamin C.

44 **Tuna**—Besides being a good choice for omega-3s, tuna is high in vitamins B6 and B12 as well as protein. If you buy canned tuna, opt for water-packed, not oil-, and resist the impulse to mix it with fatty mayo; try low-fat mayo or mayonnaise mixed with low-fat yogurt.

45 **Turkey breast**—Like its poultry cousin, chicken, skinless turkey breast delivers plenty of protein—38 percent of daily needs in a three-ounce portion—without a lot of fat (five grams, including 1.5 grams of saturated fat). Turkey is also rich in B vitamins and selenium. Besides making a good main dish, sliced turkey breast can substitute for processed meats in your sandwiches.

46 **Walnuts**—Remember what we said about almonds? The same goes for walnuts: They're low in saturated fat, free of cholesterol and high in unsaturated fats, but only a good idea when replacing foods packed with saturated fat. Although a quarter-cup of walnuts contains four grams of protein, you're also consuming 160 calories. Walnuts are relatively high in essential minerals and in folate.

47 **Watermelon**—A good source of lycopene, a cup of watermelon also gives you about 20 percent of your daily vitamin C and 15 percent of vitamin A, in a sweet treat with only 45 calories.

48 **White fish**—While fatty fish such as salmon have the added benefit of omega-3s, they needn't be the only fish in your repertoire. White fish such as flounder, cod and sole, although not high in heart-healthy fats, are also outstanding choices. A three-ounce serving of cod, for example, offers 30 percent of your daily protein with only 68 calories and less than one fat gram. Fish sticks and fish sandwiches don't count as healthy choices, however—go with baked, broiled or grilled fish.

49 **Whole-grain bread**—The new federal dietary guidelines encourage Americans to consume the whole-grain equivalent of at least three one-ounce slices of bread daily. Switching from white to whole-grain bread is an easy way to get started—but check the label to make sure the first ingredient listed is "whole wheat" or another whole grain. Don't be fooled by terms such as "multi-grain," "100 percent wheat," "cracked wheat" or "seven-grain."

50 **Whole-grain pasta**—If you've been put off by tough, grainy whole-wheat pasta in the past, it's time to give it another try. In the first quarter of 2005 alone, more than 28 new whole-grain pastas were introduced, taking advantage of new technology to make tastier products.

51 **Yogurt (non- or low-fat)**—Here's a delicious way to get your daily dairy. Besides calcium, yogurt gives you protein, magnesium and a variety of vitamins including B12. It's even been linked to better breath. (Yogurt doesn't have vitamin D, however, so it's no substitute for milk.) Instead of sugared varieties, control calories by adding your own fresh fruit to plain, low-fat yogurt.

Getting Personal With Nutrition

Some of us have personal trainers, monogrammed towels, vanity license plates, or at least value our "personal" space, but are we ready for "personalized nutrition?"

Well, at least 130 delegates from 17 countries who attended the Second International Conference on Nutrigenomics in Amsterdam, The Netherlands in early November think we might be. A wealth of information about the role of genes in determining our health has become available with the deciphering of the human genome. The concept of "personalized nutrition," or "nutrigenomics" as some scientists call it, takes this information one step further. Personalized nutrition involves the establishment of individual dietary recommendations based on knowledge of nutritional requirements, nutritional status, and each person's unique genetic makeup to potentially reduce risk of disease. Many speakers emphasized that, although this new knowledge is very intriguing, we are still at early points on the learning curve despite the tremendous potential of nutrigenomics.

Shedding Light on the Science

According to Dr. Jose Ordovas of Tufts University, society has often embraced a "one-size-fits-all" approach to current dietary recommendations, such as low-fat and low-cholesterol diets for the entire population. Although this broad approach to recommendations will likely benefit the majority of people, research indicates that a number of complicated genetic factors may minimize the benefits of such dietary changes, potentially harm some individuals, or have no effect for some.

Different species, such as mice and humans, have particular genes in common; however, the genome, or an entire set of genes in a particular arrangement, is unique to each individual. Dr. Ben van Ommen, of TNO Nutrition and Food Research in The Netherlands, stated that it is now possible to determine the sequences of a whole genome and determine how the genes in that genome are expressed; rather than focus on one gene as a single datum point. "Nobody is equal, and neither are our genes, since every gene has at least ten variants," van Ommen said. He also emphasized that nutrition provides more subtle changes to gene expression than do pharmaceuticals.

Robert Kushner, MD, Medical Director of the Wellness Institute at the Northwestern Feinberg School of Medicine and Northwestern Memorial Hospital, shared his perspectives on how physicians may provide information on personalized nutrition to have better quality discussions with their patients. "Nutrigenomics has the potential to spark interest among physicians in seeing that nutritional needs are more clearly determined for individuals," Dr. Kushner stated.

Professor Michael Muller, of Wageningen University in the Netherlands, defined nutrigenomics as an attempt to study the genome-wide influences of nutrition by combining nutrition at the molecular level with genomics. He asked, is it possible that someday we might move from our broad-beam flashlight-approach to adopt more of a fine-tuned laser beam-approach to nutrition recommendations, making them very specific to an individual's needs?

Consumers Lead the Way

The conference featured an impressive array of scientific findings and experts showing great enthusiasm about future possibilities, but what do consumers think about all of this?

Unveiling highlights from a comprehensive, landmark survey of US consumer attitudes toward the broad area of genomics, including nutrigenomics, Christy White, principal of Cogent Research in Cambridge, Massachusetts, indicated that consumers are ready to learn more.

Three-fourths of Americans are interested in obtaining their personal genetic information to identify their risk of diseases like cancer, osteoporosis, and heart disease, and nearly half of Americans are prepared to use diet-related products tailored to their health needs on the basis of their genetic makeup, according to Cogent's October 2003 survey of 1,000 Americans. "Americans are ready and willing to buy products based upon their genetic information, but the science is only in the early stages of being able to deliver," said White. "The good news is consumers aren't looking for complete diet regimens, but for individual approaches and basic recommendations."

The survey reveals that more than 90 percent of Americans are aware of the connection between diet and health, and 71 percent believe that genetics play a crucial role in health

Examining the Ethical Issues of Nutrigenomics

New research designed to help consumers create customized diets on the basis of their genetic make-up could create ethical and legal challenges with serious implications for the scientific and medical communities, according to a panel of international experts.

Dr. David Castle of the University of Guelph presented a paper in Amsterdam, *Nutrition and Genes: Science, Society and the Supermarket,* a joint project of the University of Toronto Joint Centre for Bioethics (JCB) and the University of Guelph philosophy department, the study examines the ethical questions surrounding nutrigenomics, the study of how nutrients and genes interact, and how genetic variations can cause people to respond differently to food nutrients. Castle cautioned against a rush to embrace nutritional genomics before there has been a detailed examination of its moral and ethical implications, backed by national awareness campaigns and public consultations.

The paper, prepared by a nine-member panel of international experts, stops short of prescribing specific ethical guidelines for the development and implementation of nutritional genomics technology. Rather, it is designed to foster public debate, setting out the issues that must be considered as consumers begin customizing diets to prevent and mitigate chronic health conditions. The panel wants input from professional groups, citizens' organizations, and individuals before it issues recommendations. Which it will do in 2004.

Environmental and lifestyle factors are thought to play a large role in the development of many diseases. However, science has determined, for example, that most people's genetic predisposition to cardiovascular disease is dependent upon variations in scores of genes, each of which appears to lead to small increases in susceptibility. As well, it appears that one gene can be involved in a number of conditions. Genetic testing may be able only to indicate an increased susceptibility to cardiovascular disease, rather than the certainty of future disease, the paper says.

The paper identifies the following as principal concerns:

• When is the science strong enough to market genetic tests in a widespread way?

• Who should have access to nutritional genomics information, who should not, and how should improper access be prevented?

• How should nutritional genomics information be delivered to consumers?

• How can society prevent potential nutritional genomics-related inequities, especially those created between developed and developing countries?

• Which nutritional genomics concerns should be the subject of regulation and oversight?

Use of Nutritional Genomic-Related Information

"As more is learned about individual genetic susceptibility to disease, information from genetic tests may become increasingly attractive to outside parties who stand to gain from it," the paper says. "There is a concern that employers or insurers could use genetic information to the unfair disadvantage of some people." Two-thirds of respondents in a 1997 survey said that they would not undergo genetic testing if they thought that health insurers and employers would have access to the results.

One of the most important issues is whether private genetic information should be treated as confidential in nature and not communicated to others without consent. Personal medical information usually remains private, but genetic tests may be relevant to blood relatives. Physicians may therefore face situations in which they must choose between patient confidentiality and providing potentially useful information to other members of the same family.

The main purpose of looking for food-gene interactions is to prevent or reduce the risk of disease; so the sooner useful dietary changes are made, the better the chances of avoiding nutrition-related diseases are. This suggests that testing children early would provide the widest range of health benefits. However, a balance must be maintained between acting in the interests of children before they are mature enough to make decisions and interfering with their right to the confidentiality of their genetic information. "This raises the question of whether the decision to administer a nutritional genomics test to a child falls within the legitimate range of parental discretion," says Dr. Castle.

"The collection, storage, and use of genetic information will be one of the most hotly debated medical issues of the coming decade," says Dr. Abdallah Daar of JCB and director of the Program in Applied Ethics and Biotechnology. "Even at this early stage, scientific progress is outstripping the public's ability to make informed choices about what kind of regulations should be introduced to address ethical and privacy concerns."

For more information go to the JCB Web site (**http://www.utoronto.ca/jcb**).

---

throughout life. However, 73 percent are concerned about how personal genetic information would be stored and who would have access to that information (see "Examining the Ethical Issues of Nutrigenomics" above).

In October 2003, the US Senate unanimously passed the Genetic Privacy Bill, which would prevent health plans from providing access to insurance companies on the basis of genetic information and from using such information to underwrite policies. Employers would be allowed to collect genetic information only to determine overall workplace exposures but could not use the information in hiring. Although the

Bush administration supports the bill, the House must still approve it.

Cogent Research also found that consumers most strongly preferred the term "personalized nutrition" with the term "nutrigenomics" being the least-liked term among the terms tested to describe this emerging area. Other terms tested included "nutrigenetics," "individualized nutrition," and "nutritional genomics." Cogent's conclusions on terminology are consistent with research that the International Food Information Council Foundation commissioned Cogent to conduct in December 2002. The findings of Cogent Research are from a broader, syndicated research study on genomics that explored applications including pharmaceuticals, health and beauty products, and nutrition. The study marks one of the largest efforts to understand consumers' acceptance of the use of their genetic information to influence the balance between health and disease.

What will it take to bring the promise of personalized nutrition to reality? Dr. Bruce German of the University of California at Davis painted the big picture for the delegates in Amsterdam. He sees this new knowledge as an opportunity to empower individuals to make informed and personal choices for their diet and lifestyle. According to German, "Scientists can enable the joys of life but not tell people what to do with their lives. We don't want to be the same—we want to be as healthy as we want to be. Success will involve personalizing health and delight simultaneously!"

Reprinted from the International Food Information Council Foundation, (December 2003).

The Slow Food Movement Picks Up Speed

Forsake fast food and convenience cuisine. Savor the enjoyment of ripe, locally grown produce and freshly prepared foods that have made a short, simple field-to-plate journey.

Sharon Palmer, RD

There's a slower, gentler food movement afoot. People are talking about slowing down our food supply and enjoying the pure taste of food that isn't weighed down with processing and chemicals. They are buying fresh, ripe produce from local farms that wasn't picked green, polished with wax, and trucked across the country. People are remembering the way their grandparents and great-grandparents ate, when they harvested apples in the fall and made jars of applesauce for the winter. The buzz is about wondering how your lunch was produced instead of inhaling a burger in the car while fielding cell phone calls. It's essentially the antithesis of fast food. Welcome to the slow food movement.

Food professionals, chefs, and foodies are embracing this concept and now dietitians are joining their ranks. It's no surprise, as slow food includes the message that dietitians have been preaching for decades—a focus on whole foods, such as fruits, vegetables, whole grains, nuts, and legumes. The slow food philosophy digs deeper into the food system, tracing foods all the way back to the very soil in which they were grown. According to Melinda Hemmelgarn, MS, RD, columnist and a Kellogg Foundation Food and Society Policy fellow, the message of slow food is about "thinking beyond your plate."

As the food supply became increasingly centralized and mega food companies started feeding a growing percentage of American bellies, people lost touch with the food supply and the flavors of real food. These days, it's easy to find food products that boast maltodextrin as the first ingredient and families gathered around the dinner table for a packaged, convenience meal with a long list of ingredients from all over the country. Ask a classroom of urban kids whether they've ever picked a fresh strawberry and let the juice run down their chins. Then, for extra credit, ask them how strawberries are cultivated.

"With the globalization of food, we are no longer eating food in season or fresh. We want to bring it back to people's consciousness. We don't want our palates dulled, we want to eat only when it's ripe and at its fullest," said Alice Waters recently at the Association of Food Journalists conference in San Francisco. Founder and owner of Chez Panisse in Berkeley, Calif., Waters is widely regarded as the mother of the local, sustainable food movement.

The Birth of Slow Food

Slow Food, an international organization, was founded in 1986 in Italy by Carlo Petrini, who maintained that the industrialization of food was standardizing taste and leading to the extinction of thousands of food varieties. With 83,000 members worldwide, the network is organized into local groups called *convivia* that are engaged in organizing dinners, tastings, and promoting campaigns. Slow Food's mission is to help motivate people to come back to kitchens and tables to nurture culture and community. By doing so, the organization hopes to invigorate regional and seasonal culinary traditions and celebrate taste while promoting ecologically sound food production.

"Carlo Petrini, the father of Slow Food, spoke at the Food and Society Policy conference last spring. He described quality food as meeting three criteria: 1) It tastes great; 2) It is produced sustainably, with care for the environment; and 3) The food is produced in a humane and socially just manner," explains Hemmelgarn. "For example, a food may be delicious and grown organically, but if the people working in the fields are treated like slaves, then it doesn't fit with the Slow Food philosophy. Individuals who embrace the concept of Slow Food believe it is important to critically question the food we eat and ask, Who grows or produces it and under what conditions? Where was the food produced and how many miles did it have to travel to reach my plate? How were the animals treated in life and in death, and how will the growing practices impact our environment?"

Measuring Food Miles

In the slow food world, people throw around the term *food miles* almost as frequently as dietitians use the word *calories*. A food mile is the distance food travels from where it is grown or raised to where it is ultimately purchased by the consumer. In the United States, food typically travels 1,500 to 2,500 miles to get to our plates, according to a recent study by the Worldwatch Institute.[1]

Most Americans don't realize that much of food production and processing happens far from where they live and rarely consider the costs of food related to production, processing, storage, and transportation. The environmental costs are the increased amount of fossil fuel used to transport food long distances and the increase in greenhouse gas emissions resulting from the burning of these fuels. According to USDA Agricultural Marketing Service produce arrival data from the Chicago terminal market, produce arriving by truck traveled an average distance of 1,518 miles. Data from three Iowa local food projects where farmers sold to institutional markets found that the food traveled an average of 44.6 miles to reach its destination. A conventional system used four to 17 times more fuel and released five to 17 times more carbon dioxide from the burning of the fuel than the Iowa-based regional and local food systems.[2]

Fresh From the Farm

Slow food has helped save small farms that may have been swept up by the big food industry. By supporting local farms, proponents help preserve the bucolic scenery of faded barns and patchwork farms that have been woven into the American landscape, as well as genetic diversity in crops.

In Marin County, California, 25 years ago dairy woman Ellen Straus and biologist Phyllis Faber sensed that agriculture was in danger of being lost forever to non-agricultural land development. They set out to protect the land through the Marin Agricultural Land Trust, which is now a model for farmlands across the country. This preservation compensates farmers and ranchers for the development value of their land while perma-

nently protecting the land for agriculture. Now the region is studded with small farms and ranches, such as the James Grossi Ranch and the McEvoy Olive Ranch.

One of the best ways to support slow foods is to frequent farmers' markets, which promote locally grown, organic fruits and vegetables, and small family farms. The number of farmers' markets has doubled in the last five years. A recent study from the Leopold Center for Sustainable Agriculture showed that farmers' markets produced $20.8 million in sales and more than 325 jobs for the Iowa economy, turning out to be the No. 1 marketing channel for Iowa's vegetable and fruit growers.[3]

Artisan Foods Move in Quickly

The artisan movement, in which purveyors craft foods on a small scale with a dedication to quality ingredients, is walking hand in hand with slow foods, creating a whole new market. People are willing to pay a higher price for food not prepared by the food giants. With 38 workers, The Straus Family Creamery (Marin County, Calif.) sells 27 million pounds of milk per year for as much as 50% more than major brands. Stores like Whole Foods Market and Wild Oats, whose philosophies support slow food, have seen double annual revenue in the past five years. Whole Foods not only stocks a plethora of specialty foods, they have started their own Authentic Food Artisan program in which foods are labeled with a special sticker indicating artisan status. Chefs in elegant restaurants now spell out artisanal products and sources of food ingredients on their menus by name.

Laura Chenel, founder and owner of Laura Chenel's Chevre, Inc., credits her affinity for goats as motivation for starting her artisan goat cheese production company, considered to be the originator of American goat cheese. Chenel claims that she is extremely involved with her herd of 500 goats, even down to calling them by name. "For me, an artisan is a craftsperson. It is all about care and attention to detail, pride, and ownership," says Chenel. Her goats are on a healthy

schedule of grain and alfalfa feedings intermixed with grazing and play times in the pasture that may put mothers of human kids to shame.

Even meat purveyors are becoming part of the slow and artisan food movements. Oregon Country Natural Beef raises their meat without antibiotics and hormones. At Marin Sun Farms in Northern California, David Evans watches over his family's herd of Hereford-Angus cows and more than 1,000 laying hens, becoming known for his innovative and humane ranching techniques.

Seasonal Celebration

One tenant of slow foods is eating seasonally, the way people did generations ago. Our ancestors never dreamed of eating raspberries in January. Preservation was necessary and traditional dishes evolved that celebrated the seasons. Celebrity chefs and Martha Stewart have helped make the lost art of preservation en vogue again. A slow food advocate before it had a name, Waters says, "This is an idea that has been around since the beginning of time. We rigidly follow seasons. When we got into winter vegetables, we discovered the flavor and varieties of the winter palette."

Simply in Season (*World Community Cookbook*) [Herald Press, 2005], cowritten by Mary Beth Lind, RD, and Cathleen Hockman-Wert is packed with inspiration for eating seasonally. The book lists six reasons to eat simply in season, which include freshness, taste, nutrition, variety, environment, and local health, as farmers' markets support the local economy.

Slow Roots in Culinary Arts

Slow food gained momentum in the culinary arts community. Waters opened Chez Panisse in 1971 with a dedication to local, seasonal products. Today's chefs follow in her footsteps by boasting their own organic gardens to supply their kitchens, even picking fresh salad greens on their way to work. They frequent farmers' markets and change their menus daily to incorporate the latest harvest. They are starting to develop personal relationships with farmers. Dishes on restaurant menus have become simpler so they celebrate the

Out of Africa

Dietitians such as Stacia Nordin, RD, nutrition consultant in sustainable food and nutrition security specialist, have found ways to fit the slow food philosophy into their careers. Nordin has been working in Malawi, Africa, to improve food and nutrition security, partly through reviving the knowledge of indigenous foods and integrating them into modern diets. In the past, the diet of the people of Malawi revolved around a variety of local fruits, vegetables, nuts, seeds, millets, sorghums, roots, and animal foods. But such foods began to vanish because of the push to supply year-round maize and the interest in western foods. With more than 90% of people living in Malawi fulfilling their nutrition needs through subsistence agriculture, if the environment around them doesn't supply the necessary food, there is nothing to eat.

— SP

flavor of one particular food, whether it's a fresh peach or Neiman Ranch beef. Slow food followers are searching Web sites to discover which restaurants are slow food-friendly before they make a reservation. Hemmelgarn reports that she asks waiters which foods on the menu are local before ordering.

Chefs Collaborative is an organization directed to chefs and the food community with a mission to foster local foods and a sustainable food supply. With their Seafood Solutions, Meat of the Matter, and Farmer-Chef Connection programs, Chefs Collaborative offers helpful information about making decisions in the food supply and hopes to be a catalyst for change in the country. "We provide tools for purchasing decisions for chefs and guidelines for sustainable, healthful food," says Nancy Civetta of Civetta Comunicazioni, the public relations company for Chefs Collaborative.

Edible Gardens for Kids

As it becomes painfully clear that our kids do not have enough face time with real food, slow food has started to take root in school gardens. Dan Desmond, 4-H Youth Development Advisor in El Dorado County, California, says, "In recent years with poor nutrition seen in children, the garden offers one solution. Early research shows that when children garden, they include fruits and vegetables more regularly into their diet." The National Farm to School Program is listed as a resource in the School Wellness Policy Web site.

"We need to develop the relationship between the child and food products. Taking junk food out of schools is great, but you need to change the whole culture. If you want to change the culture, you have to start with children," says Desmond. He reports that the school garden is alive and well in many parts of the United States and that there are approximately 3,000 school gardens in California, ranging from half wine barrels to 20-acre farms. Desmond believes California First Lady Maria Shriver will probably jump on the school garden bandwagon to help promote the Live Deliciously campaign.

Waters created the Chez Panisse Foundation, which started the Edible Schoolyard, a garden and kitchen classroom at Berkeley's Martin Luther King, Jr. Middle School. Last year, the Berkeley Unified School District signed an agreement with the Chez Panisse Foundation to create a formal curriculum that includes organic gardening, cooking, and eating healthy lunches for the district's 9,000 students. "We're trying to reach kids who aren't eating with their parents and don't know about food," says Waters. "I want them to come to foods and fall in love, to have a whole new relationship with food that is connected to nature, tradition, and culture."

The Food Project in Massachusetts has a mission to help grow a community of youth and adults from diverse backgrounds to work together to build a sustainable food system. Since 1991, the Food Project built a model of getting young people to change through sustainable agriculture. They work with hundreds of teens and thousands of volunteers to farm on 31 acres of rural Lin-coln and on several lots in urban Boston, growing nearly a quarter-million pounds of food without chemical pesticides, one-half of which is donated to local shelters.

Dietitians Move Slow

It seems that dietitians can benefit from learning more about slow food, whether they work in wellness or manage a school foodservice program. "The philosophy behind slow food is part of my DNA, a part of how I was raised, but the principles of slow food have not generally been a part of the dietetic curriculum. Many dietitians need help understanding these ideas and translating them into practical recommendations," says Amanda Archibald, RD, founder of Field to Plate, a company that aims to teach the principles of local, seasonal, and regional foods. Archibald reports that her workshops reveal that dietitians are often curious and hungry for new ideas in food and nutrition education and are becoming more motivated to learn about slow food. "There are Dietary Guidelines for Americans, but I believe that we are ready for something more sustainable in our approach to nutrition education. We're ready to 'green' the guidelines," says Archibald, who recommends that dietitians join the Hunger and Environmental Nutrition Dietetic Practice Group, whose motto is that all people should have access to food from a healthy, sustainable environment.

"There is growing interest and awareness in the importance of how local agriculture methods are impacting our food system and the health of our region and the people in it, from an economic, environmental, and medical perspective. This interest and awareness does not originate from the conventional healthcare community, sadly enough. It comes from the general public recognizing the impact and interconnection of their medical concerns with what is happening in the greater world," says Lynn Mader, MBA, RD, food system consultant. Mader is involved with a farm-to-school initiative to identify local, seasonal foods that can be used by schools.

Slow Food is Moving

Slow food is inching its way across the country, even though it currently resides mostly in the well-educated, high-income strata of society. Since slow food typically costs more, plenty of people simply can't afford it. "Slow food remains an amazing philosophy, but it's out of reach to so many people," adds Archibald. Some experts predict that slow food will trickle down to all walks of life, as do many trends.

Some food professionals argue that slow food is not realistic, as consumers are still just as pressed for time as ever. After all, new products keep rolling out that conveniently fit into car cup holders. But new companies are proving that slow foods may not be just a pipe dream. Take Burgerville, a chain of 39 fast-food restaurants in the Pacific Northwest that features a McDonald's-like menu, but most ingredients come from local farms. Sodexho is starting to offer regionally sourced meals to their university and corporate clients and Kaiser Permanente is hosting farmers' markets at some facilities. It looks like the future of food may be moving more slowly for a change.

References

1. Halweil B. Homegrown: The Case for Local Food In A Global Market, November 2002. Available at: http://www.world-watch.org/pubs/paper/163

2. Pirog R, Van Pelt T, Enshayan K, et al. Food, Fuel, and Freeways: An Iowa perspective on how far food travels, fuel usage, and greenhouse gas emissions. Leopold Center for Sustainable Agriculture. June 2001. Available at: http://www.leopold.iastate.edu/pubs/staff/ppp/food_mil.pdf

3. Study Shows Positive Economic Impact of Iowa Farmer's Markets, 5-10-05, Leopold Center for Sustainable Agriculture. Available at: http://www.leopold.iastate.edu/news/newsreleases/2005/markets_051005.htm

---

—Sharon Palmer, RD, is a freelance food and nutrition writer in southern California.

Who's filling your grocery bag?

James E. Tillotson, PhD, MBA

Eight of our largest US food companies sell overwhelming amounts of the snacks that many Americans overeat. In all snack categories—soft drinks, candy, salty snacks, cookies, crackers, ice cream—1 or 2 mega-food companies dominate the market, selling from 50% to 75% of each type of fun food. What effect, if any, does this overarching market concentration have on Americans' obesity?

Nearly two thirds of American adults are overweight or obese, and many of our children are also getting unpleasantly plump. Therefore, it is important to examine all the factors in our food world, including the industry, that could contribute to overeating. In the last column, we saw that a few of the largest food companies—Pepsi, Mars, Coca-Cola, Nabisco, Frito-Lay—have dominant shares of fun-food markets—soft drinks, candy, ice cream, crackers, cookies, and salty snacks. Overwhelming marketing concentration means that these companies have a lot of clout in determining what products and marketing practices rule in the snack categories. Current industry structure and marketing practices deserve a searching look because of the role they *may* play in overeating. Any meaningful analysis must be *based on objective research, not on opinion or emotion.*

Table 1 shows the 8 leading fun-food companies discussed in part 1 of this article, the specific snacks marketed by each, and the estimated combined market share (in either sales or volume) of the 1 or 2 leading companies in each category (candy, carbonated beverages, etc.), as well as each company's total retail sales (2001). Several companies market more than one type of snacks. Some of these companies (Nestle, Unilever, Mars, Kraft, and Kellogg) market a broader range of branded foods than just snacks; others (Coca-Cola, PepsiCo, and Hershey) concentrate their marketing efforts predominantly on snack foods and beverages. Six of the companies are among our 10 largest food companies (sales), and the other 2 are among our 20 largest companies.

If public information is correct, 1 or 2 mega-food companies in each snack category have between 50% and 75% share of the market (based on either dollar or product volume). These are all tasty tempting snacks, which most of us eat in varying amounts. My immediate reaction, on finishing this chart, was to wonder if I had stumbled on one of the leading causes of American obesity.

Then I read a headline about a study by Gladys Block, Professor of Epidemiology and Public Health Nutrition, University of California Berkeley, which read: "Of the food Americans eat, sugary snacks and soda reign supreme over healthier options such as vegetables and fruits."[1] In her analysis of population-based data from the National Health and Nutrition Examination Survey (NHANES) data, she found that on average, *one-third of all Americans' calories* now come from what she defines as "junk food" (with sweets and desserts, soft drinks, and alcoholic beverages supplying many of the calories Americans consume).

One third of all Americans' calories now come from "junk food."

Is that it? Maybe the answer to the obesity problem is to ban, tax, or ration fun foods, and then we will all be svelte. (Except, of course, for those of us who will go to our neighborhood snack speakeasy for our daily fun food fix!). I suppose it's only a natural impulse to blame the marketing efforts of these mega-fun foods, with their outsized market shares and many customers, as "the" problem, simply because they supply so many of the treats we eat so much of so often. However, even 25 or 30 years ago snacks contributed approximately one quarter of all calories in diets, so there are probably other factors involved as well.

In examining the possible causes of heavily eating these leading snacks, we need to remember that we have an inherent liking for sweet, fatty, and salted fun foods (and many that contain alcohol, as well). By catering to this natural taste proclivity, it is likely that eaters will be highly attracted to these manufacturers' treats. Do snacks

Table 1. Major Food and Beverage Companies Selling Snack Categories in the United States

Snacks	Companies	Combined Category Market Share	2001 Sales,* $ Billion
Carbonated beverages	PepsiCo	Approximately 75% volume	26.9
	Coca Cola		20.1
Ice cream	Unilever	Approximately 50% sales	23.8
	Nestle		13.2
Candy	Mars	Approximately 70% sales	15.5†
	Hershey		4.6
Cookies	Nabisco (Kraft)	Approximately 50% sales	33.9
	Kellogg		8.9
Crackers	Nabisco (Kraft)	Approximately 60% sales	33.9
	Kellogg		8.9
Salty snacks	Frito-Lay (PepsiCo)	Approximately 56% sales	26.9
Non carbonated Beverages	PepsiCo	Approximately 75% volume	26.9
	Coca Cola		20.1

Sources: Food Institute, Food Processing, and assorted newspaper articles.
*Total company sales (all products) excluding food/beverage fast-food restaurants and food service subsidiaries.
†Sales for 2000.

produced by megacompanies pose greater risks of over-eating just because of these companies' great size? Is the high fun-foods market concentration *alone* a factor in the increased consumption of snacks? *If these companies didn't offer these snacks, wouldn't there be other companies in their place equal in size who would do so?*

I have found no proof that such market concentration, *by itself*, and devoid of other potential advantages, is any more conducive to greater individual consumption than a greater number of medium-sized marketers or even many small companies. *Size alone apparently is not the source of the health problem.*

Are the *megafuns* answering consumers' unfilled natural desires for high levels of foods that contain sweets, fat, and salt that are high in calories, or are they driving consumption beyond people's natural desire levels by some sort of marketing trickery? Are major snack producers creating an *unnatural* demand by tricking our taste buds into overconsuming? Is the latter condition even physiologically or psychologically possible? It is unlikely; *you can't sell people what they don't want to buy.*

Not all people who are obese eat the same foods or even the same commercially prepared food. There are plenty of people who are obese who eat few of the fun foods—soft drinks, candy, salty snacks, ice cream, and fast foods—daily, whereas other people who are equally obese seem to eat nothing but snacks. No question that you can be overweight without fun foods; snacks *aren't the only culprits in obesity.*

Well then, if commercial snack and fun foods are not always a factor in obesity and there is no proof that market concentration, *by itself*, is a factor in increased con-

sumption, then maybe high market share firms are just more adept at catering to people's desires (product, price, and convenience) in snacks, and because of this, people eat a little more of their snacks a lot of the time. The big 8 in snacks didn't get there by just being run-of-the-mill organizations; they got there by being the best in their snack categories over decades. *Plainly and simply, they are better marketers than the other guys!*

We know carbonated beverages have doubled in annual average consumption in recent decades. What caused this to happen? Do we know how much of this increased consumption is the result solely of mega-beverage companies' superior marketing, distribution, and promotional efforts? How much can be attributed to answering unfilled consumer desire for more sweetened drinks? Are the marketers driving the consumer market, or is the consumer market driving the marketers? Are these trends compensated for by decreases in other categories, or is there a net increase overall in calories consumed? *Again, we have no answers.*

Perhaps extreme market concentration of the major snack producers allows for other avenues of influence on consumer consumption, and these, in turn, have an effect on overconsumption of snacks. Here are some, but not all, of the factors that have been suggested and may be involved:

- *Heavy marketing and high profit margins of snack and fun foods.* Industry sources report that among the product mix of these large fun-food companies, food and beverage snacks are commonly their most profitable products. Thus, there is an economic rationale for these companies to place their heaviest marketing emphasis and persuasive skills on their fun-food products. *Suspicion, but lack of proof.*

- *Megacompanies sell more than snack foods alone, so their marketing practices dominate supermarket shelves and consumer purchases.* If we focus our inquiry only on the snacks marketed by these food companies, we limit our understanding of the potential impact that these large companies may be having on Americans' diets. The 8 food and beverage companies listed had an estimated all-product retail sales total of $147 billion (2001), including their top snack brands. Obviously, as shown by their total sales number, the big 8 products in both fun and other types of foods are a significant part of the food purchases of many Americans. *Suspicion, but again lack of proof.*

- *Retail channels demand fun-food giants' products because of consumer demand.* The total US all-products food retail sales (supermarkets, non-food outlets, convenience stores, etc.) were $408.2 billion in 2001. These 8 food-fun giants combined with their other type of food products were apparently the source of 36% of all retail food sales. These mega-8 are a significant source of Americans' food purchases—*one third of all retail sales* (2001). As a result, our supermarkets and other retail outlets may be *required* to preferentially offer their products, both fun and otherwise, to satisfy their customers' everyday product demands. Does the high concentration of major sources of fun foods today in a few megacompanies combined with the broader range of other foods marketed result in retail-purchase condition, favoring purchase and consumption of their snacks?

- *Retailers favor category captains and vice versa.* Do retail channels (supermarkets and other retail outlets) favor these megacompanies because they offer a wider range of foods and thus increased efficiencies for the retail trade in handling and selling both their snack and other food products? Or *do the megas serenade the retailers harder to get what they believe is their rightful Lebensraum of retail shelf space?*

- *Heavy advertising.* Do the economies of scale resulting from market-category consolidation (into a few large companies) result in increased promotional, marketing, and distribution capacities and efficiencies and favor increased sales of the megabrand snacks and fun foods? *The leading snack and fun foods are among our leading advertisers (all-products) and have unbelievably large advertising budgets* (Table 2).

All of these characteristics are structure-related factors of the industry that may result in market conditions (price, product sizes, availability, product shelf space access, pref-

Table 2. Major Food and Snack Companies 2003 Advertising and Ranking

Snack Companies	Us Advertising, $ Millions	Ranking, Top Ten Advertisers
Unilever	1,332	17*
Altria (Kraft)	1,311	18
PepsiCo	1,212	23
Nestle	1,113	27
Mars	813	41
Kellogg	570	57
Coca Cola	473	69
Hershey	NA	†

Source: Advertising Age, June 18, 2004.

* Includes personal care products and food.

†Company not in Top 100 (2003) in advertising spending.

erential product displays) that could be particularly favorable to motivating increased consumer purchase and consumption of snacks. *Suspicion, but lack of proof.*

I pointed out in the first part of this article that in addition to the high market concentration in the fun-food categories, there is wide market concentration throughout the entire consumer food sector; our 10 largest food companies supply more than 40% of each dollar's worth of all food Americans purchase annually at retail; expanding this number to the largest 40 companies, the figure comes up to 80% of all retail food sold. Never in recent times has our nation of some 300 million people been as narrowly commercially sourced by as few food companies.

There could be a silver lining to this market structure. If this high market concentration into megafood firms offers consumers overall the choice of readily available and more balanced dietary choices (in line with the Dietary Guidelines for Americans), this could be a good thing for diet and health.

Today, the prominent business strategy for large food companies is to increasingly concentrate on a limited number of their food brands, where the company's brands are the market leaders or a close competitor to the category leaders, seeking the higher profitably of leading national brands.

This trend has resulted in many large companies getting out of the business of selling low profit-margin commodity-type foods in favor of branded added-valued highly processed foods. For example, companies such as Kraft, Unilever, Nestle, and others have recently discontinued hundreds of second-tier brands, seeking greater overall company profitability.

A cursory search of big-food's product lines today shows a heavy offering of high-caloric-density low-nutrient-density products, as well as other foods of varying degrees of nutritional worth. Moreover, unlike the past, when our largest food firms marketed a broad range of foods, megacompanies today offer a much narrower range of foods. The megacompanies tend to stakeout a more re-strictive and a narrower line of products today for all the reasons I mentioned. Then they aggressively market and promote these *fortress brands* because of the competitive advantage such brands offer in the marketplace, as well as the greater profitability that concentrating predominantly on top brands offer.

How about their role in marketing fruits and vegetables? Today, these megacompanies have a negligible market presence (excepting in the fruit-juice beverage categories). The trend in recent years has been for them to divest businesses producing fruit and vegetable products (Birdseye) because of their lower profitability compared to other more profitable leading added-value food products. Some interesting new products are now in place (calcium-fortified orange juice), and others are on the horizon or already doing well in some markets (juices with sterols to lower serum cholesterol). The question is whether consumers will pay for these new bells and whistles.

Bottom Line

The role of our largest fun-food and beverage companies, the 8 giants, and their marketing, their branded snacks, and the resulting structural ramifications not on the market economics but on our overweight problem is far from settled, let alone what to do about if they are proven to be a significant negative factor.

My own personal take, formed by 2 decades in the consumer food industry and my recent time in the academic world studying the food industry, is that megafood companies' activities are certainly not the root cause of the obesity problem. There is a large dollop of personal behavior (*diet, behavior, and physical activity*) and plenty of other environmental factors as well in the causation of obesity.

However, I don't believe that we can let the concentrated structure of the food industry into megafood companies (and also large chain restaurants) totally off the hook. These companies combine their great economic power, marketing muscle, sales strategies, and tasty products to play a dominant role in shaping our daily diets by supplying too many of the discretionary calories we consume.

As a result of this market clout, I believe that there is great likelihood that these few large companies are an important factor in determining what, when, and how much many Americans eat or overeat today. This makes the mega-snack companies among environmental factors suspected as contributing to obesity risk, at least among those who eat a lot of their products. Obesity is similar to cancer in that its causes are complex and multiple and depend on a web of environmental and inborn factors. It follows that tackling this problem must involve the megafood companies as part of the solution. (Could you feed yourself today without these companies?) Therefore, just don't blame them, help fix them!

REFERENCES

1. Yang S. *Nearly One-Third of the Calories in the US Diet Come From Junk Food, Researcher Finds.* Berkeley, Calif: Media Relations; 2004.
2. Block G. Food contributing to energy intake in the US: data from NHANES III and NHANES 1999-2000. *Composition Analysis.* 2004;17:439-447.

James E. Tillotson, PhD, MBA, is currently Professor of Food Policy and International Business at Tufts University. Before returning to the academic world, Dr Tillotson worked in industry, holding various research and development positions in the food and chemical sectors. Correspondence: James E. Tillotson, PhD, MBA, PO Box Ten, Cohasset, MA 02025-0100 (e-mail: james.tillotson@tufts.edu).

Moving Toward Healthful Sustainable Diets

Nutritionists have increasingly been focusing on the challenge of moving consumers toward healthful diets and simultaneously helping them to make the connection between healthy food and a healthy environment. Simply stated, to foster food sustainability, consumers will need to choose minimally processed and minimally packaged foods. In addition, when possible, they should buy locally produced foods to support regional agriculture and local economies, preserve farmland, and use less energy and other natural resources.

BARBARA STORPER, MS, RD

Nutritionists have increasingly been focusing on the challenge of moving consumers toward healthful diets and simultaneously helping them to understand that what's good for their health may well be good for the health of the planet. Promoting food sustainability and ecologic harmony as an essential function of the nutrition professional was first proposed more than 20 years ago by Dr Joan Gussow, Mary Swartz Rose Professor Emeritus of Nutrition Education at Teachers College, Columbia University, and Dr Kate Clancy, Director of The Agriculture Policy Project at the Henry A. Wallace Institute for Sustainable Agriculture. Today, their message falls on receptive ears, as nutritionists better understand the connection between agriculture, the environment, hunger, health, and, ultimately, food security.

Drs Gussow and Clancy first introduced the term "food sustainability" to the nutrition profession in an article published in 1986 by the *Journal of Nutrition Education* entitled, "Dietary Guidelines for Sustainability."[1] They explained how the US Dietary Guidelines, the government's model for promoting health, can also be used as the framework by which nutritionists can promote sustainable diets. The article still serves today as a seminal treatise, calling the profession to promote a diet that is healthy for the individual, the rest of the world, and the planet.

Dr Gussow is still on the forefront of this mission today, promoting the sustainability advantages of "whole foods"—foods that are minimally processed and packaged. Nutritionally, whole foods fit more easily into a healthful diet than their processed and packaged counterparts because they are naturally higher in fiber and lower in fat, sodium, sugar, and additives. Globally, whole foods also bypass the high energy costs of food processing. In general, more profit stays with the farmer, helping farmers to make a livable income, thus staving off the alarming decline of the small and family farm in this country. Last, but far from least, Gussow claims that whole foods taste

better, give people more opportunity to prepare them the way they like, and allow people to feel more connected to the food's origin.

To foster sustainability, consumers should choose minimally processed and minimally packaged foods and, when possible, buy locally produced foods to support regional agriculture that preserves farmland and is less energy intensive

---

What's even better, she proclaims in her newest book, *This Organic Life: Confessions of a Suburban Homesteader*[2] is for people to eat locally produced food, and whenever possible, grow their own. The important current issue, says Gussow, is learning how to produce food for everyone in a way that's sustainable, and we are not doing that. What we are doing, she continues, is overproducing food globally while destroying the environment and our capacity for future food production. Supermarkets "trick" the consumer by selling foods from around the world all year long so that consumers on the East Coast expect summer produce in the winter, such as strawberries in January. The economic and environmental costs associated with these practices, however, are invisible to most consumers.

For Gussow, localization of the food supply remains the optimal approach to foster sustainability. The need to relocalize our food supply is urgent now, according to Gussow, because of the increasing harm caused by agribusiness practices—their emphasis on monocultures (ie, growing single crops over large areas) and their continued dependence on pesticides. She claims that our present agricultural system downplays the health and environmental hazards of pesticides, which are being used today at a far greater rate than when Rachel Carson's[3] *Silent Spring* first exposed their alarming consequences.

SUSTAINABILITY AND MODERN FARMING PRACTICES

Gussow uses the example of a potato to explain why current farming practices are not sustainable. There are 5,000 known varieties of the potato plant. Peruvian Indians in the Andes knew and used 3,000 of them. Yet, today, only 6 are grown commercially in the United States. Why? According to Gussow, it is to meet the demands of a processing industry that requires uniformity. The fast-food industry, in particular, prefers a single variety, the Russet, for its shape. The Russet potato is long enough so that when made into French Fries, the fries can extend beyond the edges of the cardboard container, creating the visual appearance consumers expect. Yet, she claims that limiting a nation's reliance on a few varieties of a crop is precisely what devastated Ireland's economy in the 1840s, when blight struck the two varieties of potatoes on which the entire nation depended for its food supply.

She also argues that monoculture also depletes the soil, creating an increased dependence on fertilizers and pesticides, manufactured from nonrenewable fossil fuels. This overdependence on pesticides, in turn, increases the health problems for growers and consumers of pesticide-ridden produce here and abroad.

Returning to a more locally produced food supply will not only help the environment but also, according to Gussow, make the public more aware of the link between their food and the health and environmental consequences of modern farming methods. Buying locally not only supports small farms and helps to maintain local economies but also helps neighbors stay in business and ultimately promotes sustainable communities.

It is surprising, according to Gussow, that the United States ranks as one of the leading food importers in the world! She believes that emphasizing local agriculture here may also help poor people in other countries who are steadily being pushed off their own lands when large agribusiness firms establish production sites for luxury and out-of-season foods for US tables. Ironically, she notes, the fruits and vegetables we eat out of season are often produced in countries with poor sanitation and questionable hygienic practices. Why eat a fruit from a country where one would not drink the water? Eating locally may offer a safe and healthy alternative to the consequences of a global marketplace.

MOVING TOWARD SUSTAINABLE DIETS

Here are some ways nutritionists can help to promote sustainability:

- Recommend that a certain portion of the weekly grocery money be used exclusively for foods that are produced locally and sold in farmers markets or through farms that establish memberships with local residents.

- Learn about and promote seasonal foods that can be grown locally in the consumer's own region and teach people how to cook these foods—or how to cook at all!

- Have your own backyard garden and encourage public organizations, schools, hospitals, etc, to build community gardens and use the foods grown for feeding programs.

Here are some creative resources nutrition educators can use to promote food sustainability with school-age children:

- LIFE Program (Linking Food and the Environment) a project of Teacher's College, Columbia University promotes the "Food Triangle"—a take-off on the Food Pyramid. Using a triangle, the project staff divide foods into three groups— "plant foods," "animal foods," and "man-made foods"—to help children learn about how their food choices affect their environment and their health. They also use hands-on activities such as gardening, cooking, shopping, composting, and recycling.

- "Earth Friends" is a minidiscovery museum housed at Teacher's College where classes from New York City schools visit and learn about food from farm to table in a series of games, exhibits, and cooking activities. Contact David Russo, Project Coordinator, 212-678-3955.

- "Cookshop" is a classroom curriculum designed by the New York Community Food Resource Center to help students and teachers cook a variety of locally grown wholesome foods that will then be introduced in the school cafeteria. Evaluations show dramatic increases in consumption of these previously unfamiliar foods when students learn about them first in class. Contact Toni Liquori at 212-894-8074 or tliquori@cfrcnyc.org.

- "Close Encounters with Agriculture," a Cooperative Extension Service of the University of Maryland Program links elementary school children with class activities and field trips to agricultural areas to learn about animals, horticulture, and farming.

- "Field to Table," a Cornell University Extension Project helps students to identify and increase their consumption of locally grown fruits and vegetables based on the Northeast Regional Food Guide.

- "From Land to Landfill" is a program developed by nutritionists at Purdue University using a systems approach to integrate health and nutrition into core subject areas.

- "FOODPLAY" is this author's traveling nutrition theater show that tours schools nationally and uses juggling, theater, music, magic, and audience participation to encourage children to make food choices that are good for their health and the health of the planet. Contact Barbara Storper at 800-FOODPLAY or http://www.foodplay.com.

Barbara Storper, MS, RD, is the Director of FOODPLAY Productions, an Emmy Award-winning nutrition media organization that produces national touring school theater shows, video kits, media campaigns, and resources to improve children's health. Ms Storper holds degrees in both journalism and nutrition and has received the first Outstanding Young Nutrition Educator in the Country Award and Media Partnership from the Society for Nutrition Education.

Corresponding author: Barbara Storper, MS, RD, FOODPLAY Productions, 221 Pine St, Florence, MA 01062 (e-mail: barbara@foodplay.com).

REFERENCES

1. Gussow JD, Clancy K. Dietary guidelines for sustainability. *J Nutr Edu.* 1986; 18:1–15.
2. Gussow JD. *This Organic Life: Confessions of a Suburban Homesteader.* White River Junction, Vt: Chelsea Green Publishing Company; 2001.
3. Carson R. *The Silent Spring.* Boston: Houghton Mifflin; 1994..

From *Nutrition Today*, March/April 2003, pp.57-59. © 2003 by Lippincott Williams and Wilkins. Reprinted by permission. http://lww.com

UNIT 2
Nutrients

Unit Selections

Key Points to Consider

- Keep a 24-hour food record and calculate the amount of antioxidant vitamins you consumed. Compare this amount to your daily requirements.

- Determine the glycemic index of foods you eat in one meal and classify them into high-, medium-, and low-glycemic index foods.

- Check out several labels from foods you eat frequently. Can you tell how much fat each contains?

- Determine the percentage of your average daily calories that is contributed by total fat and saturated fat. What do your results tell you about your potential health risks?

- Identify environmental sources of lead exposure you may be in contact with.

Student Website

www.mhcls.com/online

Internet References

Further information regarding these websites may be found in this book's preface or online.

Dole 5 A Day: Nutrition, Fruits & Vegetables
http://www.dole5aday.com

Food and Nutrition Information Center
http://www.nal.usda.gov/fnic/

Nutrient Data Laboratory
http://www.nal.usda.gov/fnic/foodcomp/

NutritionalSupplements.com
http://www.nutritionalsupplements.com

U.S. National Library of Medicine
http://www.nlm.nih.gov

Fish Contamination Resource
www.epa.gov/waterscience/fishadvice/advice.html

This unit focuses on the most recent advances that have been reported on nutrients and their role in health and disease. With the onset and development of new technologies in the area of nutrition—the plethora of information on the role of certain nutrients and the speed with which information is printed and disseminated—even the professional has a very hard time keeping up with the advances. The media reports sensational, even erroneous data, that confuses the public and creates misunderstandings. Preliminary reports have to undergo rigorous testing in animal models and clinical trials before they are accepted and implemented by the scientific community.

Additionally, how individuals will respond to dietary changes will depend on their genetic make-up in addition to other environmental factors. Thus, the National Academy of Science has a difficult task in establishing the exact amounts of nutrients that will cover human requirements but not create toxicity for the majority of the population.

The articles of this unit have been selected to present current knowledge about nutrients resulting from state-of-the-art research and controversies brewing at the present time. Articles related to nutrient function and their effects on chronic disease such as cardiovascular disease, obesity, diabetes mellitus, and osteoporosis are included.

An area of perennial controversy concerns fats and the types of fat. Americans have focused on single nutrients attempting to exclude them from the food they eat. This has resulted in the proliferation of low-fat products that are not necessarily low in calories. Two articles present current scientific finding about types of fats. Trans fatty acids that arise from food processing, which convert liquid oils to solid margarines, are as harmful to heart health as saturated fat. Current scientific findings on trans-fat are discussed and labeling for trans-fat became mandatory by the FDA beginning in 2006. As research evolves, a diet moderate in total fat is advised, especially incorporating omega-3 fatty acids found in fish such as tuna and salmon. Omega-3-fatty acids promote heart health and eye health and have beneficial effects on the immune system. Ways to incorporate them into our diet and recommendations to prevent methyl mercury toxicity from supplement use and fish consumption are discussed in some articles.

The heavy metal, lead, is another area of concern for nutritionists and other scientists because it has been linked to hypertension, kidney and cognitive dysfunction, and cataract formation. Additionally, once it accumulates in the body there is no mechanism to get rid of it. One of the articles in this unit provides information as to sources of lead in the environment, how to test for lead, and how to prevent your exposure.

The importance of vitamins is of great interest to consumers since vitamins have been touted to cure and/or prevent disease.

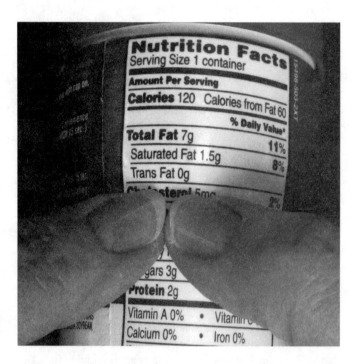

As the baby boomers are aging, diseases that affect their eyes—such as macular degeneration and cataracts—are on the rise. Several antioxidant vitamins such as vitamins C and beta-carotene and phytochemicals such as lutein and zeaxanthin may have a protective effect. Another vitamin whose deficiency produces irreversible neurological damage is vitamin B12. Populations vulnerable to this deficiency, how it precipitates, and solutions to preventing the deficiency are discussed.

The role of dairy products on health and their use as a functional food is described in another of the articles in this unit. A review of the scientific evidence as to their mechanism of action on bone health, hypertension and heart disease, cancer, weight loss, and the immune system is offered.

With the rise in obesity and diabetes mellitus in recent years, Americans are going on low carbohydrate, high-fat, and high-protein diets. The misconceptions about carbohydrates and the differences between "good" and "bad" carbohydrates based on the glycemic index and the glycemic load, are explained. The food industry as always, has been eager to fill consumer demand by developing low-carbohydrate containing products. Added sugars have been decreased and new products are fortified with fiber in form of lignin, arabinogalactosan, gums etc. for weight maintenance, cardiovascular and gastrointestinal health.

Omega-3 Choices:
Fish or Flax?

What are the health benefits of the fatty acids found in fish and flax?

BY ALISON J. RIGBY, PhD, MPH, RD

Fish consumption has been advocated on the basis of its lean high biological value protein, vitamin and mineral content, and "good" fat value from the omega-3 fatty acids found in fish. The health benefits of eating fish were essentially discovered by epidemiological studies of the Northern Inuit population, who were shown to have reduced rates of myocardial infarction as a result of their consumption of marine omega-3 fatty acids, compared with Western control subjects.[1] European countries have been supplementing their baby formulas for some time with omega-3 fatty acids for brain health. A recent American Heart Association (AHA) Scientific Statement on fish consumption, fish oil, omega-3 fatty acids, and cardiovascular disease amplified the benefits of eating fish and recommended the AHA guidelines of at least two servings of fish per week and the use of omega-3 supplementation for patients with coronary heart disease (1 gram per day) and larger doses (2 grams per day to 4 grams per day) for those patients with hypertriglyceridemia.[2]

REVIEW OF THE OMEGA-3 FATTY ACIDS

The omega-3 fatty acids are polyunsaturated fatty acids (missing many hydrogen atoms), with the last double bond located three carbons away from the methyl end. Eicosopentaenoic acid (EPA), or 20:5n-3, and Docosahexaenoic acid (DPA), or 22:6n-3, are the omega-3 fatty acids found in oily fish, with mackerel, salmon, trout, sardines, and herring being excellent sources. Approximately 1 gram of EPA/DPA can be obtained from 100 grams (3.5 ounces) of oily fish. Although this quantity of EPA/DPA can vary depending upon the degree of oiliness of the fish (Atlantic mackerel = 2.5 grams omega-3 per 100 grams; salmon = 1.2 grams omega-3 per 100 grams;

tuna = 0.5 grams omega-3 per 100 grams; and red snapper = 0.2 grams omega-3 per 100 grams).

The average intake of total omega-3 fatty acids in the United States is approximately 1.6 grams per day (0.7% of energy intake), with actually only 0.1 grams per day to 0.2 grams per day coming from EPA/DHA (the rest from alpha-linolenic acid [ALA]).[2] ALA (18:3n-3) from plant sources can desaturate and elongate in the human body to form EPA and DHA. Sources of ALA include oils from flaxseed, canola (rapeseed), soybean, walnut, and wheat germ, with flaxseed (linseed) being the most abundant source.

HEALTH BENEFITS OF OMEGA-3 FATTY ACIDS

A selection of epidemiological studies with important clinical trials have outlined the benefits of the omega-3 fatty acids.

The Diet and Reinfaction Trial supported the role of fish or fish oil in decreasing total mortality and sudden death in patients with myocardial infarction.[3] The Lyon Diet Heart Study[4] added canola oil as a source of ALA to the diet; the Singh study[5] added fish or mustard oil; and the GISSI-Prevenzione trial[6] added 850 grams to 882 grams of omega-3 fatty acids to a Mediterranean diet for a large 11,324-participant study, resulting in a decrease in mortality for these groups.

In the Cardiovascular Health Study,[7] a population-based prospective cohort study among 3,910 adults, the consumption of tuna and other broiled or baked fish was associated with a lower risk of ischemic heart disease (IHD) death, especially arrhythmic IHD death. In the Nurses' Health Study,[8] the relative risk of total stroke was lower among women who regularly ate fish than among those who did not. A significant decrease in the risk of thrombotic stroke was observed in women who ate fish at least twice per week, compared with women who ate fish less than once per month, after adjustment for age, smoking, and other cardiovascular risk factors.

The omega-3 fatty acids have been associated with having anti-inflammatory, antithrombotic, antiarrhythmic, hypolipidemic, and vasodilatory properties.[9] Some of the health benefits that have been associated with omega-3 fatty acids include the secondary prevention of chronic diseases and an association with the following:

- Inflammatory conditions: Improves rheumatoid arthritis, psoriasis, asthma, and some skin conditions
- Ulcerative colitis and Crohn's disease: Reduces the severity of symptoms
- Cardiovascular disease: Lowers triglycerides and raises high-density lipoprotein cholesterol levels, improves blood circulation, reduces clotting, improves vascular function, and lowers blood pressure
- Type 2 diabetes mellitus: Reduces hyperinsulinemia and insulin resistance
- Renal disease: Preserves renal function in IgA nephropathy; potentially reduces vascular access thrombosis in hemodialysis patients and is cardioprotective
- Mental function: Reduces severity of several mental conditions such as Alzheimer's disease, depression, and bipolar disorder; improvement in children with attention deficit hyperactivity disorder and dyslexia also noted
- Growth and development: Neurodevelopment and function of the brain and also the retina of the eye where visual function is affected

FITTING OMEGA-3 FATTY ACIDS INTO THE DIET

Western diets are characterized by low intakes of EPA and DHA relative to linoleic acid (LA; 18:2n-6) and arachidonic acid (AA; 20:4n-6). The high intake of trans fatty acids in our diets can interfere with the desaturation and elongation of LA and ALA. A high intake of LA leads to decreased production of AA and interferes with the desaturation and elongation of ALA to EPA and DHA. The high intake of LA also promotes a prothrombotic and proaggregatory state, characterized by increased blood viscosity and vasoconstriction, and potentially decreased bleeding time.

The omega-3 fatty acids have been associated with having anti-inflammatory, antithrombotic, antiarrhythmic, hypolipidemic, and vasodilatory properties.

Therefore, the required intake of long-chain polyunsaturated omega-3 fatty acids needed for optimal effects depends on the intake of other fatty acids. The Western diet ratio of omega-6 to omega-3 fatty acids ranges from 20:1 to 30:1[9] and is probably even higher with the increased intake of vegetable oils, historically rec-

ommended as a substitute for saturated fat. The competing omega-6 vegetable oils include corn, safflower, cottonseed, sesame, and sunflower seed oils.

FISH VS. FLAX

The optimal intake of LA compared with ALA appears critical for the metabolism of omega-3 fatty acids. An increase in AA, EPA, and DHA leads to an increase in membrane fluidity, alters the structure of the membrane receptors, and can have other beneficial effects associated with the omega-3 fatty acids. They also play a role in the regulation of cell surface expression, cell-cell interactions, and cytokine release.[10] A ratio of 1:4 (LA:ALA) or less is recommended for conversion of ALA to longer chain metabolites (EPA and DHA).[9] This is an important concept for vegetarians, whose diets are often much richer in LA. The intake of 3 grams per day to 4 grams per day of ALA is equivalent to 0.3 grams per day of EPA with optimal elongation.

The increased consumption of flaxseed, canola, soybean, walnut, and wheat germ oils should be supported. However, ALA does not appear to be comparable with its biological effects, compared with EPA and DHA found in fish oil. It appears that the EPA and DHA from marine oils are more rapidly incorporated into plasma and membrane lipids. Algae and some fungi are also capable of forming omega-3 fatty acids de novo, and the DHA from algae supplements needs to be explored further for the vegetarian.

THE METHYL MERCURY SCARE

A recent local survey in the Bay Area of California found several varieties of fish to contain toxic levels of mercury: swordfish (containing the highest concentration), Chilean sea bass, and ahi tuna. Mercury is the environmental pollutant largely from coal-fired power plants that is at the highest concentration in the large predator fish.

The FDA has an advisory warning that swordfish, shark, king mackerel, and tilefish consumption should be limited by pregnant women and women of childbearing age, and this warning is apparent in many fish markets. Mercury can damage the nervous, cardiovascular, immune, and reproductive systems, and symptoms include tremors, memory loss, and fatigue. Subtle symptoms of methyl mercury toxicity in adults have included numbness or tingling of the hands and feet or around the mouth.

A high dietary intake of mercury from the consumption of fish has been hypothesized to increase the risk of coronary heart disease.

According to the FDA, consumption of fish with methyl mercury levels of one part per million, such as shark and swordfish, should be limited to approximately 7 ounces per week. The FDA states that consumption advice is unnecessary for the top 10 seafood species, which makes up approximately 80% of the seafood market: canned tuna, shrimp, pollock, salmon, cod, catfish, clams, flatfish, crabs, and scallops. The methyl mercury levels in these species are at less than 0.2 parts per million, and not many people eat more than the suggested weekly limit of 2.2 pounds of fish. Canned tuna, which is composed of smaller pieces of tuna, such as skipjack and albacore, typically have lower levels of methyl mercury compared with large fresh tuna, sold as steaks or sushi.

A high dietary intake of mercury from the consumption of fish has been hypothesized to increase the risk of coronary heart disease. In a study that investigated the association between mercury levels in toenails and risk of coronary heart disease among male health professionals with no previous history of cardiovascular disease (40 to 75 years of age), there was no association between total mercury exposure and risk of coronary heart disease.[11] Adjustment with the intake of omega-3 fatty acids did not substantially change the results from this study.

RECOMMENDING OMEGA-3 SUPPLEMENTS

A low rate of coronary heart disease has certainly been shown in fish-eating populations. Studies have highlighted reduced cardiovascular risk with a higher intake of ALA, and the omega-3 fatty acids have also consistently been shown to decrease serum triacylglycerol concentrations in studies in humans. A meta-analysis[12] suggested that dietary and nondietary intake of omega-3 fatty acids reduces overall mortality, mortality due to myocardial infarction, and sudden death in patients with coronary heart disease.

Based on the AHA Scientific Statement, it seems reasonable to recommend at least two servings of fish per week in the diet and the use of omega-3 supplements for patients with coronary heart disease up to 1 gram per day and larger doses (2 grams per day to 4 grams per day) for those patients with hypertriglyceridemia.[2] The exact ratio of EPA:DHA needs to be explored further in clinical trials.

As a cautionary safety note, a dose of 1.8 grams per day of EPA has not been documented as having any prolongation of bleeding time. The use of 4 grams per day has shown increased bleeding time and decreased platelet count, but no overall adverse effects.[13]

A fish oil supplement that is "clean" and has been processed by molecular distillation is important. A good place to start when deciding which brand of fish oil supplement to select is *Consumer Reports* magazine (www.consumerreports.org), which tests the top-selling brands of fish oil capsules. The 16 top-selling brands of fish oil capsules they tested found that the products "all contained roughly as much omega-3s as their labels claimed," and none were contaminated with pollutants.

REFERENCES

1. O'Keefe JH, Harris WS. From Inuit to implementation: Omega-3 fatty acids come of age. *Mayo Clin Proc.* 2000; 75:607–614.

2. Kris-Etherton PM, Harris WS, Appel LJ. Fish consumption, fish oil, omega-3 fatty acids, and cardiovascular disease. *Circulation.* 2002; 106:2747.

3. Burr ML, Fehily AM, Gilbert JF, et al. Effect of changes in fat, fish and fiber intakes on death and myocardial reinfaction: Diet and reinfaction trial (DART). *Lancet.* 1989; 2:757–761.

4. de Lorgeril M, Renaud S, Mamelle N, et al. Mediterranean alpha-linolenic acid-rich diet in the secondary prevention of coronary heart disease. *Lancet.* 1994; 343:1454–1459.

5. Singh RB, Rastogi SS, Verma R, et al. Randomized controlled trial of cardiovascular diet in patients with recent acute myocardial infaction: Results of one year follow up. *Br Med J.* 1992; 304:1015–1019.

6. GISSI-Prevenzione Investigators. Dietary supplementation with n-3 polyunsaturated fatty acids and vitamin E after myocardial infaction: Results of the GISSI-Prevenzione trial. *Lancet.* 1999; 354:447–455.

7. Mozaffarian D, Lemaitre RN, Kuller LH, et al. Cardiac benefits of fish consumption may depend on the type of fish meal consumed: The Cardiovascular Health Study. *Circulation.* 2003; 107(10):1372–1377.

8. Skerrett PJ, Hennekens CH. Consumption of fish and fish oils and decreased risk of stroke. *Prev Cardiol.* 2003; 61(1):38–41.

9. Simopoulos AP. Essential fatty acids in health and chronic disease. *Am J Clin Nutr.* 1999; 70(suppl):560S–569S.

10. Grimm H, Mayer K, Mayser P, Eigenbrodt E. Regulatory potential of n-3 fatty acids in immunological and inflammatory processes. *Br J Nutr.* 2002; 87(1):S59–S67.

11. Yoshizawa K, Rimm EB, Morris JS, et al. Mercury and the risk of coronary heart disease in men. *N Eng J Med.* 2002; 347(22):1755–1760.

12. Bucher HC, Hengstler P, Schindler C, Meier G. N-3 polyunsaturated coronary heart disease: A meta-analysis of randomized controlled trials. *Am J Med.* 2002; (4):298–304.

13. Saynor R, Verel D, Gillott T. The long term effect of dietary supplementation with fish lipid concentration on serum lipids, bleeding time, platelets and angina. *Atherosclerosis.* 1984; 50:3–10.

— Alison J. Rigby, PhD, MPH, RD, is a researcher at Stanford University, where she is currently investigating the use of fish oils in the diet. She also teaches nutrition/dietetics classes at San Francisco State University.

Revealing Trans Fats

Scientific evidence shows that consumption of saturated fat, trans fat, and dietary cholesterol raises low-density lipoprotein (LDL), or "bad" cholesterol, levels that increase the risk of coronary heart disease (CHD). According to the National Heart, Lung, and Blood Institute of the National Institutes of Health, more than 12.5 million Americans have CHD, and more than 500,000 die each year. That makes CHD one of the leading causes of death in the United States.

The Food and Drug Administration has required that saturated fat and dietary cholesterol be listed on food labels since 1993. With trans fat added to the Nutrition Facts panel, you know how much of all three—saturated fat, *trans* fat, and cholesterol—are in the foods you choose. Identifying saturated fat, *trans* fat, and cholesterol on the food label gives you information you need to make food choices that help reduce the risk of CHD. This revised label is of particular interest to people concerned about high blood cholesterol and heart disease.

However, everyone should be aware of the risk posed by consuming too much saturated fat, *trans* fat, and cholesterol. But what is *trans* fat, and how can you limit the amount of this fat in your diet?

What is *Trans* Fat?

Basically, *trans* fat is made when manufacturers add hydrogen to vegetable oil—a process called hydrogenation. Hydrogenation increases the shelf life and flavor stability of foods containing these fats.

Trans fat can be found in vegetable shortenings, some margarines, crackers, cookies, snack foods, and other foods made with or fried in partially hydrogenated oils. Unlike other fats, the majority of *trans* fat is formed when food manufacturers turn liquid oils into solid fats like shortening and hard margarine. A small amount of *trans* fat is found naturally, primarily in dairy products, some meat, and other animal-based foods.

Trans fat, like saturated fat and dietary cholesterol, raises the LDL cholesterol that increases your risk for CHD. Americans consume on average 4 to 5 times as much saturated fat as *trans* fat in their diets.

Although saturated fat is the main dietary culprit that raises LDL, *trans* fat and dietary cholesterol also contribute significantly.

Are All Fats the Same?

Simply put: No. Fat is a major source of energy for the body and aids in the absorption of vitamins A, D, E, and K, and caro-

tenoids. Both animal- and plant-derived food products contain fat, and when eaten in moderation, fat is important for proper growth, development, and maintenance of good health. As a food ingredient, fat provides taste, consistency, and stability and helps you feel full. In addition, parents should be aware that fats are an especially important source of calories and nutrients for infants and toddlers (up to 2 years of age), who have the highest energy needs per unit of body weight of any age group.

While unsaturated fats (monounsaturated and polyunsaturated) are beneficial when consumed in moderation, saturated and *trans* fats are not. Saturated fat and *trans* fat raise LDL cholesterol levels in the blood. Dietary cholesterol also raises LDL cholesterol and may contribute to heart disease even without raising LDL. Therefore, it is advisable to choose foods low in saturated fat, *trans* fat, and cholesterol as part of a healthful diet.

What Can You Do About Saturated Fat, *Trans* Fat, and Cholesterol?

When comparing foods, look at the Nutrition Facts panel, and choose the food with the lower amounts of saturated fat, *trans* fat, and cholesterol. Health experts recommend that you keep your intake of saturated fat, *trans* fat, and cholesterol as low as possible while consuming a nutritionally adequate diet. However, these experts recognize that eliminating these three components entirely from your diet is not practical because they are unavoidable in ordinary diets.

Where Can You Find *Trans* Fat on the Food Label?

Although some food products already have *trans* fat on the label, food manufacturers have until January 2006 to list it on all their products.

You will find *trans* fat listed on the Nutrition Facts panel directly under the line for saturated fat.

How Do Your Choices Stack Up?

With the addition of *trans* fat to the Nutrition Facts panel, you can review your food choices and see how they stack up.

Don't assume similar products are the same. Be sure to check the Nutrition Facts panel because even similar foods can vary in calories, ingredients, nutrients, and the size and number of servings in a package.

How Can You Use the Label to Make Heart-Healthy Food Choices?

The Nutrition Facts panel can help you choose foods lower in saturated fat, *trans* fat, and cholesterol. Compare similar foods and choose the food with the lower combined saturated and *trans* fats and the lower amount of cholesterol.

Although the updated Nutrition Facts panel will list the amount of *trans* fat in a product, it will not show a Percent Daily Value (%DV). While scientific reports have confirmed the relationship between *trans* fat and an increased risk of CHD, none has provided a reference value for *trans* fat or any other information that the FDA believes is sufficient to establish a Daily Reference Value or a %DV.

Saturated fat and cholesterol, however, do have a %DV. To choose foods low in saturated fat and cholesterol, use the general rule of thumb that 5 percent of the Daily Value or less is low and 20 percent or more is high.

You can also use the %DV to make dietary trade-offs with other foods throughout the day. You don't have to give up a favorite food to eat a healthy diet. When a food you like is high in saturated fat or cholesterol, balance it with foods that are low in saturated fat and cholesterol at other times of the day.

The FDA's *trans* fat labeling regulations don't take effect until Jan. 1, 2006, but some manufacturers are already listing the amount of *trans* fat in their products.

Do Dietary Supplements Contain *Trans* Fat?

Would it surprise you to know that some dietary supplements contain *trans* fat from partially hydrogenated vegetable oil as well as saturated fat or cholesterol? It's true. As a result of the FDA's new label requirement, if a dietary supplement contains a reportable amount of *trans* or saturated fat, which is 0.5 gram or more, dietary supplement manufacturers must list the amounts on the Supplement Facts panel. Some dietary supplements that may contain saturated fat, *trans* fat, and cholesterol include energy and nutrition bars.

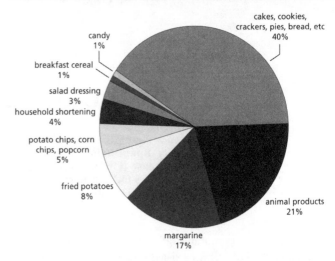

Major Food Sources of Trans Fat for American Adults
(Average Daily Trans Fat Intake is 5.8 Grams or 2.6 Percent of Calories)

- cakes, cookies, crackers, pies, bread, etc 40%
- candy 1%
- breakfast cereal 1%
- salad dressing 3%
- household shortening 4%
- potato chips, corn chips, popcorn 5%
- fried potatoes 8%
- margarine 17%
- animal products 21%

Data based on FDA's economic analysis for the final *trans* fatty acid labeling rule, "*Trans* Fatty Acids in Nutrition Labeling, Nutrient Content Claims, and Health Claims" (July 11, 2003)

Fat Tips

Here are some practical tips you can use every day to keep your consumption of saturated fat, *trans* fat, and cholesterol low while consuming a nutritionally adequate diet.

- **Check the Nutrition Facts panel** to compare foods because the serving sizes are generally consistent in similar types of foods. Choose foods lower in saturated fat, *trans* fat, and cholesterol. For saturated fat and cholesterol, keep in mind that 5 percent of the daily value (%DV) or less is low and 20 percent or more is high. (There is no %DV for *trans* fat.)

- **Choose alternative fats.** Replace saturated and *trans* fats in your diet with monounsaturated and polyunsaturated fats. These fats do not raise LDL cholesterol levels and have health benefits when eaten in moderation. Sources of monounsaturated fats include olive and canola oils. Sources of polyunsaturated fats include soybean oil, corn oil, sunflower oil and foods like nuts and fish.

- **Choose vegetable oils** (except coconut and palm kernel oils) and soft margarines (liquid, tub, or spray) more often because the amounts of saturated fat, *trans* fat, and cholesterol are lower than the amounts in solid shortenings, hard margarines, and animal fats, including butter.

- **Consider fish.** Most fish are lower in saturated fat than meat. Some fish, such as mackerel, sardines, and salmon, contain omega-3 fatty acids that are being studied to determine if they offer protection against heart disease.

- **Ask before you order when eating out**. A good tip to remember is to ask which fats are being used in the preparation of your food when eating or ordering out.

- **Watch calories**. Don't be fooled! Fats are high in calories. All sources of fat contain 9 calories per gram, making fat the most concentrated source of calories. By comparison, carbohydrates and protein have only 4 calories per gram.

To keep your intake of saturated fat, *trans* fat, and cholesterol low:

- Look at the Nutrition Facts panel when comparing products. Choose foods low in the combined amount of saturated fat and *trans* fat and low in cholesterol as part of a nutritionally adequate diet.

- Substitute alternative fats that are higher in mono- and poly-unsaturated fats like olive oil, canola oil, soybean oil, corn oil, and sunflower oil.

Highlights of the Final Rule on *Trans* Fat

- Manufacturers of conventional foods and some dietary supplements will be required to list *trans* fat on a separate line, immediately under saturated fat on the nutrition label.
- Food manufacturers have until Jan. 1, 2006, to list *trans* fat on the nutrition label. The phase-in period minimizes the need for multiple labeling changes, allows small businesses to use current label inventories, and provides economic savings.
- FDA's regulatory chemical definition for *trans* fatty acids is all unsaturated fatty acids that contain one or more isolated (i.e., nonconjugated) double bonds in a *trans* configuration. Under the agency's definition, conjugated linoleic acid would be excluded from the definition of *trans* fat.
- Dietary supplement manufacturers must also list *trans* fat on the Supplement Facts panel when their products contain reportable amounts (0.5 gram or more) of *trans* fat. Examples of dietary supplements with *trans* fat are energy and nutrition bars.

From *FDA Consumer*, September/October 2003. U.S. Food and Drug Administration.

Good Carbs, Bad Carbs

BY RITA SCHEFRIN, MA, RD

The nutrition armies continue to battle, wielding words and theories, each camp claiming it possesses the weapon to win the weight war and promote health. The purported great debate is this: Should we be eating a diet high in protein (often accompanied by high saturated fat) and low in carbohydrate, high in unrefined carbohydrate and low in fat, or should mundane moderation be the maxim? Further, could it be conceivable that there is a reconciling bridge, a common thread, between these three seemingly opposing theories? Such a bridge—increasingly gaining acceptance, though still controversial—exists: the glycemic index and glycemic load.

Glycemic index and glycemic load are two measurements that have been developed to rate the effect of carbohydrate-containing foods on blood sugar, also called blood glucose. Foods containing carbohydrates cause blood glucose to rise. The pancreas responds by releasing insulin into the blood to restore a normal blood glucose level—the higher the rise in blood glucose, the more insulin the pancreas releases into the blood. So, by measuring the effect that a carbohydrate-containing food has on blood glucose, scientists can indirectly gauge the body's insulin response to that food.

One reason that the high-protein camp advises a severe restriction of carbohydrate consumption is to prevent this blood glucose and insulin rise. Now, some scientists who advocate a diet of moderation and those who advocate a diet high in unrefined carbohydrates and low in fat are also advising minimizing this glucose and insulin response, believing that the degree and speed with which a carbohydrate-containing food increases the level of blood glucose and subsequent insulin response may dramatically impact health and weight.

These researchers are recommending restriction or elimination of the carbohydrates that quickly increase blood glucose with a subsequent insulin rush and advocating consumption of the carbohydrates that affect blood glucose more moderately. The carbohydrate-containing foods that produce a small blood glucose rise and subsequent small insulin reaction are those from which glucose is absorbed slowly into our bodies: most fruits, vegetables (nonstarchy), and legumes and many whole, intact grains. The carbohydrate-containing foods that produce a large blood glucose rise and subsequent large insulin reaction are those from which glucose is absorbed quickly into our bodies: refined foods high in starch, including many baked flour products.

What Is a Carbohydrate?

Carbohydrate is an essential nutrient that provides our bodies and brains with the energy needed to function. The National Academies' Institute of Medicine recommends that carbohydrates contribute 45% to 65% of an adult's daily calories.

Carbohydrates are divided into two groups: simple carbohydrates (simple sugars) and complex carbohydrates (starches). Simple carbohydrates are composed of one (monosaccharides) or two (disaccharides) molecules and include glucose (a monosaccharide) also called dextrose, which is found in most plant foods; fructose, or fruit sugar (a monosaccharide), which is found in fruit, some vegetables, honey, and saps; sucrose, or table sugar (a disaccharide), which is also found in honey, maple syrup, fruits, vegetables, and grains; and lactose, or milk sugar (a disaccharide), which is found in dairy products. Fruits, nonstarchy vegetables, and dairy products are simple carbohydrates.

Complex carbohydrates consist of long chains of glucose and are found in grains, such as rice and wheat; legumes (dried beans), such as chick peas and lentils; and tubers, such as potatoes and yams. Glucose is the form of sugar that our bodies use for energy and is the form of sugar found in our blood. After a carbohydrate-containing food is digested and absorbed, the body (liver) converts all of the other forms of carbohydrate in that food to glucose.

Scientists measure carbohydrates in grams. Meats and fats such as oils and butter contain almost no carbohydrates. To learn the carbohydrate content of fruits, vegetables, grains, legumes, and dairy, a table of food values is needed. The following are some examples to keep in mind: one small apple contains approximately 15 grams; one slice of bread contains approximately 15 grams; ½ cup of cooked beans contains approximately 15 grams; 1 cup of milk contains approximately 12 grams; and ½ cup of cooked carrots contains approximately 5 grams.[1] Different fruits and vegetables contain different amounts of carbohydrates. In general, fruits contain more carbohydrates than vegetables, with dried fruits containing the most.

So Simple, Yet So Complex

Today, some experts claim that complex carbohydrates are healthier than simple carbohydrates because complex carbohydrates contain fiber. However, a complex carbohydrate can be refined, such as white breads, white rice, and white flours. These refined complex carbohydrates have had vitamins, minerals, and most of their fiber removed.

Fiber is healthy because it lowers blood cholesterol, aids elimination, is filling, and slows the absorption of glucose into our bodies. Alternatively, simple carbohydrates can be unrefined and contain fiber, such as the simple carbohydrates in whole fruits and vegetables. Instead of "complex," the term to describe the healthier carbohydrates should be "unrefined"—the carbohydrates as they are found in nature, such as fruits, vegetables, legumes, and whole, intact grains.

The Origin of the Theory

Until the early 1980s, scientists assumed that all simple carbohydrates and all complex carbohydrates had the same effect on blood glucose levels. Then, a group of scientists, led by Dr. David Jenkins at the University of Toronto, began questioning this belief and, in order to help people with diabetes, started testing many common carbohydrate-containing foods. The results confirmed their hunches, and the glycemic index was born.

Slow and Steady Should Be the Pace

Why should you care how quickly your body converts carbohydrates to glucose? After eating carbohydrates, which raises blood glucose, the pancreas pours insulin into the blood to restore a normal blood glucose level. Insulin lowers blood glucose by "escorting" glucose from the blood into the cells, where the glucose is used. A rapid rise of blood glucose causes the pancreas to pour out an excessive amount of insulin.

So, what's the problem with high blood glucose and insulin levels? First, they may play a role in the development of heart disease and hypertension (high blood pressure). Another problem may be type 2 diabetes, which has reached epidemic proportions. One theory of the cause of type 2 diabetes is that the pancreas, after years of spewing out insulin, wears out and stops producing insulin. In other words, one of the causes of type 2 diabetes may be an exhausted pancreas, possibly caused by years of overwork due to a diet of high-glycemic-index carbohydrates. In the past, type 2 diabetes occurred mostly in adults, but the number of children with type 2 diabetes is on the rise. Obesity, which has also reached epidemic proportions, may be yet another problem. An abundance of insulin significantly lowers blood glucose (hypoglycemia), causing hunger. Insulin, a fat-favoring hormone, also helps our bodies produce and store fat.

Insulin Resistance and Syndrome X (Metabolic Syndrome)

When the body's cells need more insulin to accept glucose from the blood, that is insulin resistance. This condition overworks the pancreas, forcing it to produce more insulin. The factors that contribute to insulin resistance are obesity, physical inactivity, a diet that promotes insulin production, a diet low in monounsaturated and polyunsaturated fatty acids and high in trans fatty acids, and genetics. In addition to possibly leading to diabetes, insulin resistance may also cause Syndrome X or metabolic syndrome, a cluster of risk factors associated with heart disease: insulin resistance, abdominal obesity, high blood pressure, high blood triglyceride levels, low high-density lipoprotein levels, high blood insulin levels, and elevated fasting blood glucose levels. In *Syndrome X*, author Dr. Gerald Reaven states that approximately 25% to 30% of Americans are insulin resistant and that the high-carbohydrate, low-fat diets are perilous for this population.[2]

Our Paleolithic Past

While most of our stone-age relatives did not live long enough to suffer from any of the chronic diseases that plague us today and that we now believe are at least in part diet-and-lifestyle-related, a look at our ancestral "table" is interesting and perhaps instructive.

In *The Paleolithic Prescription*, Dr. S. Boyd Eaton writes that before the inception of agriculture (8,000 B.C. to 10,000 B.C.), we were hunter/gatherers eating a diet consisting of approximately one-third wild game (according to Eaton, this meat was closer in quality to poultry, fish, and shellfish, having much less total and saturated fat than domesticated meat), with the remaining two-thirds of the diet comprised mostly of a wide variety of fruits and vegetables, with occasional honey. Absent from this diet were grains, dairy (skeletal remains indicate denser bones than we have today, probably due to calcium-rich vegetables and plenty of exercise), legumes, and sugars, such as sucrose and molasses. Even when grains were introduced, they were unrefined—whole and intact.[3]

So, the foods of our ancestors, lacking in refined carbohydrates, did not produce an intense increase of blood glucose with a consequent insulin rush. The diet was "pancreas-friendly." However, as the agricultural age progressed, grains were ground into flours, which became more and more refined until, as is the case of today's white bread and white flour, the fiber almost totally disappeared. Eventually, refined sugars were also introduced.

The Glycemic Index

The glycemic index measures a person's blood glucose response to a carbohydrate-containing food, independent of the number of carbohydrate grams in a portion of that food. The glycemic index is lowest for foods that raise blood glucose levels slowly and moderately; foods with a low glycemic index are converted to glucose slowly because they are slowly digested and absorbed. The glycemic index is highest for foods that raise blood glucose levels quickly and high; foods with a high glycemic index are converted to glucose quickly because they are quickly digested and absorbed. In other words, the harder that your body has to work to convert the starch and sugar in a food to glucose, the lower that food's glycemic index will be. So, anything that slows the digestion and absorption of a carbohydrate-containing food will lower its glycemic index.

The glycemic index of a food is affected by: 1) particle size—larger particle sizes found in stone-ground flour as opposed to finely processed flours slow digestion and lower the glycemic index;

2) soluble, or viscous, fiber—this type of fiber, found in some fruits and vegetables, legumes, oat bran, and oatmeal, slows digestion and lowers the glycemic index; 3) fibrous covering—foods with a fibrous cover, such as beans and seeds, are digested more slowly and have a lower glycemic index; 4) acidity—the acid found in more acidic foods, such as some fruits, pickled foods, and vinegar, slows digestion and lowers the glycemic index; 5) the ratio of different sugars—fructose, for example, has a lower glycemic index than glucose because it is absorbed more slowly since the liver must convert it to glucose; 6) the ease of digestibility of the starch in a food—gelatinized starches and starches with a high amylopectin content are more easily digested and raise the glycemic index; and 7) fat content—fat slows digestion and lowers the glycemic index.

Scientists are now compiling tables of the glycemic index of carbohydrate-containing foods with Dr. Jennie Brand-Miller at the University of Sydney, Australia, who is doing much of the research. (This article cites figures from the book, *The New Glucose Revolution*, by Brand-Miller, Wolever, Foster-Powell, and Colagiuri.)[4] Because the glycemic index is an approximate value, values may differ somewhat from one table to another.

Here is how the scientists unlock the secret: They test foods on volunteers to determine each food's effect on blood glucose. They take a test food that contains carbohydrate, such as a carrot, and compare its effect on blood glucose with the effect of a reference food on blood glucose. They measure the reference and test food's effect on the rise and subsequent fall of a person's blood glucose. The portion size of the reference food and the food being tested must contain identical amounts of available carbohydrates ("available" carbohydrates do not include fiber, a carbohydrate, because the body cannot digest fiber). Usually, the amount of food needed to provide 50 grams of available carbohydrates is used.

To complicate matters, two measurements of glycemic index exist. Some researchers are comparing foods with pure glucose (one reference food), while other researchers are comparing foods with

white bread (the other reference food). Pure glucose is 100% carbohydrates, while white bread is not. (White bread also contains water, protein, fat, fiber, vitamins, and minerals, which add to its weight.) Three tablespoons of pure glucose provides 50 grams of available carbohydrates, and approximately 3½ slices of white bread provides 50 grams of available carbohydrates.

How is this done? A healthy volunteer fasts overnight. The next morning, the volunteer ingests the chosen reference food. He or she drinks either 50 grams of pure glucose dissolved in water or eats enough white bread to provide 50 grams of available carbohydrates. Blood samples measuring the rise and fall of the volunteer's blood glucose are taken several times over the next two or three hours (in people with diabetes). Another day, also after an overnight fast, the volunteer eats a test food—enough to provide 50 grams of available carbohydrates. Again, blood samples are taken over the next two or three hours. The volunteer's response to the reference and test foods are repeated several times, and an average for each is calculated. The reference food receives a value of 100. The glycemic index of the test food is calculated by dividing the volunteer's blood glucose response to the test food by the volunteer's blood glucose response to the reference food (glucose or white bread).

> Today, some experts claim that complex carbohydrates are healthier than simple carbohydrates because complex carbohydrates contain fiber. However, a complex carbohydrate can be refined, such as white breads, white rice, and white flours. These refined complex carbohydrates have had vitamins, minerals, and most of their fiber removed.

Because we all respond to a glucose "challenge" a little differently and may respond to individual foods a little differ-

ently, these tests are performed on eight to 10 people. An average is calculated to establish the glycemic index of each food.

You can convert a glycemic index value compared with white bread to a glycemic index value compared with glucose and vice versa. Here is how: With glucose as the reference food, white bread has a glycemic index of 70, or 70%. This means that glucose causes a 30% higher increase of blood glucose than white bread does. Because the reference food gets a value of 100, or 100%, the conversion factor between white bread and glucose is approximately 1.4: $100/70 = 1.43$.

For example, spaghetti has an average glycemic index of 38, or 38%, when compared with glucose. Multiply this glycemic index by 1.4, and you get a glycemic index of 53 when spaghetti is compared with white bread. So, to convert a glycemic index compared with glucose to a glycemic index compared with white bread, multiply the value by 1.4. To convert a glycemic index compared with white bread to a glycemic index compared with glucose, divide the value by 1.4. Because white bread has a glycemic index 1.4 times lower than that of glucose, a test food will have a glycemic index 1.4 times higher when compared with white bread than when compared with glucose.[5] Because the glycemic index numbers differ depending upon the reference food employed, you should always know if glucose or white bread was used as the reference food when looking at the figures.

While the glycemic index is a relative scale, when measured against glucose, a glycemic index less than 55 is considered low, a glycemic index between 55 and 70 is considered intermediate, and a glycemic index more than 70 is considered high.[6]

When measured against white bread, a glycemic index less than 77 is considered low, a glycemic index between 77 and 98 is considered intermediate, and a glycemic index more than 98 is considered high.

The Glycemic Load

The problem with the glycemic index is that the portion size of the test food is the portion size that contains 50 grams of available carbohydrates from that food. With some foods, however, a portion providing 50 grams of available carbohydrates does not represent an average portion. For example, to analyze the glycemic index of the amount of carrots providing 50 grams of available carbohydrate, 1½ pounds of carrots had to be consumed—not exactly the amount that most people eat at one sitting. The problem then becomes how to measure the effect of a specific portion size on blood glucose.

Enter the glycemic load. Glycemic load is a measure conceived by researchers at Harvard University that takes into account the portion size of food being consumed. To calculate the glycemic load of a portion of food, multiply that food's glycemic index by the number of grams of carbohydrate contained in that portion.

For example, to calculate the glycemic load of ½ cup of boiled carrots, multiply the glycemic index of carrots (49, or 49%, when compared with glucose) by the number of carbohydrate grams contained in ½ cup of carrots, or five grams. The glycemic load for 1 ½ cup of boiled carrots is 2.45 (.49 X 5). (Glycemic load numbers for the same food will differ, depending upon which reference food was used to calculate the glycemic index used.) The glycemic load for one cup of boiled carrots is 4.9 (.49 X 10); 9.8 (.49 X 20) for two cups of boiled carrots; and 14.7 (.49 X 30) for three cups of boiled carrots.

In contrast, consider spaghetti. When measured against glucose, white spaghetti has a glycemic index of 38. One and one-half cups of spaghetti contains 48 grams of carbohydrates. The glycemic load for 1½ cups of the spaghetti is calculated by multiplying .38 X 48, which provides a glycemic load of 18.24. Think about what a 1-cup measuring cup looks like. When you eat spaghetti, do you think that you are eating only ½ cups? Perhaps you are eating 2, 3, or maybe even 4 cups? If you eat three cups, you are eating a glycemic load of 36.48 (.38 X 96). You can see that 3 cups of boiled carrots has a lower glycemic load than 3 cups of spaghetti. So, a food with a higher glycemic index may have a

lower glycemic load when portion size is considered.

What glycemic load should we aim for? In *The New Glucose Revolution*, Brand-Miller et al advise that a person eating 250 grams of carbohydrates daily (which translates into 1,000 calories of carbohydrate) averages a glycemic load between 138 and 163, depending upon whether that person's goal is to eat all or only one-half of his or her carbohydrates from low-glycemic-index carbohydrates.[7]

Glycemic Surprises

The glycemic index and glycemic load values for a food are sometimes more different than you might expect. For example, whole-wheat bread made from finely ground, whole-wheat flour has nearly the same glycemic index as refined white bread because the fiber is so finely ground. (But, whole-wheat bread is a better nutritional bet because of its superior vitamin and mineral content.) And, would you believe that the average baked potato has a higher glycemic index than ½ cup of 16%-fat vanilla ice cream? The starch in the potato is swollen, easily digested, and quickly converted to glucose, while the sucrose (a disaccharide consisting of glucose and fructose) in the ice cream is less easily converted to glucose (fructose must be converted to glucose in the liver), and the fat lowers its glycemic index. The glycemic index of the baked potato, when compared with glucose, is 85, while the ice cream has a glycemic index of 38. These numbers translate into a glycemic load of 25.5 for the potato (multiply the potato's glycemic index by the number of carbohydrate grams in one potato, or .85 X 30) and 5.32 (.38 X 14) for ½ cup of ice cream. However, if you eat 1 cup of the ice cream, the glycemic load increases to 10.64 (.38 X 28). And, alas, because of its high-caloric, sugar, saturated fat, and cholesterol content, this lower glycemic index does not make ice cream a food to eat indiscriminately.

Because we eat foods in combination, each meal or snack has its own glycemic index and load. Adding fat or fiber to a meal lowers its glycemic load. For example, juice will probably have a higher glycemic index and glycemic load than the fruit or vegetable from which it was made

because the fiber has been lost; so, adding foods high in soluble fiber such as green, leafy vegetables or broccoli to a meal will lower that meal's glycemic load. Likewise, adding foods high in monounsaturated or polyunsaturated fats such as nuts or oil to a meal is another healthy way to lower a meal's glycemic load.

Be Your Own Detective

Short of testing your own blood glucose—which may not even be accurate because blood glucose response can vary daily—you can get a table of glycemic indexes and loads on the Web or from a book.[8] Or, you can try to be your own detective. If you consistently get hungry ½ hour to 3 hours after eating a certain carbohydrate-containing food, that food may be excessively raising your blood glucose, thus causing an exaggerated insulin response.

What to Eat?

No one can foretell how future nutrition advice might change as knowledge advances. However, the most recent recommendations of the National Academies' Institute of Medicine's Food and Nutrition Board advise that healthy adults eat in percentages of total daily calories a diet of 45% to 65% carbohydrates (with at least 130 grams to avoid ketosis); 20% to 35% fat, limiting saturated fat, cholesterol (animal foods provide almost all dietary saturated fat and all dietary cholesterol), and trans fats (manmade fats, also known as partially hydrogenated fats, found in many commercially processed foods) to the lowest levels possible while maintaining a healthy diet; and 10% to 35% protein (the Recommended Dietary Allowance for protein is 0.8 grams of protein per kilogram of body weight). A healthy diet is rich in fruits and especially vegetables (nonstarchy are low in calories), which provide needed vitamins, minerals, fiber, and phytochemicals (plant substances manifested through the succulent colors of the foods of the plant kingdom that include some of the antioxidants and may protect against disease), and is low in saturated fat, cholesterol, and trans fat. And, studies suggest that whole, intact grains (not refined grains) are protective against diabetes, heart disease, and perhaps cancer.

In his book *Eat, Drink, and Be Healthy*, Dr. Walter Willett, chairman of the department of nutrition at the Harvard School of Public Health and a proponent of the glycemic index and load theories, recommends daily physical activity and weight management as the basis for a healthy lifestyle. For food choices, he advises intact or coarsely ground whole grains; use of monounsaturated oils (such as canola, olive, and peanut oils) and polyunsaturated oils (such as corn, soybean, and sunflower oils); plenty of vegetables; fruits; protein foods that contain less saturated fat than red meat (such as poultry) and that provide beneficial unsaturated fats (such as fish) and are also high in fiber, vitamins, minerals, and phytochemicals (such as beans and nuts); and strict limits on the consumption of foods high in saturated fat (such as butter and red meat) and on foods with a high glycemic index or that produce a high glycemic load (such as refined grains and breads, potatoes, and sweets). Dr. Willett believes that a diet with more than 30% of its calories from fat is fine if the fats are unsaturated and that calcium supplements are the best means of insuring adequate calcium intake.[9]

While some scientists do not accept the glycemic index and load theories, others would advise that most of the carbohydrate-containing foods that you choose have a low glycemic index or that your portion sizes or meals provide a low glycemic load. Brand-Miller, Wolever, Foster-Powell, and Colagiuri believe that only one-half of one's carbohydrates need to come from low-glycemic-index foods.[10] Perhaps individual sensitivity will prove more critical than currently recognized. And, remember: "portion portion"—for weight control, calories (thus, portion sizes) count, no matter what foods are eaten.

—**Rita Schefrin, MA, RD, has taught nutrition at Montclair State University. She has a special interest in weight control and has completed the ADA/CDR Certificate of Training in Adult Weight Management program.**

Notes

1. American Diabetes Association and American Dietetic Association Exchange Lists.

2. Reaven G, Strom TK, Fox B. *Syndrome X*. New York, N.Y.; 2000.

3. Eaton SB, Shostak M, Konner M. *The Paleolithic Prescription*. New York, N.Y.; 1988.

4. Brand-Miller J, Wolever TMS, Foster-Powell K, Colagiuri S. *The New Glucose Revolution*. New York, N.Y.; 2003.

5. Brand-Miller J, Wolever TMS, Colagiuri S, Foster-Powell K. *The Glucose Revolution.* New York, N.Y.; 1999.

6. Brand-Miller J, Wolever TMS, Foster-Powell K, Colagiuri S. *The New Glucose Revolution*. New York, N.Y.; 2003.

7. Ibid.

8. Brand-Miller J, Wolever TMS, Colagiuri S, Foster-Powell K. *The Glucose Revolution*. New York, N.Y.; 1999.

9. Willett W. *Eat, Drink, and Be Healthy*. New York, N.Y.; 2001.

10. Brand-Miller J, Wolever TMS, Foster-Powell K, Colagiuri S. *The New Glucose Revolution*. New York, N.Y.; 2003.

Are you getting enough of this vitamin?

If you're a vegetarian or over age 60, you need to be concerned about getting enough vitamin B₁₂.

Lately, there's been increased concern about going overboard with vitamins. Researchers have found that a high intake of vitamin A in its retinol form is associated with a high rate of fractures. Other studies have cast a cloud of suspicion over vitamin E supplements.

Vitamin B_{12}, though, is different: It is easier than once thought to get too little. Studies have found that 20% of Americans ages 65 and over have low levels of the vitamin in their blood. Sometimes the only symptoms are subtle cognitive and neurological changes. More serious shortages can result in dementia or anemia, because B_{12} is essential for the production of red blood cells in the bone marrow. Breast-fed infants of mothers with a B_{12} deficiency are at risk for severe developmental abnormalities and irreversible neurological damage. Some experts say that it's the most common nutritional deficiency in the developing world and possibly in the United States as well.

In this country (and other prosperous places) the problem isn't hard to solve. A multivitamin or a vitamin-fortified breakfast cereal (B_{12} is usually included) will do the trick. In fact, the crystalline form of the vitamin contained in pills and breakfast cereals is more readily absorbed than the "natural" form found in food.

Solving nutrition problems in poor countries is never easy, but inexpensive programs that involve adding milk or meat to school meals have been effective in correcting B_{12} deficiencies.

The carnivore's vitamin

When we think about natural sources of vitamins, we usually think of fruit and vegetables. But plants neither use nor contain vitamin B_{12}, so the only dietary sources are animal-derived: meat, fish, shellfish, poultry, eggs, milk, and milk products. Beef liver and several varieties of fish contain high amounts, dairy products and eggs not so much. Vegetarians can eat tempeh, which is made from fermented soybeans (the bacteria produce B_{12}).

Four ways deficiencies develop

In normal digestion, stomach juices pry B_{12} loose from animal protein. But the small intestine can't absorb the vitamin in this liberated, solo state. To be absorbed, it must be combined with a protein called intrinsic factor that is produced by cells in the lining of the stomach.

It may take quite a while for a deficiency to develop. A healthy person's liver can store up to a five-year supply of B_{12}. And the small intestine does a marvelous job of B_{12} recycling, reabsorbing it from bile made by the liver. Of course, a deficiency will develop sooner if reserves are low to begin with.

Diets without food derived from animals. In poor countries, people often have to eat this way. In richer ones, many people choose animal-free diets. Vegans, the strict vegetarians who avoid all animal products, are most at risk for developing a full-fledged B_{12} deficiency. But even lacto-ovo vegetarians, who eat eggs and dairy products, may have low levels. Studies have found that the average lacto-ovo vegetarian consumes less than 1 microgram (mcg) daily, which is less than half the adult Recommended Dietary Allowance (RDA) of 2.4 mcg.

Lack of stomach acid. Up to 30% of people ages 50 and over suffer from atrophic gastritis, a thinning of the stomach lining. This condition reduces the acid secretions that free B_{12} from animal protein, so much less is absorbed by the small intestine.

Lack of stomach juices may also allow the overgrowth of bacteria in the small intestine. The bacteria grab B_{12} for their own purposes, leaving less for the intestine to absorb.

Theoretically, drugs like lansoprazole (Prevacid) and omeprazole (Prilosec) could cause B_{12} problems because they suppress gastric secretions. But so far, B_{12} deficits have not been linked to long-term use of these or other drugs that reduce stomach acid.

Lack of intrinsic factor. Some people's stomachs don't make enough intrinsic factor, so they can't absorb enough B_{12}. The cause is an autoimmune disorder: The body's immune system gets confused and produces antibodies, which, instead of chasing down germs as they should, pounce on the stomach cells that produce intrinsic factor. The result can be anemia. This consequence was recognized long before the cause, so the condition is called pernicious anemia (pernicious because, until it was identified, it was inevitably fatal). It runs in families, suggesting a genetic component, and usually develops after age 40. Less than 1% of the population is affected.

Gastrointestinal disorders and surgeries. Crohn's disease might cause a B_{12} shortage because it interferes with the functioning of the small intestine. Some people develop a B_{12}

shortage after a surgical procedure that shrinks the stomach, such as gastric bypass, because a smaller stomach means far fewer of the cells secreting stomach acid and intrinsic factor.

Solutions

Vegetarians and older people with atrophic gastritis can get all the B_{12} they need from a multivitamin pill, fortified breakfast cereal, or both. Most multivitamins contain 6 mcg, which is 100% of the Daily Value set by the FDA. (The RDA of 2.4 mcg was set by the Institute of Medicine. The difference between the two amounts is probably not important.) Fortified breakfast cereals have varying amounts of B_{12}.

People with pernicious anemia have a more difficult problem. Because they're short on intrinsic factor, they don't benefit from the extra B_{12} in vitamin pills and fortified cereal. At least initially, most need B_{12} injections. After that, some do fine with pills alone, but others need additional injections every few months.

Some researchers think high-dose pills (2,000 mcg or more) could be just as effective as injections for pernicious anemia. There's some evidence that about 1% of the B_{12} in pills is absorbed by simple diffusion, regardless of intrinsic factor or the state of the intestine. Recent studies suggest that even if they don't have pernicious anemia, older people with fairly mild deficits may need to take similarly large doses of B_{12} to bring their levels up to normal. More research is needed, though. Fortunately, even very large doses of the vitamin don't seem to pose any danger.

People with Crohn's disease and other malabsorption problems may also need B_{12} injections depending on the severity of their condition. Gastric bypass patients may need them, too.

Should you be tested?

Those at risk for B_{12} deficits include older people and strict vegetarians. Research also suggests that long-term use of metformin, the diabetes drug, may lower B_{12} levels. Although a severe deficiency is fairly unlikely, lesser shortfalls may affect balance, memory, or perhaps mood. If you have these problems and you're in an at-risk category, ask your doctor about ordering a B_{12} test. It's a common, inexpensive blood test that could make a big difference in your life.

Excerpted from Vol. 30, No. 10, the August 2005 issue of *Harvard Health Letter,* pp. 1-2. Copyright © 2005 by Harvard Health Publications Group. www.health.harvard.edu Reprinted with permission via Copyright Clearance Center.

Feast For Your Eyes

Nutrients That May Help Save Your Sight

Research is uncovering yet another reason to eat with health in mind—our eyes. Going beyond the vitamin A in carrots that help us to see well in the dark, other nutrients may protect vision, particularly for aging eyes, including vitamins C and E, beta-carotene, two related carotenoids (lutein and zeaxanthin), zinc, and even certain types of fats.

Age-Related Eye Diseases

Age brings about changes that can lead to two common sight-robbing disorders, cataracts and age-related macular degeneration (AMD).

A cataract is a cloudy area in a part of the eye lens or the entire eye lens that keeps light from passing through the lens. As a cataract develops, it can cause blurred vision, sensitivity to light, increased nearsightedness, and distorted images, eventually causing partial or full loss of eyesight. Cataracts are also associated with diabetes, other systemic diseases, alcoholism, premature birth or birth defects, heredity, smoking, eye injuries, exposure to ultraviolet (UV) rays, and certain medications.

Macular degeneration involves damage to the macula; an area of the retina in the back of the eye responsible for the sharp central vision needed to read, drive, and perform other daily activities. Although the causes of macular degeneration are not known, risk factors include family history, smoking, high blood pressure, high blood cholesterol, and exposure to sunlight.

Visionary Research

Research is shedding rays of hope for individuals suffering from age-related eye disease, and for those at

Focus on Food

Although nutrients from supplements may help slow the progression of AMD—mainly for people with intermediate and advanced stages of AMD—data on the benefits of supplementation of these nutrients is still preliminary. A strong body of evidence, however, points to foods that can be consumed to reduce the risk of both AMD and cataracts.

In a study that looked at the intakes of carotenoids and antioxidants from food, people who ate the most antioxidant-rich dark, leafy greens, particularly those rich in lutein and zeaxanthin, had about a 40 percent lower risk of macular degeneration than those who ate the least amount of these vegetables.

The project examined food records and cataract development in women between 50 and 70 years old. The results confirm that antioxidant nutrients, particularly vitamin C, at daily intakes of about three times the Daily Value for vitamin C (60 mg/day), reduced the odds for the development of cataracts by nearly half. With higher intakes, easily attained by five to nine daily servings of fruits and vegetables, the odds were reduced even more.

risk of eye disease. Emerging evidence suggests that risk of certain eye changes associated with aging may be reduced by dietary components.

Antioxidant Vitamins and Zinc

The Age-Related Eye Disease Study (AREDS), launched by the National

Institutes of Health's National Eye Institute, is an ongoing study aimed at evaluating various combinations of high-dose antioxidant vitamins (beta-carotene and vitamins C and E) and zinc supplements on eye health. One published analysis of a 6-year period in the double-blind study examined these effects on nearly 3,600 people between the ages of 55 and 80. Subjects included men and women with varying macular status ranging from no evidence of AMD in either eye to relatively severe disease in one eye.

Study results related to AMD were impressive, although somewhat limiting. Only individuals with the intermediate and advanced stages of AMD appeared to benefit. Nevertheless, the benefit was such that the study's authors urged high risk individuals with no contraindications such as smoking, to consider taking daily supplements similar to those used in the study: 500 mg vitamin C, 400 International Units vitamin E, 15 mg beta carotene, 80 mg zinc, and 2 mg copper (copper needs are increased with high doses of zinc). The effectiveness and safety of routine use of this regimen by individuals with early AMD or persons at risk for developing AMD remain unclear. It is also important to note that this is a single study and further research is needed.

The high-dose formulations used in the AREDs study had no significant effect on the development or progression of age-related cataracts. Nevertheless, other studies have found that antioxidants have favorable effects, especially vitamin C in larger amounts and for a longer duration (>10 years).

Lutein and Zeaxanthin

The yellow-colored carotenoids, lutein and zeaxanthin, are found in a variety of vegetables, including leafy greens, broccoli, zucchini, corn, peas, and brussels sprouts to name a few. Highly concentrated deposits of lutein and zeaxanthin are also present in the macula. Here they are referred to as macular pigment.

Research has shown that the macular pigment density, or the amount of lutein and zeaxanthin in the macula, appears to be associated with AMD. Dr. Richard Bone, a professor of biophysics at Florida International University, has been studying macular pigments for more than 20 years. In a postmortem study of the eyes of people who had AMD and those who did not, Bone found that those with the highest concentrations of lutein and zeaxanthin had an 82 percent lower incidence of AMD.

Bone and colleagues also studied how lutein and zeaxanthin in the diet affect macular pigment density. "These results suggest an association between dietary intake of lutein and zeaxanthin and macular pigment density," said Bone. "But we don't know yet how much lutein and zeaxanthin are needed to raise the macular pigment density to a protective level." Currently Bone is conducting a dose-response study to determine the appropriate doses.

Dietary Fats

Several studies have hinted at an association between the amount and type of dietary fats consumed and the risk for AMD. Findings from the ongoing Beaver Dam Eye Study suggest that higher intakes of saturated fats and cholesterol may confer an increased risk for AMD.

The high level of polyunsaturated fatty acids in the retina supports the possibility that certain fats may have a protective effect against the development of AMD. Although some results have linked higher intakes of omega-3 fatty acids and fish with a decreased risk for advanced AMD, the majority of population studies have failed to establish a clear connection.

More recently, a case-control population study led by Dr. Johanna Seddon, an eye expert at Harvard University, found that diets high in vegetable (mono- and polyunsaturated) fats were associated with a higher risk for advanced AMD. Although polyunsaturated fats are considered protective against cardiovascular disease, the study's authors suggest that consumption of high levels of unsaturated fats may increase the susceptibility of the macula to oxidative damage. However, an optimal balance of high levels of omega-3 fatty acids (found in fatty fish such as salmon and mackerel) and lower levels of linoleic acid (an omega-6 fatty acid found in various vegetable fats) in the diet appeared to offer a protective effect.

Seeing is Believing

Although some of the results of studies related to the maintenance of eye health through diet are compelling for specific populations, it is too early in the study of nutrition and eye disease to draw general conclusions, advises Julie Mares-Perlman, PhD, associate professor in the Department of Ophthalmology and Visual Sciences at the University of Wisconsin-Madison.

"There are holes in the evidence that need further study," contends Mares-Perlman. As with any research, one or two studies showing a tendency are not enough. "What we do know is that a large body of evidence supports the fact that diet is important in maintaining eye health. How specific nutrients from food or supplements affect the types and stages of eye disease is yet to be defined," she said.

Get the Lead Out

WHAT YOU DON'T KNOW CAN HURT YOU

David Schardt

"If you want to know about the effects of lead exposure over a lifetime, the amount of lead circulating in the blood may not be the most relevant measure," says Brian Schwartz, a professor of environmental health science at Johns Hopkins University.

Blood levels represent your average exposure during the last three or four months, he notes. "They're used mainly because they're easy, convenient, and cheap to measure."

It's far more revealing to look at the amount of lead in your bones. That's where your body deposits 90 to 95 percent of the lead it has absorbed over the years.

In Schwartz's Baltimore Memory Study, which is tracking 1,000 men and women in their 50s, 60s, and 70s, the average bone lead level of the participants is 19 parts per million (ppm).

"To put that into context," says Schwartz, "we've also studied about 1,000 former lead workers in New Jersey who haven't worked with lead for at least two decades. Their average bone lead level is about 15 ppm."

In other words, older residents of Baltimore—from all socioeconomic and racial groups—who were merely exposed to lead from paint, gasoline, and plumbing have at least as much lead in their bones as people in their 50s who once worked with the metal.

"By contrast, people who are now in their 20s and 30s grew up at a time when there was much less lead in the food they ate, the water they drank, and the air they breathed," Schwartz points out. They have little or no lead in their bones.

Lead is toxic to just about every tissue in the body. And it doesn't just do its damage when you breathe, eat, or drink it.

Over the years, "stored lead can be released back out of the bones and possibly cause more damage in the body," Schwartz notes. The half-life of lead in the tibia (the larger of the two lower leg bones) is about 25 years, which means it takes that long to release half of the lead stored there.

"That's especially significant for some middle-aged and older women who have osteoporosis," says Schwartz. "As their bones thin and lose calcium and other minerals, the lead is released into their blood and is circulated throughout the body."

In a recent study, women aged 40 to 59 who had gone through menopause had blood lead levels that were 25 to 30 percent higher than women of the same age who hadn't yet undergone menopause[1]. And the less dense their bones were, the more lead they had in their blood.

"Preventing bone loss may lessen or prevent this exposure to lead," says study co-author Ellen Silbergeld of Johns Hopkins.

Heavy Metal

Lead is linked to a host of potential health problems.

"We don't know that high levels of lead in the bones will cut years off your life," says Schwartz. "But it might decrease the quality of your life."

- **Blood pressure**. "Lead increases your risk of hypertension," says Schwartz. Men with the highest levels of lead in their bones were nearly twice as likely to be diagnosed with high blood pressure over a six-year period as men with the lowest bone lead levels, according to the Normative Aging Study, which looked at 833 veterans living in the Boston area[2]. The same researchers found similar results in women[3].

- **Kidney function**. The kidneys filter toxins and other harmful compounds out of the blood. In the Normative Aging Study, that ability deteriorated earlier and faster in men with higher levels of lead in their blood[4]. The researchers found a faster decline even in men with modest lead levels—10 micrograms per deciliter, which is above optimal but not high.

"High levels of lead could push someone with compromised renal function into dialysis," warns Harvard's Howard Hu, who is a professor of occupational and environmental medicine. "The effect of lead on the kidney is 15 times worse in individuals who have Type 2 diabetes. And diabetics with kidney disease are a huge cost to the nation in terms of Medicare payments for dialysis."

- **Cognitive function**. "Lead accelerates declines in memory and mental abilities," says Hu. In the Normative Aging Study, men with the most lead in their bones were twice as likely to score lower on the Mini Mental Status Examination as those with the least lead[5]. The exam tests memory, awareness, and mental agility.

Scores deteriorated four times faster over a six-year period in men with the highest lead levels. And those men were more likely to score below 24 points out of a possible 30.

"The 24 score is important," Hu points out, "because that's the screening cutoff that clinicians often use for sending somebody to the neurologist to be assessed for dementia and Alzheimer's."

"I can't say that lead is a cause of Alzheimer's," cautions Hu. "But it seems to be a risk factor for cognitive declines that could push some people over the edge into more of the clinically senile state."

In the Johns Hopkins studies of lead workers, "we call it 'accelerated aging,'" says Brian Schwartz. "When we look at the impact on cognitive function, we find that high levels of lead in bone are equivalent to three to six more years of aging in the brain."

"In the Baltimore Memory Study we're trying to see if something similar is happening in the general population," he adds, "since they have bone lead levels just as high as the lead workers."

- **Cataracts**. "Lead accumulation is a major risk factor for developing cataracts," says Hu. In the Normative Aging Study, men with the most lead in their tibias were three times more likely to develop cataracts as men with the least lead[6].

"Lead accelerates oxidative damage, binds to proteins, and also causes changes in calcium balance, all of which can affect the clarity of the lens," Hu explains.

Gulp!

While there's far less lead in the environment today than there was 30 years ago, the U.S. isn't exactly a lead-free zone. Young children can still get it if they eat peeling or chipped lead-based paint, and everyone can get it from contaminated drinking water.

"About 15 percent of the homes in the U.S. probably have enough lead contamination in their drinking water for us to be concerned about its effect on the health of both children and adults," says Richard Maas, co-director of the Environmental Quality Institute at the University of North Carolina at Asheville.

"We've tested the water in over 130,000 homes and we see problems all over the country," says Maas. "We would be hard put to find any town where the incidence of lead contamination is so low that households don't need to get their water tested."

That's true even if your local water utility tells you otherwise.

"When your water utility sends you a letter saying that you don't need to worry because your water doesn't exceed the action level for lead, that's often dangerously misleading," says Maas.

Fourteen years ago, the U.S. Environmental Protection Agency (EPA) set an "action level" of 15 parts per billion (ppb) for lead in water. That meant that if at least 11 of 100 samples exceeded 15 ppb, the utility had to reduce the lead in its water.

"The first thing to understand is that this 15 ppb level was never intended to be a health standard," says Maas. "When you pin the EPA down, they'll admit that it's not a standard based on any health effects that occur only at 15 ppb and higher."

In other words, an action level of 15 parts per billion doesn't mean that water with 14 ppb or 13 ppb of lead is safe.

Maas knows firsthand how the EPA set the action level for lead.

"In 1990, when the EPA was told by Congress to control the lead in drinking water, the agency wanted to identify those utilities with the most corrosive water," he recalls.

Water that's corrosive is more likely to draw lead out of pipes. If the EPA was going to force utilities to spend hundreds of millions of dollars on additives that coat the inside of pipes and other corrosion treatments, it wanted to target the systems with the worst problems.

Test, Don't Taste

Since you cannot see, taste, or smell lead dissolved in water, testing is the only sure way of telling whether or not there are harmful quantities of lead in your drinking water," says the U.S. Environmental Protection Agency.

"You should be particularly suspicious if your home has lead pipes (lead is a dull gray metal that is soft enough to be easily scratched with a house key)," says the EPA, or "if you see signs of corrosion (frequent leaks, rust-colored water, stained dishes or laundry)."

Testing is especially important in high-rise buildings, where running the water for a minute or more might not get rid of enough lead, says the EPA.

Your local water authority or health department should have a list of certified laboratories. You can also look under "Laboratories" in the yellow pages. You should have two samples tested—a "first draw" (taken first thing in the morning) and a "fully flushed" sample (taken after you've run the water for one minute). Expect to pay between $20 and $200, says the EPA.

A cheaper alternative: you can get the test for $17 from the nonprofit Clean Water Lead Testing Inc.—a certified lab run by the Environmental Quality Institute at the University of North Carolina at Asheville that has tested 130,000 homes in North America for lead.

The lab sends you two small plastic vials, a shipping envelope, and a short questionnaire about your house and its plumbing system. Follow the directions for filling the vials with your drinking water, fill out the questionnaire, and mail it all back. Within a couple of weeks you'll receive a report showing the level of lead in your first draw of water in the morning and how much remains after running the line for one minute.

"Once you do that," says the Institute's Richard Maas, "you've empowered yourself with all the information you need to protect yourself from lead in your household drinking water."

"So the EPA came to our Institute and asked where they would have to set the level for lead in drinking water so that about 25 percent of the utilities in the U.S. would exceed it," Maas explains. "We went through our data on 100,000 homes and told them 15 parts per billion."

"If that action level is anywhere near any kind of health standard," says Maas, "it's totally by coincidence."

"The second point to remember," he adds, "is that just because your local utility says that its water doesn't exceed the action level for lead, that doesn't really tell you anything about the levels in your own household." It just means that if the utility did the testing the way it's supposed to—and that's a big if—no more than 10 percent of its customers had lead levels over 15 ppb.

"But we know from all the testing we've done that if the 11th highest sample in a water district is 10 ppb, for example," says Maas, "then it's still very likely that the highest home out of the 100 they tested is probably 150 ppb." The next-highest family probably has about 85 ppb, the third highest probably 60-something, and so on down to where the 11th highest is 10 ppb, he adds.

"The action level wasn't exceeded, but you've still got 10 percent of homes with high lead levels. And those families are just out of luck. What's more, there's just no telling from these tests if you're one of them."

And you can't always trust water utilities to properly test their water for lead, says Maas. "They have tremendous motivation to try to game the system."

Utilities are supposed to sample water from 100 customers who they suspect have high lead levels. If the 11th highest one contains more than 15 ppb, the utility has to notify all its customers that it's a high-risk system and that the customers should consider getting their water tested for lead. The company will have to spend millions of dollars to make its water less corrosive, and it will have to keep testing homes.

"It's nothing but money and bad publicity for them if that 11th highest sample is 15 parts per billion, or more," says Maas. But if it's just 14 ppb, then they don't have to spend any of that money and don't have to endure that bad publicity. "In fact, they can send out a letter to their customers saying everything is hunky-dory, which is often wrong."

The temptation to cheat is apparently too hard to resist for some water companies. The *Washington Post* reported last October that dozens of utilities around the country, including those in Philadelphia, New York, and Boston, were manipulating the results of their lead testing, in some cases by discarding results from samples they knew to be high.

An additional 274 utilities, which together serve 11.5 million people, have reported unsafe lead levels since 2000. Few companies have been fined or held accountable by the EPA.

"It's time to reconsider whether water utilities can be trusted with this crucial responsibility of protecting the public," former EPA drinking water chief Jim Elder told the *Post*. "I fear for the safety of our nation's drinking water."

What to Do

If you're 50 or older, you probably have a fair amount of lead in your bones. (Don't bother trying to get tested. Instruments that measure lead levels in bone are currently available only to researchers.) Other than letting the water run and using a water filter, here are some things you can do to protect yourself.

• **Bones.** When your bones get thinner, they release not just calcium, but lead and other minerals, into your bloodstream. So anything you can do to ward off osteoporosis—getting enough calcium, protein, potassium, and vitamins D and K, and doing plenty of walking or other weight-bearing exercise, for example—might help minimize your exposure to lead. "If you want to prevent lead from being released from your bones, you have to prevent osteoporosis," says Johns Hopkin's Brian Schwartz.

• **High blood pressure.** "Hypertension that's induced by lead might be particularly amenable to treatment with dietary calcium," says Harvard's Howard Hu, who lowered blood levels of lead in breastfeeding women by giving them calcium supplements. Because calcium and lead are metals that are often interchangeable, Hu explains, the body sometimes confuses one with the other. "Keeping calcium levels high might counteract some of the harmful effects of lead in the body," he speculates. Chalk up another reason to make sure you get enough calcium.

• **Cataracts.** "Maximizing your intake of fruits and vegetables might mitigate the risk of cataracts," says Hu. "That's because their natural antioxidants might suppress some of the oxidative reactions that lead can cause that can contribute to the formation of cataracts." (In the best study to date, antioxidant supplements—vitamins C and E and beta-carotene—didn't prevent cataracts.) Other ways to lower your risk: don't smoke, eat leafy green vegetables like spinach and broccoli at least twice a week, eat fish at least once a week, take a multivitamin for insurance, and lose excess weight.

• **Memory.** "Until we know more about lead's effect on the brain, it makes sense to try to protect your memory and thinking skills," says Schwartz. That means keeping your blood pressure low, avoiding diets high in saturated and trans fat, reducing your risk of diabetes by keeping your weight down and your exercise level up, and keeping a lid on homocysteine levels by taking a multivitamin with 100% of the Daily Values for folic acid (400 mcg), vitamin B-6 (2 mg), and vitamin B-12 (6 mcg). Brain-challenging activities like crossword puzzles, reading, and square dancing may also help.

• **At the faucet.** Use only cold tap water for drinking, cooking, and making baby formula. Hot water is likely to leach more lead out of pipes.

Plumbing the Depths

Lead builds up in plumbing systems when water sits. "The good news is that most of the time you can flush it down to a safe level, if not completely out, by running the line for one minute," says Maas.

"Because we've done so many tests, I can tell you what's likely to happen," he adds. "If the first draw in the morning is over 10 parts per billion, then in 80 percent of the cases the second draw after a minute of running the water will be no more than 3 ppb. So, it's a pretty good solution for most households."

But running the water may not get lead levels low enough and some households may need to use a filter:

• **Lead service lines.** About two percent of U.S. residences have lead service lines that bring water in from the street. Many are in older East Coast cities like New York, Boston, and Washington, D.C. "If you have one," says Maas, "running the water for a minute or more probably isn't going to work. It's iffy at best."

• **Lead from solder.** "Until it was banned in 1988, 50-percent-lead solder was used for joints in copper plumbing systems," Maas explains. "So if your home was built before 1988, which is over three-quarters of the homes in the U.S., you definitely have that to worry about."

• **Lead from brass.** Another major source of lead: leaded brass components of the plumbing system that come in contact with water. The brass is five to seven percent lead, which is "enough to put quite a bit of lead in the water, depending on how corrosive the water is," cautions Maas.

Since most of the lead in faucet fixtures was banned in 1997, "if your faucet was purchased since then, there's a 95 percent chance that it doesn't have lead in it," says

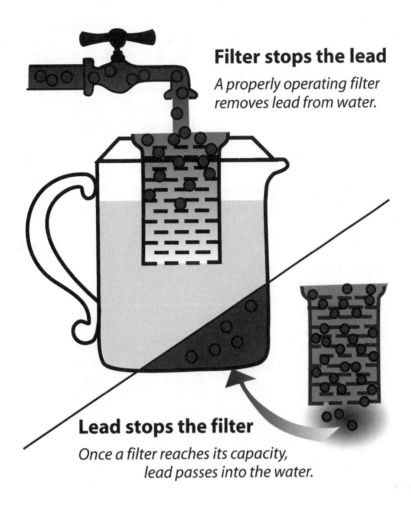

Filter stops the lead

A properly operating filter removes lead from water.

Lead stops the filter

Once a filter reaches its capacity, lead passes into the water.

Maas. "But if it was purchased before 1997, it is virtually sure to have lead in it."

Filter, Filter on the Wall

Even if you have a lead problem that can be solved by running the water for a minute, "most people eventually will turn to using a water filter," says Maas, "because flushing gets to be a nuisance after a while."

Another reason for getting a water filter: since lead quickly builds up in water that sits, if you have a lead problem, "you really need to flush the line every single time you use the water," says Maas.

"We've found that if you take water that's been sitting in the pipes overnight for eight hours, about 75 percent of the lead in it built up in the first two hours." More disturbing: "About 25 percent of the lead was deposited in the first 10 minutes."

So if your water is contaminated with lead, you may need to run the line for a minute or more every time you use it. A water filter might be more convenient.

(Lead isn't easily absorbed through the skin, so bathing or showering shouldn't pose any problems, says Johns Hopkins's Ellen Silbergeld. Neither does using water to brush your teeth with.)

Which brand of filter is best? As long as the filter claims to get rid of lead, it doesn't matter.

"We've tested hundreds of brands of water filters over the years, not only for our own research but also on behalf of companies who want to compare their products with their competitors' products," says Maas. "If a product claims to remove lead, then it's almost certainly quite effective at removing lead."

How often should you change cartridges or filters?

"We find that they last longer than their manufacturers say they do," says Maas. "They want to sell more cartridges and more filters, as you can imagine."

So if you follow the manufacturer's instructions for changing filters, you may be spending a little more money than you need to, but you'll be safe.

"The bad news," says Maas, "is that somewhere between 55 and 70 percent of the water filters out there are no longer removing lead because their owners have gone months or years past the manufacturers' recommendations."

If a filter becomes completely filled with lead, it can't take any more out of your water.

Testing 1, 2

Is there a safe level for lead in water?

"It's hard to set an exact level because any amount of lead causes some neurological damage in a child," says Maas.

But he does offer a rule of thumb: "If your first draw of water in the morning is over 10 parts per billion, you'd want to be doing something about the problem." Maas estimates that some 15 percent of U.S. households fall into that category.

"For the water you're going to be drinking all the time and using for cooking," he adds, "you probably don't want more than 3 ppb."

There's only one way to know if you have a lead problem and whether you can solve it by running the water for one minute. And that's to get a two-sample lead test of your household water, says Maas. (See "Test, Don't Taste.")

If there's a problem with the first draw, the results of the second will tell you whether purging the line for one minute will reduce the lead level to 3 ppb or less. If it does, you should run the water for a minute every time you use it for drinking or cooking.

Another option, suggests Maas, is to fill a gallon jug in the morning after you've run the water for a minute and to use that water for drinking and cooking during the day. If you're not willing to do either of those things or if running the water for a minute doesn't remove enough lead, a water filter is your best bet.

Notes

1. *Amer. J. Epidemiol. 160*: 901,2004.
2. *Amer. J. Epidemiol. 153*: 164, 2001.
3. *Amer. J. Public Health 89*: 330, 1999.
4. *J. Amer. Med. Assoc. 275*: 1177, 1996.
5. *Epidemiology 14*: 713, 2003.
6. *J. Amer. Med. Assoc. 292*: 2750, 2004.

Fortifying with Fiber

Linda Milo Ohr

Dietary fiber has been shown to aid in cardiovascular health, gastrointestinal health, cancer prevention, and weight management. Yet Americans fall short in their consumption of this important nutrient. The American Dietetic Association (ADA) recommends consumption of 20–35 g of dietary fiber/day, but the average American currently eats only 12–17 g. Since about one-fourth of this is soluble fiber, the average American is only consuming 3–4 g of soluble fiber/ day, below the recommended 5–10 g. This is a shame, because a growing body of research supports fiber's various health benefits.

• **Cardiovascular Health.** Soluble fiber has been proven to reduce blood cholesterol levels, thus helping to reduce the risk of heart disease. The heart-health benefits of fiber are acknowledged in the Food and Drug Administration's approved health claim for the relationship between dietary fiber and cardiovascular disease, which is applicable for beta-glucan in oats and psyllium husk.

• **Gastrointestinal Health.** Fiber increases stool weight and improves laxation, maintaining regularity. Dietary fiber also functions as a prebiotic, increasing the number of beneficial microflora in the gut and enhancing the gastrointestinal system and immune system.

• **Weight Management.** Fiber-rich meals are processed more slowly, and nutrient absorption occurs over a greater time period. This aids in the feeling of satiety. In addition, a study on more than 74,000 female nurses in the United States (Liu et al., 2003) showed that those with the greatest increase in intake of dietary fiber gained an average of 1.52 kg less than did those with the smallest increase in intake of dietary fiber. Women in the highest quintile of dietary fiber intake had a 49% lower risk of major weight gain than did women in the lowest quintile.

• **Cancer.** Fiber has been associated with preventing certain types of cancer, such as bowel and breast. A study published last year (Bingham et al., 2003) examined the association between dietary fiber intake and incidence of colorectal cancer in 519,978 individuals age 25–70 years taking part in the European Prospective Investigation into Cancer and Nutrition study. Dietary fiber in foods was inversely related to the incidence of large bowel cancer. The authors concluded that in populations with a low average intake of dietary fiber, an approximate doubling of total fiber intake from foods could reduce the risk of colorectal cancer by 40%.

To obtain these benefits, it is clear that people need to consume more fiber. "Modest increases in intakes of fruits, vegetables, legumes, and whole- and high-fiber grain products would bring the majority of the North American adult population close to the recommended range of dietary fiber intake of 20–35 g/ day," stated ADA in its position on dietary fiber (ADA, 2002). The majority of consumers, however, do not have balanced diets, resulting in inadequate fiber consumption.

This is where fiber-fortified foods can help. Food formulators can use gums, polydextrose, inulin, fructooligosaccharides, and resistant starch to create foods that offer another option for consumers to get more fiber. Here's a run-down of some ingredients that contribute to a food's dietary fiber content.

Inulin

Inulin is a plant-derived carbohydrate with the physiological benefits of soluble dietary fiber. It is not digested or absorbed in the small intestine, but is fermented in the colon by beneficial bacteria. Functioning as a prebiotic, inulin has been associated with enhancing the gastrointestinal system and immune system. In addition, it has been shown to increase the absorption of calcium and magnesium, influence the formation of blood glucose, and reduce the level of cholesterol and serum lipids.

"When used as an ingredient in food products, inulin can be measured and added to foods as a source of dietary fiber," said Bryan Tungland, Vice President of Scientific and Regulatory Affairs at Sensus America, Monmouth Junction, N.J. (646-452-6140)."The entire inulin molecule, due to its solubility in the 80% alcohol step in some older AOAC methods (985.29; 991.43, etc.), has resulted in the requirement to use newer AOAC methods (997.08 and 999.03) to measure the total amount of inulin in a food or food product," he explained. "I should note that the AOAC method 999.03 does not measure fructooligosaccharides (FOS) appropriately and should only be used for inulin of plant origin," he added.

"Using either 997.08 or 999.03 accurately measures inulin's contribution to fiber in various foods," he said. "A total dietary fiber measurement in a food containing inulin can be accomplished by first measuring the food using the standard AOAC method 991.43 and using a specific enzyme to destroy the inulin, and then running the food for total inulin by either of the two specific methods. Totaling the two results provides a measure of the total dietary fiber, including the inulin content."

Sensus America offers *Frutafit*® and *Frutalose*® inulin and FOS for use in a wide variety of foods and beverages. "Many applications of inulin as a health ingredient are related to its properties as a soluble, prebiotic fiber: in developing fiber-enriched and low-carbohydrate foods, improving calcium uptake in the body, and promoting a healthy microflora and immune function in the colon," said Tungland. *Frutafit* inulin, depending on the product of choice, con-

Going with the Grains

Nutritionally speaking, grains are a powerhouse of nutrients. They are a source of fiber, antioxidants, phytoestrogens, and omega-3 fatty acids. Whole grains have been linked to a reduced risk of heart disease and certain forms of cancer, such as lung, colon, and stomach. They have even been linked to aid in weight loss. Here are some nutritious grains to keep an eye on.

• **Amaranth** seed is high in protein (15–18%) and contains respectable amounts of lysine and methionine, two essential amino acids that are not frequently found in grains, according to information from the Wheat Foods Council. It is high in fiber and contains calcium, iron, potassium, phosphorus, and vitamins A and C. The fiber content of amaranth is three times that of wheat, and its iron content is five times more than wheat.

• **Barley** provides soluble fiber that has been shown to improve several cardiovascular risk factors. Kay Behall and colleagues at USDA Agricultural Research Service Diet and Human Performance Laboratory in Beltsville, Md., are investigating whether eating barley and oats can reduce the body's glycemic response and hyperinsulinemia, independent of weight loss.

• **Flaxseed** has been linked to a reduced risk of both prostate and breast cancer. In 2002, researchers from Duke University Medical Center showed that a diet rich in flaxseed appeared to reduce the size, aggressiveness, and severity of tumors in mice that have been genetically engineered to develop prostate cancer (http://news.mc.duke.edu/news/article.php?id=6041). In 3% of the mice, the flaxseed diet kept them from getting the disease at all.

A study in Minnesota among 28 postmenopausal nuns in a convent, chosen primarily because of their strict dietary practices, looked at the effect of flaxseed on breast cancer (Slavin, 2001). Consumption of 5 or 10 g of flax significantly decreased blood levels of certain types of estrogen that may increase a woman's risk of developing breast cancer.

• **Oats** were the subject of a study which found that the risk of obesity is lower for kids who eat oatmeal regularly compared to those who do not. According to the study by researchers from Columbia University and Quaker Oats who presented the results at Experimental Biology 2003, the number of 2- to 18-year-olds who are overweight or at risk of becoming overweight is almost 50% lower in oatmeal-eaters than in children who do not consume oatmeal. In addition, children who eat oatmeal are about twice as likely to meet fiber intake recommendations, with fiber intakes 17% higher than for those who do not eat oatmeal.

• **Rice** is another nutritious grain. One-half cup of cooked white rice provides 0.3 g of dietary fiber, while one-half cup of cooked brown rice provides 1.8 g. The bran layers of brown rice are rich in minerals and vitamins, especially the B-complex group, according to the USA Rice Federation. The protein in rice is considered high quality and well balanced because all eight essential amino acids are present and in proper proportion. Therefore, rice is a unique cereal grain.

tributes at least 90% dietary fiber and as much as 99.5% on a dry-weight basis.

Last year, the Dutch Public Health Ministry approved a "healthy colon" claim for *Frutafit* inulin in breads baked by Bakkerij Veenhuis, a unit of Royal Ahold. The breads are currently marketed in the Netherlands under the brand *Vitaalbrood*®. The claim states that a daily consumption of three slices of the bread with 5 g of inulin/100 g of bread creates a well-balanced intestinal flora composition, which then leads to optimal colon functioning by selectively stimulating the growth of bifidobacteria.

In May last year, FDA stated that it had no objections to the Sensus claim that inulin is Generally Recognized As Safe (GRAS). The U.S. Dept. of Agriculture also approved it for nonstandardized meat applications. "This certainly is an important step in bringing Americans closer to the many physiological and functional benefits that inulin offers," said Tungland.

Another commercial form of an enriched inulin, *Raftilose*® *Synergy1*, manufactured by Orafti Active Food Ingredients, Malvern, Pa. (610-889-9828). According to Orafti, it has been shown to improve calcium and magnesium absorption in post-menopausal

women (www.orafti.com/orafti/OraftiGr.nsf/Home?openform). The study was conducted by Anne Friedlander and colleagues at the Palo Alto VA Health Care System in California. The study involved 15 healthy post-menopausal women and used a randomized crossover design. Calcium and magnesium absorption were measured at baseline and 6 weeks after each treatment period. The study showed that the enriched inulin could enable post-menopausal women to increase both their calcium and magnesium up-take by as much as 20%. Orafti said that this research confirmed previous studies which have shown the positive effects of the ingredient on mineral absorption.

Orafti also offers the *Raftiline*® family, which consists of two main groups of products: those based on native chicory inulin (*ST, ST-Gel*, and *GR*) and those with a longer chain length for high performance applications (*HP, HP-Gel*, and *HPX*). In addition, the *Raftilose* family consists of a group of liquid and powder products composed of oligofructose and the natural sugars glucose, fructose, and sucrose in varying combinations.

Fructooligosaccharides

FOS are natural constituents of a wide variety of fruits, vegetables and grains, and can be produced in commercial quantities. They have shown positive effects on laxation, attenuation of blood cholesterol levels, and blood glucose levels. These prebiotics have found successful use in yogurts, such as *Mountain High Naturally Nutritious Yogurt*, offered by Mountain High, Englewood, Colo. The product contains *NutraFlora*®, a short-chain FOS (*sc-FOS*™) from GTC Nutrition, Golden, Colo. (800-522-4682).

Mountain High states that the fiber enhances calcium absorption. In addition, the company's Web site informs customers that "Scientific studies show that 3 grams of *NutraFlora* dietary fiber per day provide a measurable effect on improving intestinal health." Two 4-oz servings of the yogurt provide 3 g of the dietary fiber.

Colorado-based Horizon Organic also offers *Baby Yogurt* and *Yo-Yo's,* its kids yogurt enriched with the dietary fiber to enhance calcium absorption. The company's Web site states, "As a prebiotic, *NutraFlora* increases the level of good bacteria in your digestive system and promotes overall digestive health."

NutraFlora is 95% pure scFOS, meaning that the molecular structure of the fiber is always glucose terminated (important for beneficial fermentation) and has a chain length no longer than 5. Other forms of FOS may not always be glucose terminated and can have chain lengths up to 10, explained Linda Chamberlain Douglas, Manager of Scientific Affairs at GTC Nutrition. "*NutraFlora* is a prebiotic fiber that consists of a specific, defined composition, so it consistently provides significant health and functional benefits at low doses. It is derived from sugar cane or sugar beets using a natural fermentation process," said Douglas.

The main benefits of scFOS include improving intestinal integrity and function, increasing calcium and magnesium absorption, modulating intestinal immune response, supporting a healthy cholesterol and increasing isoflavone absorption. According to GTC Nutrition, a lowering effect on total and low-density-lipoprotein (LDL)-cholesterol has been demonstrated in people receiving 8 g of scFOS/day. Other studies have shown scFOS to affect the bioavailability of the soy isoflavones genistein and daidzein. For example, in overariectomized mice, scFOS increased the bioavailability of isoflavones, leading to cooperative positive effects on bone mineral density (Ohta et al., 2002).

We believe that in 2004, an increasing number of innovations with scFOS will be realized in the market. In particular, there may be more dairy formulations and nutritional foods, such as bars and shakes, that include prebiotic fiber for its health-enhancing properties," stated Douglas. "Using scFOS in dairy foods presents great opportunity for innovation due to a number of positive synergies, such as increasing calcium absorption. For cultured dairy products, such as yogurt or kefir, the synergy between probiotic cultures and prebiotic fiber results in a maximum potential for optimized health."

GTC also introduced *CalciLife*™ in 2003. This unique ingredient is a combination of calcified sea plants rich in calcium, magnesium, and trace minerals and scFOS. "The trend we are seeing is that food companies are interested in fortifying a variety of foods with calcium and want to increase their ability to make bone health claims by using the calcium–scFOS blend," said Douglas.

Arabinogalactan

Arabinogalactans are water-soluble polysaccharides found in plants, fungi, and bacteria. Dietary intake of arabinogalactans comes from foods such as carrots, radishes, tomatoes, pears, and wheat. Arabinogalactan derived from the larch tree is commercially available as a fiber ingredient and is considered a non-digestible soluble dietary fiber. It is also thought to stimulate the colonic growth of such bacteria as bifidobacteria and lactobacilli.

One commercial form of larch arabinogalactan, *FiberAid*®, from Larex Inc., White Bear Lake, Minn. (800-386-5300), is currently being used in several products on the market as a source of fiber. Affinta, Belmont, MA, sells *Delight-Full*™ snack bars that "help consumers eat less." The bars contain *FiberAid* and other fibers, which, according to the company, are lower-glycemic-index carbohydrates that cause consumers to feel full longer. Each bar offers 2.5 g of dietary fiber. Jamba Juice, San Francisco, Calif., also uses *FiberAid* in the power boost in its smoothies.

Gums

Gums such as guar and arabic also contribute to a food's dietary fiber content. Both provide more than 85% soluble dietary fiber on a dry basis, according to TIC Gums, Belcamp, Md. (800-221-3953).

Guar gum has been shown to provide important health benefits because of its soluble fiber content. Numerous studies have shown that the consumption of guar gum lowers serum LDL cholesterol and triglycerides and increases glucose tolerance. TIC Gums said that in one recent study, rats fed guar gum as a part of their diet showed a 25% decrease in plasma cholesterol. TIC Gums offers *Pretested*® *GuarNT*® *Bland*, which is specially formulated to have low odor properties in addition to its thickening capabilities.

Gum arabic (also known as acacia gum) is derived from the acacia tree. It is water-soluble and contains arabinogalactan. TIC Gums offers an array of *Pretested Gum Arabic* systems to address specific food, beverage, pharmaceutical, and cosmetic functions. Because of its low viscosity, gum arabic can be used to boost fiber levels in a food or beverage without drastically altering the finished viscosity. According to TIC, studies have shown that gum arabic, as a source of soluble dietary fiber, may provide important dietary benefits such as maintaining healthy LDL and total cholesterol in healthy men, speeding oral rehydration, and acting as a prebiotic.

Another form of acacia gum, *Fibregum*™ has been studied for its bifidogenic properties. It contains more than 80% soluble fiber (AOAC method). According to the supplier, Colloides Naturels Inc., Bridgewater, N.J. (800-872-1850), a single-blind study of ten healthy volunteers studied the bifidogenic nature of the ingredient by measuring its stimulating effect on fecal concentrations of bifidobacteria and lactobacilli. The study was conducted in the Human Nutrition Research Center of Nantes, France, in 1999. An increase in fecal concentrations of bifidobacteria and lactobacilli was observed at both dose levels of 10 and 15 g/day.

Resistant Starch

Resistant starch from corn functions as insoluble dietary fiber. Depending on how it is processed, it can be labeled as maltodextrin or cornstarch. "The portion of resistant starch that measures as dietary fiber can be included within the total dietary fiber content on the Nutrition Facts box," said Rhonda Witwer, Business Development Manager of Nutrition at National Starch and Chemical Co., Bridgewater, N.J. (800-797-4992). "For instance, the 60% portion of *Hi-maize*™ 260 that measures as dietary fiber is labeled as dietary fiber. We recommend to our customers that our *Hi-maize* branded ingredients be identified as cornstarch (Hi-maize brand) or corn-starch (low glycemic) or simply cornstarch. Our *Novelose 330* is identified as maltodextrin."

National Starch offers *Hi-maize 240* and *260* resistant starch ingredients (previously known as *Novelose 240* and *260*, respectively). As a better-for-you carbohydrate, resistant starch is used to add dietary fiber, lower the glycemic response ("net" carbs) when used as a substitute for flour, improve insulin sensitivity, and promote digestive health in foods. As a prebiotic fiber, resistant starch increases the population of beneficial bacteria within the large intestine and decreases the population of pathogenic bacteria. More than 120 published studies demonstrate the health benefits of resistant starch, ranging from reduced risk of colon cancer, restoring or healing the lining of the large intestine, to positive improvements on insulin sensitivity and the immune system, said Witwer.

For example, a study by Le Leu et al. (2003) showed that resistance starch increased the programmed cell death in intestinal cells damaged by a carcinogen. Once cells within the large intestine are damaged, they can be repaired, be killed, or progress to cancerous growth. This study showed that dietary consumption of the resistant starch increased the body's ability to kill the damaged cells by up to 30%, explained Witwer. The authors concluded that high-amylose starch may protect against the progression of mutated clones.

A human study confirmed systemic benefits from fermentation of resistant starch (Robertson et al., 2003). Two groups of people were fed diets that had the same amount of carbohydrates. The test group received 60 g of resistant starch, and their insulin sensitivity was measured a day later. The group that had consumed the resistant starch had significant increases in insulin sensitivity and lower impact on glycemic response to the test meal. "There is something about the fermentation of *Hi-maize* that impacts the body's metabolism of glucose," Witwer commented. "As reduced insulin sensitivity is a biomarker for Metabolic Syndrome (the combination of risk factors leading to increased risk of heart disease, obesity, cancer and other major health conditions), increases in insulin sensitivity are hugely important. Insulin sensitivity may also contribute to appetite control and weight loss benefits."

Another study (Morita et al., 2003) showed increases in immune biomarkers and a greater capacity of the large intestine to prevent a liver toxin from passing out of the large intestine into the blood and to the liver when resistant starch was ingested. It confirmed that a leaky gut allows toxins to damage other parts of the body and that restoring the health and strengthening the mucosal lining of the large intestine can have systemic health benefits.

Resistant starches can help create foods for the children's and carbohydrate-conscious markets and foods that offer digestive health benefits, said Witwer. For example, adding dietary fiber to white bread gives children who do not like whole-wheat or whole-grain bread another option to obtain fiber's benefits. For the carbohydrate-conscious market, substituting the resistant starch for flour significantly increases the dietary fiber content, lowers the "net" carbohydrate count, and lowers the glycemic response of a baked good, she said. "We have demonstrated that a bread containing 20% *Hi-maize* lowers the glycemic response in humans by approximately 45–50%. Scientific studies are showing that moderating the glycemic impact of food results in numerous benefits. Greater appetite control is a great benefit for the weight-control market."

Lignins

Plant lignins, which are phytoestrogens, have beneficial effects on heart health, bone health, prostate health, and some forms of cancer. For example, a study by Horn-Ross et al. (2003) linked lignins to a reduced risk of endometrial cancer, the fifth most common cancer among women worldwide. The researchers evaluated the associations between dietary intake of seven specific compounds representing three classes of phytoestrogens (isoflavones, coumestans, and lignins) and the risk of endometrial cancer in a case-control study of women age 35–79. Consumption of isoflavones and lignins, but not coumestans, was associated with a reduced risk of endometrial cancer, particularly among post-menopausal women.

Flaxseed boasts a high concentration of lignins, particularly secoisolariciresinol diglucoside (SDG). In 2002, Acatris Inc., Minneapolis, Minn. (952-920-7700), a division of the Dutch Royal Schouten Group, introduced *LinumLife™*, a concentrated form of flax lignins marketed for prostate health.

This past January, the company added a more concentrated extract, *LinumLife Extra*. It is standardized to contain 20% SDG. The concentrated phytoestrogens in the extract are thought to be capable of balancing natural hormone levels in the body and therefore have a positive role in testosterone production. The extract can be used in capsules or tablets and is also suitable for flax oil enrichment and cosmetic applications. To support existing studies showing the positive effects of flax and lignins on health, Acatris has established a clinical study program to research the extract.

Polydextrose

The polydextrose content of food is measured by AOAC method 2000.11 and can be added to the fiber determined by other methods, according to Danisco Sweeteners, Ardsley, N.Y. (800-255-6837 x2521). The company markets a fiber ingredient, *Litesse*®, manufactured from polydextrose. According to the company, 17 human, in-vitro, and animal published studies have demonstrated the fiber properties of polydextrose. Its prebiotic effects such as enhancing the growth of bifidobacteria, have been reported with consumption as low as 4 g/day (Jie et al., 2000).

FDA has approved *Litesse* for use in frozen dairy desserts, sweet baked goods and mixes, confections and frostings, salad dressings, gelatins, puddings and fillings, hard and soft candy, chewing gum, fruit spreads, peanut spread, sweet sauces, toppings, and syrups. The ingredient provides just 1 kcal/g; that is 25% of the calories of sugar and 11% of the calories of fats. It is non-glycemic, so it can be incorporated into a wide variety of foods with a reduced glycemic index.

For More Information

There are still more types of dietary fiber that the food industry can utilize in products such as baked goods, pasta, nutrition bars, beverages, and other products. For an extensive listing of dietary fiber types and suppliers, visit www.ift.org and click on the link for IFT's *Nutraceutical & Functional Food Buyer's Guide*, or see the December 2003 issue of *Food Technology*.

REFERENCES

ADA. 2002. Position of the American Dietetic Association: Health implications of dietary fiber. J. Am. Dietetic Assn. 102: 993–1000.

Bingham, S.A., et al. 2003. Dietary fibre in food and protection against colorectal cancer in the European Prospective Investigation into Cancer and Nutrition (EPIC): An observational study. Lancet 361: 1496–501.

Horn-Ross, P.L., John, E.M., Canchola, A.J., Stewart, S.L., and Lee, M.M. 2003. Phytoestrogen intake and endometrial cancer risk. J. Natl. Cancer Inst. 95: 1158–1164.

Jie, Z., Bang-yao, L., Ming-jie, X., Hai-wei, L., Zu-kang, Z., Ting-song, W., and Craig, S. 2000. Studies on the effects of polydextrose intake on physiologic functions in Chinese people. Am. J. Clin. Nutr. 72: 1503–1509.

Le Leu, R.K., Brown, I.L., Hu, Y., and Young, G.P. 2003. Effect of resistant starch on genotoxin-induced apoptosis, colonic epithelium, and lumenal contents in rats. Carcinogenesis 24: 1347–1352.

Liu, S., Willett, W.C., Manson, J.E., Hu, F.B., Rosner, B., and Colditz, G. 2003. Relation between changes in intakes of dietary fiber and grain products and changes in weight and development of obesity among middle-aged women. Am. J. Clin. Nutr. 78: 920–927.

Morita, T., Tanabe, H., Takahashi, K., and Sugiyama, K. 2003. Ingestion of resistant starch protects endotoxin influx from the intestinal tract and reduces D-galactosamine-induced liver injury in rats. J. Gastroenterol. Hepatol., in press.

Ohta, A., Uehara, M., Sakai, K., Takasaki, M., Adlercreutz, H., Morohashi, T., and Ishimi, Y. 2002. A combination of dietary fructooligosaccharides and isoflavone conjugates increases femoral bone mineral density and equol production in ovariectomized mice. J. Nutr. 132: 2048–2054.

Robertson, M.D., Currie, J.M., Morgan, L.M., Jewell, D.P., and Frayn, K.N. 2003. Prior short-term consumption of resistant starch enhances postprandial insulin sensitivity in healthy subjects. Diabetologia. 46: 659–665.

Slavin, J. 2001. Can flaxseed protect against hormonally dependent cancer? Presented at American Chemical Society Div. of Agricultural and Food Chemistry meeting, Chicago, August.

UNIT 3

Diet and Disease Through the Life Span

Unit Selections

Key Points to Consider

- How is the area of Nutrigenomics going to help the consumer lessen the risk from degenerative disease?

- Name some factors in the school environment that are going to promote children's and adolescent's health.

- How is magnesium involved in regulating blood glucose?

- Identify major food allergens you may be exposed to daily.

- Are you or your parents at risk for the Metabolic syndrome?

- Why do parents miss the signs of anorexia in their child?

Student Website

www.mhcls.com/online

Internet References

Further information regarding these websites may be found in this book's preface or online.

American Cancer Society
http://www.cancer.org
American Heart Association (AHA)
http://www.americanheart.org
The Food Allergy and Anaphylaxis Network
http://www.foodallergy.org
Heinz Infant & Toddler Nutrition
http://www.heinzbaby.com
LaLeche League International
http://www.lalecheleague.org

In Ancient Greece, Hippocrates, the father of medicine, stated in his oath to serve humanity that the physician should use diet as part of his "arsenal" to fight disease. In ancient times, the healing arts included diet, exercise, and the power of the mind to cure disease.

Since those times, research that focuses on the connection between diet and disease has unraveled the role of many nutrients in degenerative disease prevention or reversal. But, frequently the results are controversial and need to be interpreted cautiously before a population-wide health message is mandated. We have also come to better understand the role of genetics in the expression of disease and its importance in how we respond to dietary change. The decoding of the Human Genome has heralded one of the most crucial medical projects of all time and has improved our understanding of the genetics behind certain diseases. It will help "fingerprint" people, thus identifying the exact gene that makes a person susceptible to a certain disease. Thus, based on one's genotype, disease risk may be identified and population-wide statements about diet may sift to personal, custom-made diet regimens. This is the emerging science of Nutrigenomics. Additionally, research about diet and disease has enabled us to understand the importance and uniqueness of the individual (age, gender, ethnicity, and genetics) and his or her particular response to dietary interventions.

With the recent advances in research in the area of phytochemicals such as flavonoids, carotenoids, saponins, indoles, and others in foods—especially fruits and vegetables, and their potential to prevent disease, thereby increasing both quality of life and life expectancy—we are at the zenith of a nutrition revolution. The most prevalent degenerative diseases in industrial countries, which are quickly spreading in developing countries, are cancer, cardiovascular disease, diabetes, obesity, and osteoporosis. The number of people with non-insulin dependent diabetes mellitus has increased by 50 percent compared to ten years ago.

Highly processed foods have stripped many minerals from the food supply making our diets deficient in them. One of those minerals is magnesium. Magnesium nutrition is very important due to the role of magnesium in blood glucose regulation and its implications on non-insulin dependent diabetes mellitus. One of the articles in this unit describes its food sources, the quantity we need in our diet, and its benefits on regulating blood glucose levels. Additionally, phytochemicals that are found in wine, spices, and coffee are presently under study to determine their effects on degenerative diseases such as diabetes, kidney, and heart disease.

As obesity incidence increases worldwide so does the Metabolic Syndrome, which is characterized by increased blood pressure, bloods lipids, insulin resistance, and abdominal obesity—which predispose a person to degenerative diseases. Dr. Deen reviews the syndrome and offers suggestions as to its prevention and reversal.

A risk factor for heart disease is obesity. Eating excessive number of calories leads to obesity. Animal studies have shown that restricting calories prevents disease and prolongs life. If that also applies to humans, radical changes need to be instituted in

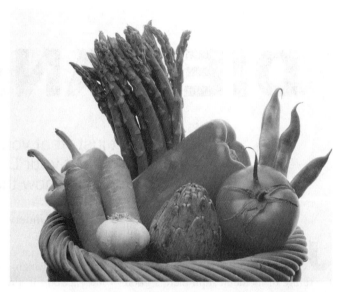

American life styles to change food-related behaviors to achieve the above. The recent obesity epidemic has not only affected adults but has also touched children. Approximately 15 percent of children in America between the ages of 6-19 are obese and 30 percent are overweight. Lack of activity and poor dietary habits are the primary contributing factors. Children are not presently eating enough fruits and vegetables or dairy foods and lack important nutrients for bone growth such as calcium and vitamin D. Children's diets also lack iron and fiber, nutrients crucial for maintenance of body weight and prevention of cardiovascular disease. Food companies have shown interest in collaborating with the American Dietetic Association and the American Academy of Family Physicians to offer healthier choices to children and provide public awareness of healthy eating habits. It has been documented that nutrition affects learning and performance. Even though unhealthy eating habits continue in young adolescents, schools have not placed student health and nutrition on high priority. The important role parents, teachers, and administrators play in developing food and nutrition policy is crucial. Developing a comprehensive health education program with nutrition as a major component should become standard in middle school curricula across America. Additionally, practicing what is preached is important in learning healthy eating behaviors and decreasing chronic diseases.

Another area of concern is that of food allergies. Recently food allergies are on the rise, especially among the younger population sometimes with lethal results. Taylor and Hefle present and discuss what the consumer should be educated about and how the food industry should control allergens through all stages of product development and processing to avoid the above.

Finally, concurrent to the rise of obesity, anorexia is also increasing among the population—regardless of gender or age. Case studies of past and present patients describing their personal stories, signs parents should be sensitive to, and treatment options are explained.

DIET AND GENES

It isn't just what you eat that can kill you,
and it isn't just your DNA that can save you—
it's how they interact.

By Anne Underwood and Jerry Adler

JOSE ORDOVAS HAS GLIMPSED the future of medicine, and there's good news for anyone who has just paid $4 for a pint of pomegranate juice. Ordovas, director of the Nutrition and Genomics Laboratory at Tufts University, believes the era of sweeping dietary recommendations for the whole population—also sometimes known as fads—may be coming to an end. Red wine may be better for your arteries than ice cream, but you can't create a diet that's optimal for everyone, Ordovas says—or, to put it another way, even Frenchmen get heart attacks sometimes. Within a decade, though, doctors will be able to take genetic profiles of their patients, identify specific diseases for which they are at risk and create customized nutrition plans accordingly. Some people will be advised to eat broccoli, while others will be told to eat … even more broccoli.

Maybe you have to be a nutritionist to appreciate the beauty of that scheme. The promise of nutritional genomics—a field that barely existed five years ago— is not to overturn a century's worth of dietary advice but to understand on the most basic level how health is determined by the interplay of nutrients and genes. The old paradigm was of a one-way process, in which "bad" foods gave you heart disease or cancer unless "good" genes intervened to protect you. New research suggests a continual inter-

action, in which certain foods enhance the action of protective (or harmful) genes, while others tend to suppress them. This supports what we know from observation, that some individuals are better adapted than others to survive a morning commute past a dozen doughnut shops. Pima Indians in the Southwest get type 2 diabetes at eight times the rate of white Americans. Individuals have widely varying responses to high- or low-fat diets, wine, salt, even exercise. Overwhelmingly, though, researchers expect that conventional dietary wisdom will hold for most people. So keep that vegetable steamer handy.

Green tea
helps silence genes that fuel breast cancer in some women.

ONE EXAMPLE:
■ **Name of gene:** HER-2
■ **Function of gene:** Triggers growth signals in cells
■ **Long-term effect:** Slows HER-2 signaling in aggressive breast tumors

The model for nutritional genomics is the work that has already been done on drug-gene interactions. Researchers are starting to unravel the mystery of why a drug may be a lifesaver for one person

while causing a fatal reaction in another, and in a third has no effect at all. Why do a third of patients fail to respond to the antidepressants known as SSRIs, including Prozac, Paxil and Zoloft? The drugs are meant to increase levels of the neurotransmitter serotonin by blocking its "reuptake," or clearance from the brain. Obviously, they can work only if serotonin is being produced in the first place. Last month researchers at Duke University discovered that some people have a variant gene which reduces the production of serotonin by 80 percent—making them both susceptible to major depression and resistant to treatment with SSRIs.

Broccoli
boosts genes that protect against heart disease.

ONE EXAMPLE:
■ **Name of gene:** GST
■ **Function of gene:** Produces the body's master antioxidants, glutathione
■ **Long-term effect:** The additional glutathione helps keep arteries healthy

But food interactions are usually far more complicated. "Normally, you take one drug at a time and for a limited amount of time," says Dr. Muin Khoury, director of the Office of Genomics and

Disease Prevention at the Centers for Disease Control and Prevention. "If you have a certain genetic variant, you stay away from a particular drug or take a different dose." But nutrients come in bulk, you consume them for a lifetime and you can get them without a prescription, even the Trucker's Pancake Special. Metabolism involves huge numbers of genes interacting in uncountable ways. There are at least 150 gene variants that can give rise to type 2 diabetes, 300 or more that are associated with obesity. Ordovas at Tufts compares the situation to an electrical panel: "We know about certain switches and how to turn them on and off. But in some people, you turn the switch but the light doesn't come on, because there are other switches upstream and downstream that we don't know about yet." It will be years before researchers have a good diagram of the circuit. That hasn't prevented the growth of a fledgling industry in personalized nutritional supplements to treat everything from osteoporosis to obsessive-compulsive disorder. At least one company will even profile your genes to take the guesswork out of choosing makeup.

Soybeans
affect 123 genes involved in prostate cancer.

ONE EXAMPLE:
- **Name of gene:** p53
- **Function of gene:** Kills mutant cells
- **Long-term effect:** A compound in soy increases activity of the p53 gene, helping to block tumor formation

But pieces of the diagram are beginning to emerge. Green tea contains potent antioxidants known to help prevent heart disease and certain cancers, but only some women seem to show a reduction in breast cancer from drinking it. A study at the University of Southern California suggests that part of the reason lies in a gene that produces an enzyme called COMT that inactivates the cancer-suppressing compounds; women with the gene variant that produces a less active form of COMT showed the most benefit from tea.

One interaction that has been studied in detail involves two categories of enzymes known as phase 1 and phase 2. These work in sequence to eliminate certain toxins from the body, such as heterocyclic amines—potent carcinogens that form, infuriatingly, in the tasty crust on broiled meat. Actually, the amines are not inherently harmful; they are dangerous only after the phase 1 enzymes have begun metabolizing them, and before the phase 2s can finish the job. So, obviously, it is desirable to have a balance of the two enzymes. But some people have a variant gene that speeds up the phase 1 enzymes, so they form carcinogens faster than the phase 2s can get rid of them. This gene is found in 28 percent of white Americans, but roughly 40 percent of African-Americans and Hispanics and nearly 70 percent of Japanese-Americans (who, as it happens, have a high rate of stomach cancer). But there are ways to tweak the system: garlic contains nutrients that slow down the phase 1 enzymes, and a substance known as sulforaphane boosts levels of the phase 2s. And sulforaphane is easy to obtain. You get it from broccoli.

Turmeric
suppresses genes that ratchet up inflammation.

ONE EXAMPLE:
- **Name of gene:** Cox-2
- **Function of gene:** Makes inflammatory compounds

- **Long-term effect:** Could help ward off colon cancer and Alzheimer's

"You can see where we're headed. We're starting to take the guesswork out of the things we eat," says Raymond Rodriguez, who heads the Center of Excellence in Nutritional Genomics at the University of California, Davis. One notable case is the gene for a protein known as Apo E, which plays a major role in regulating cholesterol. It has three major variants (or "alleles"), designated E2, E3 and E4, of which E3 is the most common. People with one or two copies of the E2 allele generally have lower-than-average cholesterol, but the E4 variety—an estimated 15 to 30 percent of the population has at least one copy of the allele—is potentially lethal. It increases the risk of diabetes, it raises total cholesterol and it reverses the usual protective effects of moderate drinking. And it vastly increases the risks of smoking. "Smoking is bad for everybody," says Ordovas, "but in a person with E4 it's a total killer. We're not talking about probabilities. It's almost certain you'll get heart disease." But, he adds, E4 is extremely susceptible to environment. The increased diabetes risk is found only in people who are overweight. If you stop smoking, give up alcohol, exercise and eat a diet low in saturated fat, "you can remove *all* the genetic predisposition for heart disease that comes with E4"—not just some, but all of it.

Patients at risk for Alzheimer's may not want to know.

On the face of it, you could make a case for universal screening for the Apo E gene. But we don't do it, and the reasons shed light on the ethical complexities of the field. One reason is peculiar to the Apo E4 allele, which also doubles the risk of developing Alzheimer's. Since there's not much that can be done to prevent it, many doctors are reluctant to give patients this news, and many patients don't want to know it themselves. More generally, there is the danger that insurance companies will discriminate against people with risk factors in their genome. Ruth DeBusk, author of "Genetics: The Nutrition Connection," thinks this concern is overblown, because by and large the risks are spread across the population. "We all have some susceptibilities," she says. "It's not as if one group has all the bad genes and the rest of us are perfect." Susceptibilities, moreover, don't necessarily amount to destiny; perhaps we can figure out what people with the E4 gene should eat to forestall dementia. But Jim Kaput, who founded a genomics-research company, wonders about people who get the correct nutritional advice for their genotype and then refuse to follow it. "Should the insurance company be obliged to pay for their health care, too?"

And—one might ask—what's the point of testing for something if the inevitable advice that comes out of it is to exercise and eat a healthy diet? Didn't we know that already? The answer lies in the "Churchill effect," people's natural inclination to believe that if Winston Churchill lived to 90 on a diet of marrow bones, champagne and cigars, why not them? "People always think the warnings don't apply to them," DeBusk says. "We hope if we can tell them 'Here's what *you're* at risk for,' it will hit home." Conversely, cardiologists now routinely put people on a low-salt diet to control high blood pressure, knowing it doesn't work for as much as half the population. Even if it doesn't work, it can't hurt, and the doctor, after all, isn't the one giving up hot dogs. But, as Dr. Victoria Herrera of Boston University says, telling patients to do something that doesn't work "makes liars out of doctors. We need to make a diagnosis based on genotype, so we can go beyond trial and error."

Not all research in the field is aimed at identifying alleles that differ among individuals. The broader purpose is to understand the interplay of nutrition and genetics. What protects Asians (at least the ones who still live in Asia and eat a traditional soy-based diet) from hormone-sensitive breast and prostate tumors? The most common explanation is that soy contains compounds that bind to estrogen receptors on cells, making them unavailable to more potent hormones. But Rodriguez has identified a soy constituent called lunasin that increases, by his count, the activity of 123 different genes in prostate cells. Among them are genes that suppress tumor growth, initiate the repair of damaged DNA and promote apoptosis, the programmed "suicide" of damaged cells before they begin to multiply. He hasn't been looking for different alleles of these genes, although it's likely they exist and may subtly affect how individuals respond to lunasin. The genetic factors predisposing men to prostate cancer can, in principle, eventually be identified and calculated for each individual. When all is said and done, though, the recommendation will probably stay the same: eat more soy. (And more fresh fruits and vegetables, and less saturated fat … and so on.)

Another compound getting a lot of study is curcumin, the yellow pigment in turmeric, an ingredient in curry spice. Curcumin reduces the action of a number of genes that promote inflammation, which is linked to heart disease, colon cancer and Alzheimer's. "It's probably no coincidence that India has the lowest incidence of Alzheimer's in the world," says Sally Frautschy, a professor of neurology at UCLA, who studies turmeric together with her husband and colleague, Greg Cole. "What I hear from the pharmaceutical industry," says Cole, "is 'What are you trying to do, ruin us?' "

> **Some people seem immune to the effects of salt on blood pressure.**

There's not much chance of that, of course. More likely, nutritional genomics will create opportunities for drug companies to isolate, concentrate, synthesize and improve on the compounds in nature, which they've been doing for a hundred years. What Cole and his colleagues seek is to shed light on the mystery of how the human body has evolved the miraculous ability to overcome, once in a while, the threat posed by the consequences of its own appetites.

Metabolic Syndrome

Time for Action

The constellation of dyslipidemia (hypertriglyceridemia and low levels of high-density lipoprotein cholesterol), elevated blood pressure, impaired glucose tolerance, and central obesity is identified now as metabolic syndrome, also called syndrome X. Soon, metabolic syndrome will overtake cigarette smoking as the number one risk factor for heart disease among the U.S. population. The National Cholesterol Education Program–Adult Treatment Panel III has identified metabolic syndrome as an indication for vigorous lifestyle intervention. Effective interventions include diet, exercise, and judicious use of pharmacologic agents to address specific risk factors. Weight loss significantly improves all aspects of metabolic syndrome. Increasing physical activity and decreasing caloric intake by reducing portion sizes will improve metabolic syndrome abnormalities, even in the absence of weight loss. Specific dietary changes that are appropriate for addressing different aspects of the syndrome include reducing saturated fat intake to lower insulin resistance, reducing sodium intake to lower blood pressure, and reducing high-glycemic–index carbohydrate intake to lower triglyceride levels. A diet that includes more fruits, vegetables, whole grains, monounsaturated fats, and low-fat dairy products will benefit most patients with metabolic syndrome. Family physicians can be more effective in helping patients to change their lifestyle behaviors by assessing each patient for the presence of specific risk factors, clearly communicating these risk factors to patients, identifying appropriate interventions to address specific risks, and assisting patients in identifying barriers to behavior change. (Am Fam Physician 2004;69:2875-82,2887-8. Copyright © 2004 American Academy of Family Physicians.)

DARWIN DEEN, M.D., M.S., Albert Einstein College of Medicine of Yeshiva University, Bronx, New York

Metabolic syndrome, also called insulin resistance syndrome or syndrome X, is a cluster of risk factors that is responsible for much of the excess cardiovascular disease morbidity among overweight and obese patients and those persons with type 2 diabetes mellitus.[1] Differences in body-fat distribution (i.e., gynecoid versus android) associated with an altered metabolic profile were documented in the medical literature 50 years ago. Given the name syndrome X in 1988,[2] each component of the syndrome has been associated with an increased risk of cardiovascular disease.[3] A report[4] from the National Cholesterol Education Program–Adult Treatment Panel (NCEP–ATP III) identified metabolic syndrome as an independent risk factor for cardiovascular disease and considered it an indication for intensive lifestyle modification.

Definition

The major characteristics of metabolic syndrome include insulin resistance, abdominal obesity, elevated blood pressure, and lipid abnormalities (i.e., elevated levels of triglycerides and low levels of high-density lipoprotein [HDL] cholesterol). Initially defined by an expert panel of the World Health Organization in 1998,[5] the NCEP–ATP III[4] has created an operational definition of metabolic syndrome: the co-occurrence of any three of the abnormalities mentioned above (*Table 1*[4,5]).

Major characteristics of metabolic syndrome include insulin resistance, abdominal obesity, elevated blood pressure, and lipid abnormalities.

Metabolic syndrome is associated with a proinflammatory/prothrombotic state that may include elevated levels of C-reactive protein, endothelial dysfunction, hyperfibrinogenemia, increased platelet aggregation, increased levels of plasminogen activator inhibitor 1, elevated uric acid levels, microalbuminuria, and a shift toward small, dense particles of low-density lipoprotein (LDL) cholesterol. Insulin resistance also has been implicated in polycystic ovary syndrome and nonalcoholic steatohepatitis (NASH).

TABLE I
Diagnostic Criteria for Metabolic Syndrome According to the WHO and the ATP III

Component	WHO diagnostic criteria (insulin resistance* plus two of the following)	APT III diagnostic criteria (three of the following)
Abdominal/central obesity	Waist to hip ratio: > 0.90 (men), > 0.85 (women), or BMI > 30 kg per m^2	Waist circumference: > 102 cm (40 in) in men, > 88 cm (35 in) in women
Hypertriglyceridemia	≥ 150 mg per dL (≥ 1.7 mmol per L)	≥150 mg per dL
Low HDL cholesterol	< 35 mg per dL (< 0.9 mmol per L) for men, <39 mg per dL (< 1.0 mmol per L) for women	< 40 mg per dL (< 1.036 mmol per L) for men, < 50 mg per dL (< 1.295 mmol per L) for women
High blood pressure	≥ 140/90 mm Hg or documented use of antihypertensive therapy	≥ 130/85 mm Hg or documented use of antihypertensive therapy
High fasting glucose	Impaired glucose tolerance, impaired fasting glucose, insulin resistance, or diabetes	≥ 110 mg per dL (≥ 6.1 mmol per L)†
Microalbuminuria	Urinary albumin to creatinine ratio: 30 mg per g, or albumin excretion rate: 20 mcg per minute	

WHO = World Heath Organization; ATP = Adult Treatment Panel: BMI = body mass index; HDL = high-density lipoprotein.

*—Insulin resistance is identified by type 2 diabetes mellitus or impaired fasting glucose.

†—The American Diabetes Association recently has suggested lowering this threshold to 100.

Adapted with permission from National Institutes of Health: Third Report of the National Cholesterol Education Program Expert Panel on Detection, Evaluation, and Treatment of High Blood Cholesterol in Adults (Adult Treatment Panel III). Executive Summary. Bethesda, Md.: National Institutes of Health, National Heart Lung and Blood Institute, 2001 (NIH publication no. 01-3670), and Alberti KG, Zimmet PZ. Definition, diagnosis and classification of diabetes mellitus and its complications. Part I: diagnosis and classification of diabetes mellitus, provisional report of a WHO consultation. Diabet Med 1998; 15:539-53.

Epidemiology/Prevalence

The prevalence of metabolic syndrome varies by definition used and population studied.[6] Based on data from the Third National Health and Nutrition Examination Survey (1988 to 1994), the prevalence of metabolic syndrome (using the NCEP–ATP III criteria) varies from 16 percent of black men to 37 percent of Hispanic women.[7] The prevalence of metabolic syndrome increases with age and increasing body weight. Because the U.S. population is aging, and because more than one half of adults are overweight or obese, it has been estimated that metabolic syndrome soon will overtake cigarette smoking as the primary risk factor for cardiovascular disease.[8] Metabolic syndrome is an even stronger predictor of risk for type 2 diabetes mellitus.[9]

Etiology

The etiology of the metabolic syndrome has not been established definitively. One hypothesis presumes that the primary cause is insulin resistance. Insulin resistance correlates with visceral fat measured by waist circumference or waist to hip ratio. The link between insulin resistance and cardiovascular disease probably is mediated by oxidative stress, which produces endothelial cell dysfunction, promoting vascular damage and atheroma formation.[10]

The second hypothesis blames hormonal changes for the development of abdominal obesity. One study[11] demonstrated that persons with elevated levels of serum cortisol (caused by chronic stress) developed abdominal obesity, insulin resistance, and lipid abnormalities. The investigators concluded that this inappropriate activation of the hypothalamic-pituitary-adrenal axis by stress is responsible for the link between psychosocial and economic problems, and acute myocardial infarction.

Clinical Evaluation

The routine medical and family history helps to identify patients at risk for cardiovascular disease or diabetes mellitus. Questions about recent or past weight changes, and a brief diet and physical activity history,[12] including occupational and leisure-time physical activity, are important. The patient should be asked to estimate how many hours a day he or she is sedentary. Questions about typical food intake and efforts to reduce dietary fat or other specific dietary changes allow the physician to estimate the patient's readiness to change lifestyle habits.

The patient's height, weight, and blood pressure should be measured. Body mass index (BMI) should be determined by calculating weight (kg)/height (m^2), and waist circumference should be measured at the narrowest point between the umbilicus and the rib cage. Waist circumference appears to be a better predictor of cardiovascular risk than waist-to-hip ratio.[13] Patients suspected of having metabolic syndrome should have a fasting glucose level and a fasting lipid profile level obtained. A euglycemic clamp or homeostasis model assessment is used in research studies to accurately assess insulin resistance, but is impractical for use in the clinical setting.[14]

Currently, no randomized controlled trials are aimed specifically at treating metabolic syndrome.

Fasting insulin levels and glucose challenge tests are indicators of insulin resistance but do not need to be measured in most situations because a fasting glucose level alone suffices for the definition of metabolic syndrome. If LDL cholesterol is normal, measuring levels of apolipoprotein B is not necessary. New tests that measure LDL particle size are expensive and unnecessary, because low HDL cholesterol levels and high triglyceride levels predict small, dense LDL particles.

The American Heart Association recommends measurement of highly sensitive C-reactive protein for risk stratification in patients at high risk of cardiovascular disease.[15] Baseline uric acid levels and routine liver function tests will screen for NASH, but abdominal ultrasonography is required to diagnose fatty liver because it may be present even in the absence of elevated liver function test results.

Treatment Strategies

Currently, no randomized controlled trials specifically examining the treatment of metabolic syndrome have been published. Based on clinical trials, aggressive management of the individual components of the syndrome should make it possible to prevent or delay the onset of diabetes mellitus, hypertension, and cardiovascular disease.[4,16,17] All patients diagnosed with metabolic syndrome should be encouraged to change their diet and exercise habits as primary therapy. Weight loss improves all aspects of the metabolic syndrome, as well as reducing all-cause and cardiovascular mortality[18] (*Table 2*). While many patients find weight loss difficult to achieve, exercise and dietary changes that can lower blood pressure and improve lipid levels will improve insulin resistance, even in the absence of weight loss.[19]

EXERCISE

Skeletal muscle is the most insulin-sensitive tissue in the body and, therefore, a primary target for impacting insulin resistance. Physical training has been shown to reduce skeletal muscle lipid levels and insulin resistance, regardless of BMI.[20] The impact of exercise on insulin sensitivity is evident for 24 to 48 hours and disappears within three to five days. Thus, regular physical activity should be a part of any effort to reverse the effects of insulin resistance.

The primary goals of dietary management for persons with metabolic syndrome are to reduce the risk of cardiovascular disease and diabetes mellitus.

EXERCISE PRESCRIPTION

Patients should be encouraged to focus on improving their personal level of physical activity. The greatest health benefits occur when sedentary persons incorporate moderate-intensity exercise into their lifestyle. Low-intensity exercise can have a significant impact on health and studies show that as the recommended frequency of exercise increases, actual participation declines.[21]

The goal for family physicians is to help patients find a level of activity that they can accomplish over the long term.[22] A combination of resistance and aerobic exercise is best, but any activity is better than none, and patients who have been sedentary need to start with walking and gradually increase duration

and intensity.[23] Use of low-weight dumbbells, elastic exercise bands, or even heavy food containers can provide the needed weight for resistance training. Walking or light jogging for one hour per day will produce significant losses of abdominal (visceral) fat in men without caloric restriction.[24]

Diet

No single diet is currently recommended for patients with metabolic syndrome; therefore, it may be best for physicians to focus on each patient's specific metabolic alterations when offering dietary advice[25] (*Table 2*). Sustained dietary changes may require referral to a registered dietitian to help implement suggestions and ensure adequate micronutrient intake (e.g., calcium, iron, folate) while reducing calories. There is debate about what proportions of macronutrients (i.e., protein, fat, and carbohydrates) will produce the best outcome (low-fat, low-carbohydrate, or Mediterranean diets). If a patient is consuming fewer calories than he or she is expending, the macronutrient composition of the diet is probably of secondary importance, because weight loss improves metabolic syndrome.

The primary goals of dietary change for metabolic syndrome are to reduce the risk of cardiovascular disease and diabetes mellitus. Two recent Cochrane Database systematic reviews support the role of dietary interventions in helping to reduce cardiovascular risk. Evidence[26] from one large and one small trial showed that a low-sodium diet helps to maintain lower blood pressure following withdrawal of antihypertensive medications. Results[27] from clinical trials of low-fat diets in which participants were involved for more than two years showed significant reductions in the rate of cardiovascular events and suggested protection from total mortality. The degree of protection from cardiovascular events was statistically significant in patients with a higher risk of cardiovascular disease.

For patients with elevated blood pressure, the Seventh Report of the Joint National Committee on Prevention, Detection, Evaluation, and Treatment of High Blood Pressure (JNC 7)[16] states that a systolic blood pressure of 120 to 139 mm Hg or a diastolic pressure of 80 to 89 mm Hg should be considered pre-hypertensive and trigger lifestyle modifications to prevent cardiovascular disease.

According to the Dietary Approaches to Stop Hypertension (DASH) study,[28] patients who consumed a diet low in saturated fat and high in carbohydrates experienced a significant reduction in blood pressure, even without weight reduction. The DASH diet emphasizes fruits, vegetables, low-fat dairy foods, whole grains, poultry, fish, and nuts, while reducing saturated fats, red meat, sweets, and sugar-containing beverages. Reducing sodium intake can further reduce blood pressure or prevent the increase in blood pressure that may accompany aging.

The Coronary Artery Risk Development in Young Adults study[29] demonstrated that consumption of dairy products was associated with a significantly reduced risk of metabolic syndrome.

Low-fat, high-carbohydrate diets have been criticized because they may raise triglyceride levels and lower HDL-cholesterol

TABLE 2
Practical Advice for Lifestyle Interventions in Patients with Metabolic Syndrome

Abnormality	Diet and physical activity interventions	Practical advice
Abdominal obesity	Reduce weight.	Reduce portion sizes to lower calorie intake.
	Increase physical activity.	30 minutes of moderate-intensity exercise daily
Hypertriglyceridemia	Reduce weight.	Reduce portion sizes to lower calorie intake.
	Increase physical activity.	30 minutes of moderate-intensity exercise daily
	Increase intake of low-glycemic–index foods.	Replace refined carbohydrates (white bread, potatoes, pasta) with legumes, whole grains, and monounsaturated fats (nuts, avocado, canola oil, olive oil).
	Reduce total carbohydrate intake.	Replace soda and juices with water, seltzer, and diet beverages.
	Increase omega-3 fatty acids.	Eat fish at least once per week.
	Limit alcohol consumption.	Limit alcohol to no more than two drinks per day for men, or one drink per day for women.
Low HDL cholesterol level	Reduce weight.	Reduce portion sizes to lower calorie intake.
	Increase physical activity.	30 minutes of moderate-intensity exercise daily
	Increase consumption of monounsaturated fats.	Eat fish, nuts, and avocados. Use olive or canola oils in salad dressing and for cooking.
	Stop smoking.	Join a smoking cessation program.
High blood pressure	Reduce weight.	Reduce portion sizes to lower calorie intake.
	Increase physical activity.	30 minutes of moderate-intensity exercise daily
	Reduce saturated fat intake.	Choose low-fat dairy products and reduce consumption of red meat, butter, and full-fat dairy products.
	Reduce sodium intake.	Reduce sodium intake to no more than 2.4 g per day or 6 g per day of salt by using more herbs in cooking; read labels for sodium content; skip the salt shaker.
	Increase consumption of fruits and vegetables.	Consume more than five servings of fruits and vegetables every day.
	Increase low-fat dairy products.	Consume three servings of low-fat dairy products daily.
	Limit alcohol consumption	Limit alcohol to no more than two drinks per day for men and one drink per day for women.
High fasting glucose level	Reduce weight.	Reduce portion sizes to lower calorie intake.
	Increase physical activity.	30 minutes of moderate-intensity exercise daily
	Reduce total carbohydrate intake; replace carbohydrates with monounsaturated fat.	Replace refined grains with whole grains (oatmeal, brown rice, corn, and whole wheat) and monounsaturated fats (nuts, avocados, canola oil, olive oil).
	Increase dietary fiber (more than 30 g per day).	Add legumes and fruit for soluble fiber.

HDL = high-density lipoprotein.

Supplied with permission by Darwin Deen, M.D., M.S., Albert Einstein College of Medicine, and Lisa Hark, Ph.D., R.D., University of Pennsylvania School of Medicine.

levels in some patients, thus aggravating the dyslipidemia of metabolic syndrome. To treat hypertriglyceridemia, or if HDL-cholesterol levels decline on a low-fat diet, carbohydrate intake can be reduced and replaced with foods high in monounsaturated fats[30] or low-glycemic–index carbohydrates. These changes create a diet similar to the Mediterranean-style diet, which also has been shown to reduce mortality from cardiovascular disease.[31]

For sedentary patients with hypertriglyceridemia and insulin resistance (particularly those who are obese or who have an abnormal waist circumference; *Table 1*[4,5]), a lower carbohydrate diet that limits sodas, juice drinks, and refined grains (such as sweetened cereals, baked goods, and desserts) may be beneficial (see http://www.ttuhsc.edu/SOM/FamMed/wholefoods.html).

One study[32] demonstrated a correlation between cardiovascular disease and the intake of refined grain products and potatoes. The investigators recommend a diet high in minimally processed plant-based foods, such as whole grains, fruits, and vegetables. Results of a recent pooled analysis of cohort studies[33] concluded that increasing dietary fiber from fruits, vegetables, and grains lowers the risk of developing cardiovascular disease.

The long-term effects of low-carbohydrate diets have not been studied adequately, but in the short-term, these diets have been shown to lower triglyceride levels, raise HDL-cholesterol levels, and reduce body weight.[34] An alternative to lowering consumption of all carbohydrates is to replace high-glycemic–index foods with less refined lower-glycemic–index foods that

TABLE 3
ATP III Guidelines for the Treatment of Patients with Metabolic Syndrome

Targeted area	Goal
Treat LDL cholesterol first.	
CHD and CHD risk equivalent (10-year risk for CHD > 20 percent)	< 100 mg per dL (< 2.60 mmol per L)
At least two risk factors and 10-year risk ≤ 20 percent	< 130 mg per dL (< 3.35 mmol per L)
Institute weight control.	−10 percent from baseline
Institute physical activity.	30 to 40 minutes per day, three to five days per week
Monitor treatment of hypertension.	< 130/85 mm Hg
Treat elevated triglyceride levels and low HDL cholesterol levels.	
Goal of non-HDL cholesterol for patients with triglyceride levels of ≥ 200 mg per dL (≥ 5.20 mmol per L) and ≥ 499 mg per dL (≤ 12.90 mmol per L)	High CHD risk: < 130 mg per dL; Intermediate CHD risk: < 160 mg per dL (4.15 mmol per L); Low CHD risk: < 190 mg per dL (4.90 mmol per L)

APT = Adult Treatment Panel; LDL = low-density lipoprotein; CHD = coronary heart disease; HDL = high-density lipoprotein.

Adapted with permission from Vega GL. Obesity, the metabolic syndrome, and cardiovascular disease. Am Heart J 2001; 142:1108-16. © 2001, Elsevier, Inc.

contain more fiber.[33] Low-glycemic–index foods produce lower levels of postprandial glucose and insulin. Current fiber intakes are below recommended levels and limiting grains will make this worse.

While alcohol consumption has been associated with elevations of serum triglyceride levels, moderate alcohol intake, defined as one drink per day for women and two drinks per day for men, need not be discouraged unless fatty liver is present,[35] because this level of alcohol intake reduces insulin resistance and cardiovascular disease.[36]

The long-term effects of low-carbohydrate diets have not been studied adequately in patients with metabolic syndrome, although short-term effects show benefit.

USING EDUCATIONAL STRATEGIES

Family physicians recognize that there are significant barriers to lifestyle counseling,[37] but patient-centered methodologies accompanied by supportive office systems can make the primary care physician more effective.[38,39] Physicians should assess patients' knowledge about the relationship of their lifestyle to their health, then provide a clear message about the importance of diet and exercise for their specific problem.

Next, physicians should try to help patients identify short- and long-term goals and barriers to change. Questions such as: "How do you think that your diet (or exercise level) affects your health?" or "What problems did you encounter in trying to change your diet (or level of activity)?" can help the physician identify effective next steps for each patient. The answers to these questions should be recorded in the medical record and reviewed at subsequent visits to help patients identify and address barriers to lifestyle changes. ICD-9 codes (97802 and 97803) are available for physician reimbursement for these counseling efforts.

PHARMACOTHERAPY

For patients whose risk factors are not reduced adequately by lifestyle changes (Table 3[1]), pharmacologic interventions to control their blood pressure and lipid levels are indicated.[40] Use of aspirin and statins lowers C-reactive protein levels, but so does weight loss. Aggressive pharmacologic management of risk factors has been shown to be more effective than routine care in preventing cardiovascular disease in patients with type 2 diabetes mellitus.[41]

Strength of Redcommendations

Key clinical recommendation	Strength of recommendation	References
The American Heart Association recommends measurement of highly sensitive C-reactive protein for risk stratification in patients at high risk of cardiovascular disease.	C	15
Evidence from a large and small trial showed that a low-sodium diet helps to maintain lower blood pressure following withdrawal of antihypertensive medications.	A	26
Results from clinical trials of low-fat diets in which participants were involved for more than two years showed significant reductions in the rate of cardiovascular events and suggested protection from total mortality.	A	27
The U.S. Preventive Services Task Force recommends intensive behavioral dietary counseling for adult patients with known risk factors for cardiovascular disease.	B	42

Prevention

The U.S. Preventive Services Task Force recommends intensive behavioral dietary counseling for adult patients with known risk factors for cardiovascular disease.[42] The evidence for counseling for physical activity is not yet strong enough to merit a recommendation.[43] Family physicians need to be more effective at helping patients adopt healthy lifestyle habits. The Diabetes Prevention Program[19] demonstrated that vigorous lifestyle intervention in patients who are prediabetic could reduce the rate of developing diabetes by more than 50 percent (from 11 to 4.8 percent).

Author note: The author indicates no conflicts of interest. Sources of funding: Nutrition Academic Award NIH 5 K07 HL0395.

The author wishes to thank Gina Lopez for her assistance with the literature review, Drs. Peter Selwyn and Janet Townsend for their review of the manuscript, and Dr. Lisa Hark for her invaluable assistance with the manuscript and the patient education handout.

REFERENCES

1. Vega GL. Obesity, the metabolic syndrome, and cardiovascular disease. Am Heart J 2001;142:1108–16.
2. Reaven GM. Banting lecture 1988. Role of insulin resistance in human disease. Diabetes 1988;37:1595–607.
3. Lamarche B, Tchernof A, Mauriege P, Cantin B, Dagenais GR, Lupien PJ, et al. Fasting insulin and apolipoprotein B levels and low-density lipoprotein particle size as risk factors for ischemic heart disease. JAMA 1998;279:1955–61.
4. National Institutes of Health: Third Report of the National Cholesterol Education Program Expert Panel on Detection, Evaluation, and Treatment of High Blood Cholesterol in Adults (Adult Treatment Panel III). Executive Summary. Bethesda, Md.: National Institutes of Health, National Heart Lung and Blood Institute, 2001 (NIH publication no. 01-3670). Accessed online March 18, 2004, at: http://www.nhlbi.nih.gov/guidelines/cholesterol/index.htm.
5. Alberti KG, Zimmet PZ. Definition, diagnosis and classification of diabetes mellitus and its complications. Part 1: diagnosis and classification of diabetes mellitus, provisional report of a WHO consultation. Diabet Med 1998;15:539–53.
6. Ford ES, Giles WH. A comparison of the prevalence of the metabolic syndrome using two proposed definitions. Diabetes Care 2003;26:575–81.
7. Ford ES, Giles WH, Dietz WH. Prevalence of the metabolic syndrome among U.S. adults: findings from the Third National Health and Nutrition Examination Survey. JAMA 2002;287:356–9.
8. Eckel RH, Krauss RM. American Heart Association call to action: obesity as a major risk factor for coronary heart disease. AHA Nutrition Committee. Circulation 1998;97:2099–100.
9. Grundy SM, Brewer HB Jr, Cleeman JI, Smith SC Jr, Lenfant C, for The American Heart Association/National Heart, Lung, and Blood Institute. Definition of metabolic syndrome: Report of the National Heart, Lung, and Blood Institute/American Heart Association conference on scientific issues related to definition. Circulation 2004;109:433–8.
10. Lopez-Candales A. Metabolic syndrome X: a comprehensive review of the pathophysiology and recommended therapy. J Med 2001;32:283–300.
11. Bjorntorp P. Heart and soul: stress and the metabolic syndrome. Scand Cardiovasc J 2001;35:172–7.
12. Hark L, Deen D Jr. Taking a nutrition history: a practical approach for family physicians. Am Fam Physician 1999;59:1521–8, 1531–2.
13. Pouliot MC, Despres JP, Lemieux S, Moorjani S, Bouchard C, Tremblay A, et al. Waist circumference and abdominal sagittal diameter: best simple anthropometric indexes of abdominal visceral adipose tissue accumulation and related cardiovascular risk in men and women. Am J Cardiol 1994;73:460–8.
14. Wallace TM, Matthews DR. The assessment of insulin resistance in man. Diabet Med 2002;19:527–34.
15. Pearson TA, Mensah GA, Alexander RW, Anderson JL, Cannon RO 3d, Criqui M, et al. Markers of inflammation and cardiovascular disease: application to clinical and public health practice. A statement for healthcare professionals from the Centers for Disease Control and Prevention and the American Heart Association. Circulation 2003;107:499–511.
16. Chobanian AV, Bakris GL, Black HR, Cushman WC, Green LA, Izzo JL Jr, et al., for the National Heart, Lung, and Blood Institute Joint National Committee on Prevention, Detection, Evaluation, and Treatment of High Blood Pressure; National High Blood Pressure Education Program Coordinating Committee. The Seventh Report of the Joint National Committee on Prevention, Detection, Evaluation, and Treatment of High Blood Pressure: the JNC 7 report [Published correction appears in JAMA 2003;290:197]. JAMA 2003;289:2560–72
17. Knowler WC, Barrett-Connor E, Fowler SE, Hamman RF, Lachin JM, Walker EA, et al., for the Diabetes Prevention Program Research Group. Reduction in the incidence of type 2 diabetes with lifestyle intervention or metformin. N Engl J Med 2002;346:393–403.
18. Gregg EW, Cauley JA, Stone K, Thompson TJ, Bauer DC, Cummings SR, et al., for the Study of Osteoporotic Fractures Research Group. Relationship of changes in physical activity and mortality among older women. JAMA 2003;289:2379–86.
19. Duncan GE, Perri MG, Theriaque DW, Hutson AD, Eckel RH, Stacpoole PW. Exercise training, without weight loss, increases insulin sensitivity and postheparin plasma lipase activity in previously sedentary adults. Diabetes Care 2003;26:557–62.
20. Goodpaster BH, He J, Watkins S, Kelley DE. Skeletal muscle lipid content and insulin resistance: evidence for a paradox in endurance-trained athletes. J Clin Endocrinol Metab 2001;86:5755–61.

21. Keller C, Trevino RP. Effects of two frequencies of walking on cardiovascular risk factor reduction in Mexican American women. Res Nurs Health 2001;24:390–401.

22. McInnis KJ, Franklin BA, Rippe JM. Counseling for physical activity in overweight and obese patients. Am Fam Physician 2003;67:1249–56.

23. Slentz CA, Duscha BD, Johnson JL, Ketchum K, Aiken LB, Samsa GP, et al. Effects of the amount of exercise on body weight, body composition, and measures of central obesity: STRRIDE—a randomized controlled study. Arch Intern Med 2004;164:31–9.

24. Ross R, Dagnone D, Jones PJ, Smith H, Paddags A, Hudson R, et al. Reduction in obesity and related comorbid conditions after dietinduced weight loss or exercise-induced weight loss in men. A randomized, controlled trial. Ann Intern Med 2000;133:92–103.

25. Szapary PO, Hark LA, Burke FM. The metabolic syndrome: a new focus for lifestyle modification. Patient Care 2002;36:75–88.

26. Hooper L, Bartlett C, Davey SG, Ebrahim S. Advice to reduce dietary salt for prevention of cardiovascular disease. Cochrane Database Syst Rev 2004;(2):CD003656.

27. Hooper L, Summerbell CD, Higgins JP, Thompson RL, Clements G, Capps N, et al. Reduced or modified dietary fat for preventing cardiovascular disease. Cochrane Database Syst Rev 2004;(2):CD002137.

28. Vollmer WM, Sacks FM, Ard J, Appel LJ, Bray GA, Simons-Morton DG, et al., for the DASH-Sodium Trial Collaborative Research Group. Effects of diet and sodium intake on blood pressure: subgroup analysis of the DASH-sodium trial. Ann Intern Med 2001;135:1019–28.

29. Pereira MA, Jacobs DR Jr, Van Horn L, Slattery ML, Kartashov AI, Ludwig DS. Dairy consumption, obesity, and the insulin resistance syndrome in young adults: the CARDIA Study. JAMA 2002;287:2081–9.

30. Grundy SM, Abate N, Chandalia M. Diet composition and the metabolic syndrome: what is the optimal fat intake? Am J Med 2002;113(suppl 9B):25S–29S.

31. Trichopoulou A, Costacou T, Bamia C, Trichopoulos D. Adherence to a Mediterranean diet and survival in a Greek population. N Engl J Med 2003;348:2599–608.

32. Liu S, Manson JE. Dietary carbohydrates, physical inactivity, obesity, and the 'metabolic syndrome' as predictors of coronary heart disease. Curr Opin Lipidol 2001;12:395–404.

33. Jenkins DJ, Kendall CW, Augustin LS, Vuksan V. High-complex carbohydrate or lente carbohydrate foods? Am J Med 2002;113(suppl 9B):30S–37S.

34. Foster GD, Wyatt HR, Hill JO, McGuckin BG, Brill C, Mohammed BS, et al. A randomized trial of a low-carbohydrate diet for obesity. N Engl J Med 2003;348:2082–90.

35. Goude D, Fagerberg B, Hulthe J, for the AIR study group. Alcohol consumption, the metabolic syndrome and insulin resistance in 58-year-old clinically healthy men (AIR study). Clin Sci (London) 2002;102:345–52.

36. Bell DS. Understanding the role of insulin resistance for the treatment of diabetes and the reduction of cardiovascular risks. J Gender-Specific Med 2002;5(suppl):1S–14S.

37. Petrella RJ, Wight D. An office-based instrument for exercise counseling and prescription in primary care. The Step Test Exercise Prescription (STEP). Arch Fam Med 2000;9:339–44.

38. Wallace LS, Rogers ES, Bielak K. Promoting physical activity in the family practice setting. Am Fam Physician 2003;67:1199–200,1202.

39. Ockene IS, Hebert JR, Ockene JK, Merriam PA, Hurley TG, Saperia GM. Effect of training and a structured office practice on physician-delivered nutrition counseling: the Worcester-Area Trial for Counseling in Hyperlipidemia (WATCH). Am J Prev Med 1996;12:252–8.

40. Ginsberg HN. Treatment for patients with the metabolic syndrome. Am J Cardiol 2003;91(7A):29E–39E.

41. Gaede P, Vedel P, Larsen N, Jensen GV, Parving HH, Pedersen O. Multifactorial intervention and cardiovascular disease in patients with type 2 diabetes. N Engl J Med 2003;348:383–93.

42. U.S. Preventive Services Task Force. Behavioral counseling in primary care to promote a healthy diet: recommendations and rationale. Am J Prev Med 2003;24:93–100.

43. U.S. Preventive Services Task Force. Behavioral counseling in primary care to promote physical activity: recommendations and rationale. Accessed online April 30, 2004, at: http://www.ahrq.gov/clinic/3rduspstf/physactivity/physactrr.htm.

The Author

DARWIN DEEN, M.D., M.S., is director of medical student education in the Department of Family and Social Medicine at the Albert Einstein College of Medicine of Yeshiva University, Bronx, N.Y. He graduated from the Albert Einstein College of Medicine and completed a residency in family medicine at Montefiore Medical Center, Bronx. Dr. Deen received his masters degree in human nutrition from Columbia University College of Physicians and Surgeons, New York City. He was co-principle investigator of a recent Nutrition Academic Award grant from the National Institutes of Health.

Address correspondence to Darwin Deen, M.D., M.S., Department of Family and Social Medicine, Albert Einstein College of Medicine, 1300 Morris Park Ave., Mazur Bldg. Suite 100, Bronx, NY 10461 (e-mail: deen@aecom.yu.edu). Reprints are not available from the author.

From *American Family Physician*, Vol. 69, No. 12, June 15, 2004, pp. 2875-2882. Copyright © 2004 by American Academy of Family Physicians. Reprinted by permission.

The *Magnesium-Diabetes* CONNECTION

Find out which foods complete the puzzle of this nutrient's link to diabetes.

Victoria Shanta-Retelny

In a gallant effort to keep the rising rates of diabetes at bay, nutrition researchers are digging deeper to uncover the role micronutrients play in glucose metabolism. A mineral commanding recent attention is magnesium. Few studies have addressed the association between specific micronutrient components of western diets and diabetes risk.[1] "A growing body of evidence," explains Jerry L. Nadler, MD, division chief of endocrinology and metabolism at the University of Virginia, "suggests that magnesium plays a pivotal role in reducing cardiovascular risk and may be involved in the pathogenesis of diabetes itself." A combination of recent research findings suggest that magnesium keeps blood sugars from rising too high, thus staving off diabetes.

Experts do not know exactly what the magical mechanism is behind magnesium's ability to decrease insulin resistance. According to Monika Waelti, PhD, of the Swiss Federal Institute of Technology in Zurich, Switzerland, "Low magnesium intake seems to play a role in the development of diabetes and insulin resistance." Waelti references three large epidemiological studies, including two Harvard studies—Nurses' Health Study (NHS) of 85,000 women and Health Professionals Follow-Up Study (HPFS) of 43,000 men, as well as the University of Minnesota's Iowa Women's Health Study of 40,000 women—which show "an inverse association between magnesium intake and the development of diabetes." These studies' findings revealed that those who ate more magnesium-rich foods, such as whole grains, vegetables, and legumes, were less likely to develop type 2 diabetes.

Food Sources of Magnesium	
Tofu, firm, ½ cup	118 mg
Chili with beans, 1 cup	115 mg
Wheat germ, toasted, ¼ cup	90 mg
Halibut, baked, 3 ounces	78 mg
Swiss Chard, cooked, 1 cup	75 mg
Peanut, roasted, ¼ cup	67 mg
Baked potato with skin, 1 medium	55 mg
Spinach, fresh, 1 cup	44 mg

—Source: USDA: Composition of Foods. **USDA Handbook No. 8 Series.** Washington, D.C., ARS, USDA, 1976-1986.

WHAT IS THE EVIDENCE?

The data from the NHS and HPFS studies are "robust and significant," according to Frank Hu, MD, MPH, PhD, associate professor of nutrition and epidemiology at the Harvard School of Public Health. With Hu's research primarily focused on the role of dietary and lifestyle factors in the development of type 2 diabetes, obesity, and cardiovascular disease, the two large ongoing cohort studies at Harvard, NHS and HPFS, comprise the majority of his research.

"It is a well-established fact that magnesium is a cofactor for insulin action and plays a critical role in insulin sensitivity," Hu explains. The Harvard research confirmed this principle by showing that increased consumption of magnesium-rich foods in both healthy men and women significantly lowered their risk of type 2 diabetes by enhancing insulin sensitivity. Increasing dietary sources of magnesium appears to be the key. Hu empha- sizes, "The research does not suggest supplementation but encourages people to eat a healthy diet, which is high in magnesium-rich foods."

The Iowa Women's Health Study found that over the six years of the study, higher consumption of total grains, whole grains, total fiber, cereal fiber, and magnesium were associated with a lower incidence of type 2 diabetes. Those with the highest intake of cereal fiber (7 to 10 grams per day) reduced their risk of developing type 2 diabetes by approx- imately 30% compared with those with the lowest intake of cereal fiber (2 to 4 grams per day).[7] Analyses from the 1989 Total Diet study of the FDA indicated that approximately 45% of dietary magnesium was obtained from vegetables, fruits, grains, and nuts, whereas approximately 29% was ob- tained from milk, meat, and eggs.[8]

> ## *"The research does not suggest supplementation but encourages people to eat a healthy diet, which is high in magnesium-rich foods."*

These findings are crucial since type 2 diabetes is on track to become one of the major global public health challenges of the 21st century.[3] The western diet is se- verely lacking in magnesium because highly processed foods are stripped of this vital nutrient. Since hypo- magnesemia is a common feature in patients with type 2 diabetes, the usual question is: What came first, the dis- ease or the deficiency? Although diabetes can induce hy- pomagnesemia, magnesium deficiency has also been proposed as a risk factor for type 2 diabetes.[4] Refined foods generally have the lowest magnesium content. With the increased consumption of refined and/or pro- cessed foods, dietary magnesium intake in the United States appears to have decreased over the years.[9] For ex- ample, the average American is getting only 6 milligrams from white bread, whereas its less consumed, unrefined counterpart, whole grain bread, has more than four times that amount at 26 milligrams per serving.

HOW MUCH MAGNESIUM IS BENEFICIAL?

The National Institute of Health describes magne- sium as a mineral needed by every cell. It is needed for more than 300 biochemical reactions in the body as it helps maintain normal muscle and nerve function and keeps heart rhythm steady and bones strong. It is also involved in energy metabolism and protein synthesis. Only 1% of the magnesium in the body is found in blood. The human body works hard to keep blood levels of magnesium constant.[2]

With the Daily Value (DV) of magnesium set at 400 milligrams, experts believe Americans do not consume nearly enough. The DV standards have been supported by the National Academy of Sciences and the Institute of Medicine after great deliberation, research, and literature review; an estimated 50% to 85% of the U.S. population is receiving inadequate magnesium intake.[5]

Nadler points out that many studies have shown that both mean plasma- and intracellular-free magnesium lev- els are lower in patients with diabetes than in the general population. The American Dietetic Association mandates that serum magnesium levels be measured in diabetes pa- tients who have the following concomitant conditions[5]:

- acute myocardial infarction;
- calcium deficiency;
- congestive heart failure;
- ethanol abuse;
- ketoacidosis;
- long-term parenteral nutrition;
- long-term use of certain drugs such as diuretics, digoxin, or aminoglycosides;
- potassium deficiency; and
- pregnancy.

In 1992, the American Diabetes Association issued a consensus statement that concluded: "Adequate dietary magnesium intake can generally be achieved by a nutri- tionally balanced meal plan as recommended by the American Diabetes Association." It recommended that "… only diabetic patients at high risk of hypo- magnesemia should have total serum (blood) magnesium assessed, and such levels should be repeated only if hypo- magnesemia can be demonstrated."[2]

In Nadler's clinical practice, all patients with existing di- abetes are seen by a dietitian. The magnesium levels are measured, and if subclinical levels are found, Nadler ex- plains, "the first line of therapy used is dietary sources to replenish magnesium stores." There are exceptions to the rule, such as in people on calorie-restrictive diets, where supplementation is necessary. Nadler emphasizes, "It is even harder to get the recommended daily allowance for magnesium when on a strict weight-loss diet." Supple- menting with wheat germ or leafy greens is a possible rem- edy mentioned by the Virginia-based endocrinologist.

Magnesium received honorable mention as a food source that can prevent the onset of type 2 diabetes in the June issue of *Nutrition Action HealthLetter*. The data indicated that women who ate 375 milligrams of magne- sium-rich foods daily (compared with 220 milligrams per day) and men who ate 450 milligrams of magne- sium-rich foods daily (compared with 270 milligrams per day) lowered their risk of diabetes by roughly 25% and 30%, respectively.[6]

> ## *The western diet is severely lacking in magnesium because highly processed foods are stripped of this vital nutrient.*

The expert consensus is that an overall healthy diet is the best prevention for diabetes since that ensures adequate intake of magnesium and other nutrients such as folate, other B-vitamins, and fiber. To meet the

DV for magnesium, the most bioavailable sources of the mineral are whole grains, avocados, squash, almonds, fruits, and leafy greens.

Magnesium is also abundant in drinking water, especially "hard" water, which typically has a higher concentration of magnesium salts. A study in Taiwan showed the risk of dying from diabetes to be inversely proportional to the level of magnesium in the drinking water. According to a study in the *American Journal of Clinical Nutrition*, since 1970, chronic mortality in Taiwan was found to be due to diabetes. The findings revealed that the chronic latent magnesium deficit caused the pathogenesis of diabetes even more so than clinical hypomagnesemia, thus suggesting that dietary magnesium—including from the water supply—is protective against diabetes.[5]

WHY IS MAGNESIUM VITAL TO BLOOD SUGAR STABILIZATION?

Physiologically speaking, there are reasons that magnesium storage and depletion are important factors, especially in people with diabetes. Magnesium depletion is found in a number of diseases of cardiovascular and neuromuscular function, malabsorption syndromes, diabetes mellitus, renal wasting syndromes, and alcoholism.[11]

Magnesium depletion in clinical observational studies has been defined by low serum magnesium concentrations as well as a reduction of total and/or ionized magnesium in red blood cells, platelets, lymphocytes, and skeletal muscle.[12] One possible cause for the magnesium depletion seen in diabetes is glycosuria-induced renal magnesium wasting.[13]

Waelti explains, "Magnesium depletion appears to have a negative impact on glucose homeostasis and insulin sensitivity, thus the impairment of insulin sensitivity seems to be related, at least in part, to a defective tyrosine kinase activity of the insulin receptor." She explains that since there are several enzymes involved in glucose metabolism that require high-energy phosphate bonds, magnesium as a cofactor is required.

As far as magnesium depletion, the Swiss researcher listed major factors for urinary losses of magnesium, such as poor metabolic control, impaired renal reabsorption, and the use of diuretics. Waelti and her colleagues' research indicates that magnesium absorption is not intrinsically impaired in patients with type 2 diabetes; however, their hypothesis (which has yet to be confirmed) is that "magnesium absorption might be decreased in people with type 2 diabetes due to enteric neuropathy and microvascular disease," explains Waelti.

Expectant mothers who have diabetes should make sure they have enough magnesium stores. Infants of mothers with type 1 (insulin-dependent) diabetes mellitus are at risk of hypocalcemia and hypomagnesemia, possibly due to magnesium deficiency in the mother.[16] Lower intracellular magnesium concentrations have been recently reported in women with gestational diabetes.[17] It

Signs of Magnesium Deficiency

- Confusion
- Disorientation
- Loss of appetite
- Depression
- Muscle contractions and cramps
- Tingling
- Numbness
- Abnormal heart rhythms
- Coronary spasm
- Seizures

—Source: http://ods.od.nih.gov

is not known whether this is a sequellae of the condition or a factor in its causation.[18]

HOW ARE MAGNESIUM LEVELS MEASURED?

Magnesium losses are measured with a magnesium tolerance test, which is based on the renal excretion of a parenterally administered magnesium load. It is considered by some to be an accurate means of assessing magnesium status in adults but not in infants and children.[14] However, the sensitivity of this method in detecting magnesium depletion may be different between subjects with and without hypomagnesemia. One of the problems in using the magnesium tolerance test is that it requires normal renal handling of magnesium. Urinary magnesium loss (related to conditions such as diabetes or drug or alcohol use) may yield an inappropriate negative test.[15] A serum magnesium concentration of less than 0.75 millimoles per liter (1.8 milligrams per deciliter) is thought to indicate magnesium depletion.[19]

Age may also be a confounding variable for measuring magnesium retention, since older subjects (73 ± 6 years) have been reported to retain significantly more magnesium than younger subjects (33 ± 10 years), despite a comparable mean daily dietary magnesium intake of 5.1 milligrams (0.2 millimoles per kilogram) of body weight.[20]

PUTTING MAGNESIUM INTO PRACTICE

Dietetics practitioners are faced with the continued task of educating patients/clients on the importance of magnesium-rich foods. Whether helping people manage diabetes or prevent its onset, it is essential to stress the importance of getting optimal nutrition from all food groups. Melissa Sujak, RD, CDE, at Northwestern Memorial Hospital Wellness Institute in Chicago knows all too well the importance of emphasizing magnesium in the diet as "these are the foods that increase insulin sensitivity," she says. With the proliferation of processed foods in the western diet, Sujak is a big advocates emphasizing the utility of magnesium-rich foods. She points to the National Health and Nutrition Examination Survey III (NHANES III) as evidence that the American diet is deficient in three food groups that are the highest in magnesium: whole grains, fruits, and vegetables.

The NHANES III study demonstrated ethnic differences in magnesium intake. In that report, non-Hispanic black subjects were found to consume less than either non-Hispanic white or Hispanic subjects. When educating patients, "let's be proactive, not reactive," Sujak states.

Everyone can benefit from magnesium-rich foods—not only for diabetes prevention but also for a decrease in risk factors. Waelti says, "A diet rich in magnesium would benefit everyone, especially people with risk factors for type 2 diabetes, such as obesity, hypertension, elevated blood lipid levels, or a family history of diabetes."

—*Victoria Shanta-Retelny, RD, LD, is a practicing dietitian at Northwestern Memorial Wellness Institute in Chicago, a freelance food and nutrition writer, and a culinary spokesperson.*

COFFEE, SPICES, WINE

New dietary ammo against diabetes?

By Janet Raloff

Non–insulin-dependent diabetes is epidemic in the United States. The potentially deadly disorder afflicts some 16 million people in this country, accounting for 95 percent of all diabetes. The number of people with non–insulin-dependent diabetes is 50 percent greater today than it was just a decade ago. Cardiovascular complications account for half of all deaths among people with this type of diabetes, commonly called type 2, and the disorder is the leading cause of kidney failure, adult blindness, and amputations in the United States. Nationally, medical expenditures associated with treating type 2 diabetes and its complications are about $92 billion per year.

The disease arises when people lose all or part of their sensitivity to insulin, the hormone that normally signals cells to move glucose from the blood into energy-hungry tissues. Because spikes in blood-glucose concentrations can damage the circulatory system and other organs, the long-term health of people with full-blown type 2 diabetes depends upon how tightly they can control their blood sugar concentrations. They do this by making lifestyle changes, such as exercising regularly, losing weight, and choosing certain foods.

People considered to be prediabetic because they have faltering blood sugar control also fare better in the long run if they follow the same lifestyle guidelines.

Restricting intake of sugar and starches is one way that people can maintain moderate blood sugar concentrations. Their diet should include primarily fibrous whole grains that release glucose slowly into the bloodstream (*SN: 4/8/00, p. 236*). That's a tough challenge in today's fast-food world, dominated by refined, highly processed foods.

WHAT A KICK—Though caffeine makes blood sugar concentrations spike, certain trace ingredients in coffee ameliorate that effect. And one study has found that decaf lowers blood sugar.

However, an assortment of new nutrition data may come as unexpectedly sweet news. Researchers are uncovering mechanisms by which a range of dietary agents—including coffee, wine, and cinnamon—appear to restore some of the body's responsiveness to insulin and control of blood sugar. Such changes seem to be transitory, however, so these foods offer no cure for diabetes. But dietary scientists now suggest that regular intake of these foods might slow the disease's onset and reduce its ravages.

COFFEE CLASH Study after study has shown antidiabetic effects of coffee. The March 10 *Journal of the American Medical Association* carries the latest epidemiological evidence—two European studies showing that people who drink 6 to 10 cups of coffee, primarily caffeinated, per day tend to develop type 2 diabetes at lower rates than individuals do who drink 2 or fewer cups a day.

For several years, scientists have been asking what constituent of java works to control blood sugar. Gradually, chlorogenic acids, a relatively minor family of chemicals in coffee beans, have emerged as prime candidates.

Much attention focused on caffeine, which has turned out to have a detrimental effect. Terry E. Graham of the University of Guelph in Ontario and his coworkers recently tested the effect of pure caffeine, caffeinated coffee, and decaf on blood sugar in lean and obese people with and without type 2 diabetes. The amount of caffeine in a mug or two of strong coffee was sufficient to disrupt control of blood sugar for several hours in any of those 67 individuals, says Graham. A paper detailing the 56 nondiabetic volunteers is due out soon in the *American Journal of Clinical Nutrition*.

Giving the volunteers caffeine in plain water followed an hour later by a slug of sugar water induced the highest blood sugar concentrations. The same amount of caffeine delivered in 2 cups of coffee before the sugar jolt raised blood sugar concentrations about 75 percent as much as the pure caffeine did. However, when the researchers gave people two cups of decaffeinated coffee and then the sugar, their blood sugar concentrations were even lower than when they drank plain water before the sugar.

That result suggests that the decaf—and, therefore, some coffee component other than caffeine—has an antidiabetic effect, says Graham.

Last year, Linda M. Morgan and her colleagues at the University of Surrey in England tested nine healthy volunteers. Each made three morning visits to Morgan's lab after fasting overnight. In the lab, they each downed 25 grains of sugar in 2 cups of a beverage. On one morning, they took the sugar in regular coffee; another morning, in decaf; and a third morning, in water. After each sugary drink, they submitted to tests of how much ingested glucose entered their blood during the next 3 hours.

Both coffee types enabled the volunteers to control blood glucose significantly better than they did after drinking the glucose-containing water, the scientists reported in the October 2003 *American Journal of Clinical Nutrition.* Once in the blood, however, glucose that was drunk with caffeinated coffee tended to stay there, as it would in a person with diabetes. The finding is consistent with other studies showing that caffeine can impair insulin's responsiveness to blood sugar.

By keeping the concentrations of chlorogenic acids the same in the decaf and caffeinated coffees, the researchers made sure that those compounds weren't the source of the effect. Earlier studies by the group had shown that low concentrations of chlorogenic acids naturally present in apples attenuated the release of glucose into the blood after volunteers ate the fruit.

Michael N. Clifford, the research team's food chemist, hypothesizes that chlorogenic acids, which are present in far greater concentrations in coffee than in fruit, reduce the efficiency of molecular-scale pumps that move glucose across the walls of cells lining the digestive tract. These acids would thereby tend to keep sugar in the gut and out of the bloodstream, reducing the chances of the high spikes of blood sugar that exacerbate diabetes.

Jane Shearer of Vanderbilt University in Nashville and her colleagues have studied the effects of pure chlorogenic acids, isolated from decaf, on enzymes that regulate the liver's release of glucose. Ordinarily, between meals, the liver sends glucose into the blood to keep it available to tissues. In people with diabetes, the liver inappropriately sends out glucose even after a meal has already boosted blood concentrations of the sugar.

The researchers showed in rats that chlorogenic acids disrupt the liver enzymes' action, bogging down glucose's release into the blood. This helps prevent blood sugar spikes after meals, the researchers reported in the November 2003 *Journal of Nutrition.*

TEA TOO? A few studies have hinted that teas—with their bounty of antioxidants called polyphenols—might also exhibit antidiabetic properties. In the latest such trial, Lucy S. Hwang of National Taiwan University in Taipei measured green tea's effect on insulin action in rats with experimentally induced diabetes.

Hwang's team substituted room-temperature tea for drinking water for half of the animals. After 12 weeks, tea-drinking rodents exhibited improved insulin sensitivity and lower blood-glucose concentrations during the 2 hours after each meal, the researchers reported in the Feb. 1 *Journal of Agricultural and Food Chemistry.*

In related test-tube studies, the group measured how well fat cells from these animals absorb glucose, an action that in the body would lower blood sugar concentrations. The cells from diabetic rats drinking green tea absorbed more than twice as much of the sugar as did cells from similar animals drinking plain water—indicating, the researchers say, that the tea had indeed improved the fat cells' insulin sensitivity.

Hwang's group has now tested other types of tea. All true teas are made from leaves from the same species of plant. Green tea is unfermented, whereas black and other teas are fermented to various extents.

Like the green tea in the original test, semifermented pouchong tea "significantly increased glucose uptake" by fat ells taken from diabetic animals that drank it, Hwang told *Science News.* However, fully fermented black tea—the favorite of most Western tea drinkers—didn't affect glucose absorption.

Since different teas contain different polyphenols that might underlie the fat-cell response, Hwang's team tested the antidiabetic effects of several polyphenols from the best-performing teas. The most effective turned out to be epigallocatechin gallate, an agent known to have anticancer properties (*SN: 7/23/94, p. 61*). In her lab tests, the compound has "insulinlike activity," Hwang says.

Hwang's team has traced the green tea's antidiabetic attributes to other mechanisms as well. In rats, green tea increased the number of insulin receptors on cells and the blood concentration of a protein—GLUT-IV—that helps move glucose out of the blood and into cells. Moreover, Hwang notes, the tea activated insulin-receptor kinase, an enzyme that makes the receptors available to bind insulin and initiate activity.

SPICE IT DOWN Scientists at the Agriculture Department's Beltsville (Md.) Human Nutrition Research Center have been studying how chromium, which is found in black pepper and some other foods, also boosts the activity of insulin-receptor kinase and related enzymes. Experiments beginning almost a half-century ago showed that chromium supplements can restore blood sugar control to some people and animals with diabetes. The question has been why that is and what might represent effective doses of chromium.

Recent studies have shown that the element chemically alters the cell-surface receptors to which insulin attaches, explains Beltsville chemist Richard A. Anderson. Without chromium, insulin can't dock at the receptors and shepherd glucose from the blood into energy-hungry cells.

When the hormone's job is done, another enzyme switches off the insulin receptor. Chromium also inhibits the shut-off enzyme's action, Anderson says. The element offers dual benefits.

Unfortunately, Anderson observes, the modern diet of highly processed foods is low in chromium. What's more, foods high in sugar stimulate the body to lose chromium.

The formulation of currently available chromium supplements doesn't permit the body to absorb the element efficiently,

Anderson says. However, his team has just received a patent for a new formulation, called chromium histidine, that in human trials results in absorption of about 50 percent more chromium than conventional supplements do, he says.

CINNAMON 'N SUGAR—The same kind of cinnamon that goes into an apple pie can boost insulin activity and blood-glucose control, studies show.

It was during tests of the new chromium supplement that Anderson and his colleagues stumbled onto an entirely different antidiabetes substance in, of all things, apple pie. During the early stages of one study, the researchers were attempting to disrupt some volunteers' blood sugar control by feeding them a low chromium diet that included pie. Surprisingly, these volunteers' blood sugar remained under control. Subsequent test-tube studies showed that cinnamon in the pie was boosting insulin activity, as chromium does, and thus controlling blood glucose. The spice turned out to be the "best thing we ever tested" for that purpose, Anderson says.

Anderson and his colleagues recently studied 60 people with type 2 diabetes. The researchers gave the participants capsules containing either cinnamon or wheat flour. The 30 people getting daily doses of l, 3, or 6 grams of cinnamon for 40 days experienced an 18 to 29 percent drop in blood glucose, compared with their values at the beginning of the study. A gram of cinnamon is about one-half a teaspoon, says Anderson. Volunteers getting wheat flour for 40 days showed no such benefit.

Cinnamon also improved Study participants' blood-cholesterol and triglycerides concentrations, Anderson's team reported in the December 2003 *Diabetes Care*.

Subsequently, the scientists found that cinnamons active ingredients are polyphenol polymers with insulinlike action. Anderson's team described those experiments in the Jan. 14 *Journal of Agricultural and Food Chemistry*.

Cloves, bay leaves, and other spices show enzymatic effects similar to those of cinnamon, Anderson has found, though none approaches cinnamons potency.

WINE SURPRISE If spices and coffee can help control blood sugar, why not wine? After all, studies have suggested that the alcohol and polyphenols that the beverage contains reduce the likelihood of heart complications among people with diabetes (*SN: 7/24/99, p. 52*). These chemicals might act by increasing cells' insulin sensitivity, reasoned wine biochemist Pierre-Louis Teissèdre of the University of Montpellier in France.

Teissèdre's team separated wine's antioxidant polyphenols from its alcohol. Diabetic mice fed one or the other type of in-

MEDICINAL?—Both the alcohol and polyphenols in red wine offer antidiabetic effects—at least in mice.

gredient showed complementary benefits, the scientists reported in the Feb. 15 *Journal of Agricultural and Food Chemistry*.

For 6 weeks, animals consumed alcohol, polyphenols, both, or neither. The maximum dose was the equivalent, taking body weight into account, of the amount that a person imbibes in three glasses of wine per day. Diabetic animals getting both alcohol and polyphenols controlled their blood sugar after a meal about as well as normal mice did. Mice getting alcohol didn't do quite as well but still had better blood sugar control than did animals getting either the polyphenols only or neither wine ingredient.

The wine components also affected the retarded growth associated with severe diabetes, which prevents cells from accessing the fuel they need to thrive. In Teissèdre's experiment, the mice getting both types of wine ingredients or only alcohol grew larger than did the animals receiving polyphenols only or no wine component.

When receiving both types of wine ingredients, "animals that had been diabetic became nondiabetic," at least temporarily, says Teissèdre. His team envisions developing wines that could be marketed as medicinal beverages—with extra polyphenols for preventing heart disease and fighting diabetes.

CAUTION ADVISED It's still too early to know the medical significance of all these tantalizing new findings, observes endocrinologist Nathaniel Clark of the American Diabetes Association in Alexandria, Va. Some may not hold up in long-term dietary tests in people. Even if they do, he notes, it would be "a tragedy" for people to think that supplementing their diets with coffee, tea, spices, or alcohol could take the place of moderate weight loss, regular physical activity, and restricted carbohydrate intake.

Moreover, Clark cautions, certain of these dietary adjustments shouldn't be adopted without advice from a physician. For instance, the caffeine in 6 to 10 cups of coffee—the amount showing an antidiabetes effect in the recent European studies—might prove too much for people with certain heart problems.

And though the diabetes association currently accepts that a daily serving or two of alcohol can fit into the diet of people with the disease, Clark warns that "the risk of overconsumption of alcohol remains, regardless of any potential benefit."

The bottom line, he says, is that people with diabetes should consider any of the potential new menu changes as an addition to existing dietary, weight-control, and exercise strategies—not as a means to avoid them.

Allergen Control

Increased awareness of food allergies is leading food companies
to develop comprehensive allergen control programs.
Here's what's involved.

Steve L. Taylor and Sue L. Hefle

Estimates of the prevalence of food allergies continue to increase. The best current estimates are that 10–12 million consumers in the United States (3.5–4.0% of the overall population) suffer from food allergies (Sicherer et al., 2004). Even as recently as the mid-1990s, the estimate of the percentage of U.S. consumers suffering from food allergies was 1–2%. Consumer perception surveys indicate that an even larger percentage (10% or more) of households believe that one or more members of the household have a food allergy. Regardless of the medical accuracy of these perceptions, these consumers are likely to make purchasing decisions based on these perceptions. So, it's no wonder that food allergies have become a serious issue for the food industry.

Is the prevalence of food allergies actually increasing? Although good baseline clinical diagnostic data from earlier decades are missing for comparative purposes, the answer to this question is probably yes. But certainly, the huge jump in the percentage of affected Americans is the result of increased awareness to a greater extent than an actual increase in the prevalence of food allergies. This increase in awareness of food allergies has resulted in increasing assertiveness on the part of food-allergic consumers. Consequently, consumer-response staffs for food companies have seen dramatic increases in the number of telephone inquiries (most are not complaints) from allergic consumers. As expected, consumer product companies are going to respond to this increasing interest in food allergies in part by implementing allergen control strategies.

The situation in the food industry with respect to food allergies continues to be muddled to some degree, however, by the poor understanding of food allergies by food industry professionals and other employees, regulatory officials, and consumers. Many consumers continue to have mistaken beliefs regarding food allergies. In those consumer perception surveys, respondents attributed other food intolerances or even food preferences to food allergies. Food allergies are abnormal responses of the immune system to specific foods that can, at least in some consumers, lead to rather serious manifestations. Other forms of food intolerance, such as lactose intolerance, also occur among many consumers, but these are not true food allergies and do not display such serious symptoms. Thus, a distinction should be made between true food allergies and other forms of food intolerances in food industry allergen management practices, but this is not yet universally happening.

This article will focus on true food allergies, including IgE-mediated reactions and cell-mediated reactions such as celiac disease, but will not cover other types of food intolerance such as lactose intolerance and sulfite-induced asthma (Taylor and Hefle, 2001a).

Designing Allergen Control Programs

The food industry began to implement allergen control programs in the early to mid-1990s. Few, if any, companies had effective allergen control programs in place in 1990, despite the likelihood that food-allergic consumers existed in appreciable numbers even then.

The increasing awareness of food allergies and their potential severity led to the development of allergen control programs, especially over the past 10 years. Many food companies have such programs in place today, although an unknown number of companies have yet to implement these programs. And the effectiveness of these programs is probably quite variable because of their complexity, including such key issues as the diversity of products and ingredients, the range of products made on shared equipment or in shared facilities, the features of processing equipment, including accessibility for allergen cleaning, and the roles of suppliers and custom processors. However, many companies have succeeded in developing highly effective allergen control programs that have lessened the likelihood of allergic reactions among consumers of their products.

The regulatory authorities also began to take notice of food allergies in the early 1990s. Before 1990, very few recalls occurred because of undeclared food allergens. Beginning in the mid-1990s, food allergen recalls became increasingly common. Of course, this regulatory attention also helped to garner the attention of the food industry. However, the number of recalls in recent years is still not an accurate reflection of the existing hazard for food-allergic consumers. Retail surveys conducted by the Food and Drug Administration indicate that about 25% of packaged food products in certain categories contain undeclared residues of peanuts (www.cfsan.fda.gov/_dms/alrgpart.html). If FDA took action on all of these products, the recall numbers could conceivably be much higher. This is also a reflection of the fact that some companies still lack effective allergen control programs.

The development of an allergen control program starts with a risk assessment focusing on some key features of true food allergies:

• True food allergies can cause very serious manifestations. Recent information suggests that 29,000 emergency room visits and 150–200 deaths occur annually from allergic reactions to foods (Bock et al., 2001). While most food-allergic consumers are not at risk of such severe reactions, industry practices should definitely be focused on prevention of severe reactions.

• The most common allergenic foods, sometimes known as "the Big 8," are milk, eggs, fish, crustacean shellfish (e.g., shrimp), peanuts, tree nuts (almonds, walnuts, etc.), soybeans, and wheat. These eight foods or food groups account for more than 90% of all food-allergic reactions (Taylor and Hefle, 2001a). While hundreds of other foods are less frequently associated with food allergies, the food industry would be wise to focus allergen control programs on the Big 8.

• All of the Big 8 foods except wheat have elicited well-documented fatal reactions. Thus, FDA considers undeclared allergens from the Big 8, with the exception of wheat, as the basis for Class 1 recalls that have the potential for severe health consequences. This regulatory stance is appropriate and serves as another reason for allergen control programs to focus on the Big 8. The U.S. Dept. of Agriculture takes a similar stance with respect to meat and poultry products containing Big 8 allergens.

• Trace amounts of the offending food can elicit allergic reactions in susceptible individuals. While the minimal eliciting doses (also known as threshold doses) are not pre-cisely known, evidence indicates that amounts as low as 1–3 mg of peanut, milk, and egg can elicit mild allergic reactions in the most sensitive individuals (Taylor et al., 2002). While a full discourse on thresholds is beyond the scope of this article, the existence of low provoking doses creates challenging issues in the development of effective allergen control programs.

By addressing the issues appropriately, food manufacturers and suppliers should be able to craft a well-focused approach to allergen management.

Components of a Comprehensive Strategy

A comprehensive allergen control strategy has many components. Quite literally, allergen control is everyone's job. This task requires total company commitment and recognition of appropriate roles by everyone in the organization. Many companies develop a core team to address the many facets of this issue. However, in smaller companies, individuals often have to play multiple roles in the implementation of a comprehensive allergen control strategy.

The most common allergenic foods are milk, eggs, fish, crustacean shellfish, peanuts, tree nuts, soybeans, and wheat.

• **Purchasing.** Food manufacturers must know the composition of all raw materials contained in their formulations (Taylor and Hefle, 2000a). While this might sound like a trivial exercise, it is not. The allergen content of all raw materials must be known. Many companies send checklists to suppliers to ascertain if the raw material contains any known allergens, ingredients derived from known allergens, or potential cross-contact allergens from use of shared equipment. This information can yield surprising results; e.g., processors have learned that flavor formulations contain known allergens. Repeated use of these checklists may be helpful to determine if any changes have occurred. Some companies audit suppliers to assess whether compliance with the checklists is satisfactory; this is especially helpful if there is some possibility of cross-contact at the supplier level. The use of allergen test kits to detect residual amounts of allergenic foods can be helpful in the auditing process. Packaging materials should be viewed as raw materials also. Recalls have occurred in the past because of mistakes made on the ingredient statements of packaging materials.

• **Receiving.** Once allergens have been identified in various incoming materials, the components must be handled appropriately once received by the manufacturing facility (Taylor and Hefle, 2000a). As pointed out by Clark (2005) elsewhere in this issue, dedication and separation are key operations issues in allergen control. However, dedication and separation are also key strategies in receiving. Many companies segregate raw materials containing allergens into distinct warehouse areas—not necessarily separate buildings but separate, divided areas. These areas then can be carefully marked; e.g., color coding together with written product identification can assure that this ingredient will be correctly identified. Allergenic materials should never be stored above non-allergenic materials where a spill might contaminate other ingredients.

Bulk tanks represent a distinct area of concern. If a bulk tank contains an allergenic component, dedication of that bulk tank is an obvious strategy. If that is not possible, then an appropriate sanitation procedure must be developed to clean the tank between allergens and non-allergens.

Care must also be taken with respect to transportation vehicles. Especially with bulk commodities, allergen contamination can occur from previous uses of these vehicles. Our laboratory at the Food Allergy Research & Resource Program (FARRP) once traced peanut contamination of a bakery product to peanut contamination of a rail car that had been used to transport wheat. Control of all such contamination is probably impossible, but gross contamination must obviously be avoided.

• **Operations.** Manufacturing facilities must often be shared by many products, some containing allergens (Taylor and Hefle, 2000b). Dedication, separation, scheduling, and sanitation are key components of an allergen control plan in such situations.

Of course, dedication of an entire facility or even an entire processing room is only possible in situations where large quantities of a product are manufactured. Some confectionery companies have dedicated certain facilities with respect to peanuts and manufacture no peanut-containing products in those facilities. A few smaller confectionery companies promote their products as peanut-free. This sort of statement requires a very high degree of vigilance. The FARRP Laboratory once traced peanut contamination of a chocolate product to the shared use of jute bags by crop harvesters in the Ivory Coast for cocoa beans and peanuts.

Separation is another widely practiced approach. If entire facilities cannot be dedicated, then perhaps individual processing lines can be. This is especially desirable in processing facilities that are not amenable to wet cleaning, such as bakeries and chocolate manufacturing. For example, cookie manufacturers could have specific baking lines that are devoted either to non-allergenic or allergenic (e.g., peanut or almond) formulations. With adjacent but separate lines, additional precautions are sometimes advisable. Dust transfer is usually not a major concern with the large volumes of material being processed. But if one of the lines is static for a period of time, cleaning may be needed to guard against dust buildup. Heavy plastic separation panels are sometimes used, too.

If neither dedication nor separation is feasible, then scheduling becomes pivotal. Ideally, allergenic products should be manufactured on shared equipment after non-allergenic products. Allergen cleanup is necessary between manufacturing of allergenic and non-allergenic formulations. Long manufacturing runs are advisable, as this practice limits the number of times that allergen cleanup is needed. Particularly potent allergenic formulations are often manufactured at the end of a shift or a manufacturing cycle, just before major cleanup. Where possible, introduction of the allergenic ingredient into the product later in the process will limit the amount of equipment that must be subjected to allergen cleanup.

Other operations strategies are also important. If in-process totes are used, then some system must be developed to allow their easy identification, such as use of color coding. Furthermore, such totes must be dedicated or effectively cleaned between uses. In some facilities, care must be taken to avoid line crossover that might allow allergen-containing material to fall into other formulations or assure that shielding/covers are in place. Lock-out, tag-out systems have been used effectively to prevent cross-contact in some manufacturing facilities.

The reuse of frying oil for more than one type of product merits some comment relative to allergen control. Shared frying oil is a common practice in the processed foods industry. We are unaware of any allergic reactions attributed to shared frying oil with processed foods, although a few episodes have occurred from similar practices in restaurants (Yunginger et al., 1988). Most companies do not now segregate frying oil, and its use for multiple products is widely practiced. Good manufacturing practices with shared frying oil include use of filtration systems. Although these filters are not designed to remove allergenic proteins, they do remove particulates which would contain allergens. As noted below in the section on sanitation, the potential allergenic hazards associated with reuse of frying oil can perhaps be evaluated by analysis of the next product fried in the oil, using specific immunoassay-based test kits.

• **Rework.** Several recalls have occurred in the past from misuse of allergen-containing rework in products that were not supposed to contain that particular allergen (Taylor and Hefle, 2000c). We advocate an "exact into exact" approach to use of rework; i.e., rework can only be used in the exact same product from which it was generated. Some companies have developed a policy whereby they either use rework on the day or shift in which it was generated or discard it. Containers for rework must be clearly labeled and easily identified. Many companies use colored totes for allergen-containing rework.

• **Sanitation.** The sanitation of shared equipment is of paramount importance (Taylor and Hefle, 2000b). Some processing equipment was never designed for easy access and cleaning; e.g., chocolate enrobers or baking ovens. Sanitation advice is particularly hard to provide, given the diversity of products and product contact surfaces in existence in the food industry.

Generally speaking, wet cleaning is preferred where it is feasible. Allergenic proteins tend to be soluble in hot water, although detergents can be useful in removing proteins, too. Cleaning companies have considerable experience with the removal of protein residues and can provide useful advice oriented toward the particular manufacturing facility. Clean-in-place systems are clearly beneficial, where feasible, because they can be made quite consistent once validated.

Dry cleaning systems are much more challenging, but the food industry is replete with examples of situations where wet cleaning is impossible (chocolate confections, baking ovens, etc.). In these situations, wipe-downs are often needed. Air hoses are not especially useful because these devices simply blow allergens from one area to another. Central vacuums are very good because they can effectively remove dry allergen materials without spreading them around.

Push-through is another useful approach in dry cleaning situations. Push-through can be accomplished with the next product or with some "inert" ingredient such as salt or flour (obviously only when undeclared wheat would not be of concern). This approach can be especially useful in places, such as piping systems, where product contact surfaces are completely inaccessible.

• **Sanitation Validation.** The validation of sanitation practices on shared equipment is highly recommended. Commercial enzyme-linked immunoassay (ELISA) kits and lateral flow devices (dipsticks) are available from several companies, among them Neogen Corp. (www.neogen.com), r-Biopharm (www.r-biopharm.com), and ELISA Systems (www.elisasystems.net). Test kits can be used to validate sanitation practices.

Quantitative ELISAs can be done to determine if detectable allergen residues exist in the first product manufactured after changeover, on the assumption that this is the product that is most likely to be contaminated if cleanup is inadequate. However, some companies are reluctant to test finished product on a regular basis. The quantitative ELISAs typically have a lower limit of sensitivity of 1–3 ppm. This level of sensitivity is likely adequate to assure that products are not potentially hazardous to allergic consumers. If the threshold dose is 1 mg of peanut for development of mild allergic reactions in the most sensitive subpopulation and the serving size is 100 g, that would equate to a level of 10 ppm.

Qualitative ELISAs and dipsticks are also available and are typically used to assess whether surfaces are clean. These tests usually have detection limits of 1–5 ppm. Of course, it is impossible to predict how much contamination might exist in the finished product based on a positive swab test of an equipment surface. It is advisable to try to swab areas that are particularly difficult to clean. For many companies, a positive swab test initiates more cleaning until a negative result is obtained.

Some companies have not validated their allergen cleaning practices with test kits. The FARRP Laboratory assisted one company that was concerned about possible allergen cross-contact from use of shared equipment. This company had instituted a very thorough approach to allergen cleanup that required about 6 hr to complete. FARRP was able to verify, using a test kit, that the 6-hr cleanup was effective (no detectable allergen in the first product manufactured after changeover), but was also able to demonstrate that a 45-min cleanup was equally effective. Clearly, the validation exercise was a cost-saving venture for this company.

As noted above, push-through can be an effective strategy in some situations. But validation is particularly important in push-through situations. For example, push-through is often used between runs of milk chocolate and dark chocolate. However, in several situations investigated by the FARRP Laboratory, dark chocolate still contained detectable residues of milk, hours after changeover, probably owing to the viscous nature of the material and concentric flow in the piping systems. Accordingly, these manufacturers appropriately decided to use advisory labeling on dark chocolate (e.g., "manufactured on shared equipment with milk"). In this case, only dedicated processing lines can reliably provide milk-free dark chocolate. In other situations, push-through has been effective, although the test kits are the only effective method to determine the volume of push-through needed to prevent allergen cross-contact.

Although some companies have developed in-house laboratory capabilities for testing, many companies rely on contract laboratories. Among others, the nonprofit FARRP Laboratory (www.farrp.org) provides testing services and has access to test methods that are not commercially available, such as those for walnut, pecan, soybean, and others. Most companies can perform the qualitative test methods easily in-house, since they do not require specialized equipment or training.

• **Allergen Auditing.** As mentioned previously, auditing has great value in assessing the adequacy of allergen control programs for food manufacturers, including custom processors and ingredient suppliers (Taylor and Hefle, 2000a). Some caution must be exercised, however, because many quality-auditing firms lack allergen training and knowledge. Variability also exists in the quality of the auditing instruments used by various quality auditors. Some companies have trained their own quality auditors, but this option is likely only viable for larger companies. FDA has also conducted some training for its inspectors, although some variability remains between individual inspectors as well.

• **Packaging Strategies.** Packaging should be viewed as another input that must be controlled as part of the overall allergen control program (Taylor and Hefle, 2001b). Steps must be taken to assure that the product ends up in the intended package and that the ingredient statement on that package is adequate in terms of allergen information. Recalls have resulted from failure to discard old packaging material that subsequently were used for a new formulation containing a new allergenic component.

Precautions should be taken to avoid mixed bundles of packaging. Companies have employed strategies such as using colored striping on the sides of packages so that mixed bundles would be readily evident to the packaging machine operator as he loads the unit.

On large packages of products, the ingredient statements on the outer wrappers should match the ingredient statements on the smaller packages contained inside—allergic consumers often complain of discrepancies in this regard.

• **Product Development.** Of course, it all starts with product development (Taylor and Hefle, 2001c). The formulation of products containing allergens will lead to the need to adopt allergen control programs in the manufacturing operations. While new products containing allergenic components will likely continue to proliferate, several strategies are worthy of consideration. Ideally, product developers should stay away from the

Examples of allergy information statements on retail packages

- Contains wheat, milk, soy and peanut ingredients.
- Corn used in this product contains traces of soybeans.
- May contain soy flour, whey, peanuts and tree nuts.
- May contain peanuts or trace amounts of allergens not listed in the ingredients.
- This product may have come in contact with peanuts or other nuts.
- Allergen information: Manufactured on equipment that processes products containing peanuts and other nuts.
- This product contains wheat, milk, eggs and soy. It is made on equipment that also makes products containing tree nuts.
- Manufactured in a facility that processed peanuts.
- Processed on equipment also used to produce products that contain milk, manufactured in a facility that processes nut products.

use of allergenic components in cases where other ingredients would work equally well.

Obviously, product developers should avoid use of allergenic ingredients in such minute amounts that they have no functional effect on the finished product. Allergic consumers are often very brand-loyal. So, the reformulation of existing products with the introduction of new allergenic components should be approached with that in mind.

The new Food Allergen Labeling & Consumer Protection Act of 2004 also raises issues regarding ingredients derived from commonly allergenic sources, i.e., the Big 8, as discussed by Trautman (2005) elsewhere in this issue.

Product developers must also be mindful of the allergenicity of ingredients derived from commonly allergenic sources. While labeling of such products is clearly required under the new Act, the need for allergen cleanup must be based on the amount of protein from the allergenic source in the ingredient. For example, if soy lecithin is the only source of soy protein in a formulation, extensive allergen cleanup between the lecithin-containing formulation and another that does not contain any sources of soy protein is probably unnecessary in most cases because the amount of soy protein in lecithin is relatively low; normal cleaning and dilution would resolve allergenic hazards.

Achieving Effective Allergen Control

The implementation of an effective allergen control program requires considerable effort and total company commitment. While this article has provided some general advice, the elements of effective allergen control vary from one food company to another, based on the nature of the products, the processes used, the ingredients, and the processing equipment.

Perhaps the most important advice is to validate the effectiveness of allergen control approaches using test kits. In some cases, advisory labeling (e.g., "may contain peanuts") will be required to alert consumers to potential allergenic risks, but FDA has indicated that such labeling cannot be a substitute for Good Manufacturing Practices. Such labeling should be considered as a last resort when other allergen control measures simply are not reliable and when extreme measures like dedicated facilities or equipment are not an economically viable option.

Many companies will need assistance in the development of allergen control programs. FARRP conducts food allergen conferences on a twice-yearly basis (see www.farrp.org for information). These conferences provide the background necessary to begin development of allergen control programs and allow companies to benchmark themselves against industry leaders in allergen control. Assistance with allergen analysis is also readily available from several sources.

REFERENCES

Bock, S.A., Munoz-Furlong, A., and Sampson, H.A. 2001. Fatalities due to anaphylactic reactions to foods. J. Allergy Clin. Immunol. 107:191-193.

Clark, J.P. 2005. Allergen-safe processing. Food Technol. 59(2): 63-64.

Sicherer, S.H., Munoz-Furlong, A., and Sampson, H.A. 2004. Prevalence of seafood allergy in the United States determined by a random telephone survey, J. Allergy Clin. Immunol. 114: 159-165.

Taylor, S.L. and Hefle, S.L. 2000a. Good manufacturing practices for the food industry—Suppliers and co-packers. Food Allergy Intolerance 1: 208-213.

Taylor, S.L. and Hefle, S.L. 2000b. Good manufacturing practices for allergenic foods—Use of shared equipment. Food Allergy Intolerance 1: 47-50.

Taylor, S.L. and Hefle, S.L. 2000c. Good manufacturing practices for the food industry—Use of rework. Food Allergy Intolerance 1:114-117.

Taylor, S.L. and Hefle, S.L. 2001a. Food allergies and sensitivities. Food Technol. 55(9): 68-83.

Taylor, S.L. and Hefle, S.L. 2001b. Good manufacturing practices for allergenic foods—Packaging and labeling strategies. Food Allergy Intolerance 2: 53-58.

Taylor, S.L. and Hefle, S.L. 2001c. Good manufacturing practices for allergenic foods—Product development strategies. Food Allergy Intolerance 2: 230-236.

Taylor, S.L., Hefle, S.L., Bindsiev-Jensen, C., Bock, S.A., Burks, A.W., Christie, L., Hill, D.J., Host A., Hourihane, J.O., Lack, G., Metcalfe, D.D., Moneret-Vautrin, D.A., Vadas, P.A., Rance, F., Skrypec, D.J., Trautman, T.A., Yman, I.M., and Zeiger, R.S. 2002. Factors affecting the determination of threshold doses for allergenic foods: How much is too much? J. Allergy Clin. Immunol 109: 24-30.

Trautman, T. 2005. Labeling food allergens. Food Technol. 59(2): 92.

Yunginger, J.W., Sweeney, K.G., Sturner, W.G., Giannandrea, L.A., Tiegland, J.D., Bray, M., Benson, P.A., York, J.A., Biedrzycki, L.,

Squillance, D.L., and Helm, R.M. 1988. Fatal food-induced anaphylaxis. J. Am. Med. Assn. 260: 1450-1452.

This work was supported by the Food Allergy Research and Resource Program (FARRP) of the University of Nebraska. A contribution of the University of Nebraska Cooperative Extension Program, Lincoln, NE 68583. Extension Journal Series No 1027.

*Author **Taylor** is Professor and Co-Director, and author **Hefle** is Associate Professor and Co-Director, Food Allergy Research & Resource Program, University of Nebraska, Lincoln, NE 68583-0919. Both are Professional Members and Fellows of IFT. Send reprint requests to author Taylor, sltaylor@unlnotes.unl.edu.*

Meeting Children's Nutritional Needs

Linda Milo Ohr

The numbers are all too well known. Nationwide, approximately 30% of children ages 6-19 are overweight and 15% are obese. In addition, 70-80% of obese adolescents become obese adults. This opens up a world of health conditions later in life, such as heart disease, diabetes, and cancer.

Childhood obesity is one of the main concerns when it comes to children's nutrition. Lack of physical activity and poor dietary habits are two overall contributing factors to the problem. Food companies have stepped up to address the growing concern with children's nutrition by offering healthier options and providing public awareness of healthy eating habits.

For example, last year, Kraft Foods, Glenview, Ill., established initiatives to address obesity. In terms of product nutrition, the company stated that it would be determining the levels at which the portion sizes of its single-serve packages would be capped, developing nutrition guidelines for existing and new products, and improving existing products and providing alternative choices, where appropriate. Nabisco 100-calorie packs, a four-item line featuring *Wheat Thins, Chips Ahoy!, Cheese Nips,* and *Oreo* brands, for example, are portion-controlled, single-serve products formulated to have 3 g or less of fat, 0 g of *trans* fat, and no cholesterol. Another new product, *Kool-Aid Jammers 10*, is made with real fruit juice, contains 100% of the daily value of vitamin C, and contributes only 10 kcal/serving.

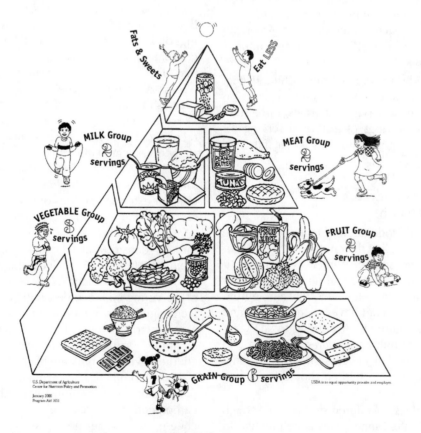

Fig. 1—The Food Guide Pyramid for Young Children is an adaptation of the original Food Guide Pyramid designed to simplify educational messages and focus on young children's food preferences and nutritional requirements.

In October 2003, Quaker Oats, a unit of PepsiCo Beverages & Foods, Chicago, Ill., in collaboration with the American Dietetic Association, introduced a five-step family nutrition program called *Quaker Oatmeal Strive for Five*. The online program teaches parents how to prevent childhood weight gain and obesity by establishing key nutrition habits at home in one month. The program was developed on the basis of a survey of nearly 1,000 ADA-member dietetic professionals who identified acting as a nutrition role model, eating mored whole-grain foods, eating breakfast daily, and understanding portion sizes as top ways that parents can help prevent weight gain and obesity in their children.

In addition to food companies' initiatives, a number of Web sites offer parents and children advice and guidelines on healthy eating.

Kidnetic.com, launched in 2002, is a site for kids 9-12 years old, parents, and health professionals. Games, a frequently asked question section, discussion boards, and recipes are among the many resources available on the site. It is part of an educational outreach program of the International Food Information Council Foundation developed in partnership with several professional associations, including ADA and the American Academy of Family Physicians.

Action for Healthy Kids (www.actionforhealthykids.org) is a nationwide initiative dedicated to improving the health and educational performance of children through better nutrition and physical activity in schools. Guidance and direction are provided by more than 40 national organizations and government agencies, including the American Academy of Pediatrics and the U.S. Dept. of Agriculture's Food and Nutrition Service.

The USDA Food Guide Pyramid for Young Children (Fig. 1) offers basic nutrition guidelines for children ages 2-6 years. They include six daily servings of grains, three servings of vegetables, two servings of fruit, two servings of milk, two servings of meat, and low intake of fats and sweets.

Foods and Nutrients Children Should Be Getting More of

"Balance, variety, and moderation of many foods is the best way for children to get all of their nutrients," said Marilyn Tanner, ADA spokesperson and clinical pediatric dietitian at St. Louis Children's Hospital and Washington University School of Medicine. However, the simple truth is that children of all ages do not have balanced diets and are not getting essential nutrients. According to ADA, intake of several important nutrients, such as calcium and iron, is less than recommended. Here is a rundown of some food groups and nutrients that children should be getting more of:

• **Fruits and Vegetables.** "Children do not eat enough fruits and vegetables," said Tanner. This is detrimental to their diets because these food groups provide fiber, vitamins A and C, B-vitamins, potassium, and complex carbohydrates for energy. Five or more servings of fruits and vegetables are recommended as part of a healthy diet. According to "State of the Plate," a study published in October 2002 by the Produce for Better Health Foundation, 90% of teen girls and 96% of kids ages 2-12 do not eat five servings per day.

The *5-A-Day for Better Health* program gives Americans a simple, positive message: Eat five or more servings of fruits and vegetables every day for better health. The National Cancer Institute and the Produce for Better Health Foundation jointly sponsor this program. The goal of the program is to increase the consumption of fruits and vegetables in the United States to 5-9 servings every day. In addition, the program seeks to inform Americans that eating fruits and vegetables can improve their health and reduce the risk of cancer and other diseases. It also provides consumers with practical and easy ways to incorporate more fruits and vegetables into their daily eating patterns.

One way to get kids to eat more fruits and vegetables is to make them more fun and portable. According to the State of the Plate study, romaine lettuce and bag lettuce are the only vegetables that Americans are eating more of than before, increasing by an average of two annual servings per person. The bagged salads are more convenient for parents to prepare for family meals. Another example of portability is baby carrots. "Everyone loves these, and they are easy and convenient," commented Tanner.

• **Dairy Foods.** Yogurt, milk, and cheese provide calcium, potassium, phosphorus, protein, vitamins A, D, and B-12, riboflavin, and niacin. USDA recommends 2-3 servings of dairy products daily, but the majority of people only consume half of this. The *3-A-Day* campaign, managed by the American Dairy Association/National Dairy Council, works to promote three servings per day. The program stresses the importance of dairy's role in children's health.

For example, a recent study by Goulding et al. (2004) recognized the importance of milk in children's diets. The study investigated the impact of milk consumption on children 3-13 years old. The investigators compared the fracture histories of 50 children who avoided drinking cow's milk for extended periods of time to a group of 1,000 children from the same city, Dunedin, New Zealand.

"Children who regularly avoided milk had lower bone mineral density and weighed more, two factors that increase fracture risk," said lead researcher Ailsa Goulding of the University of Otago, New Zealand. Nearly one in three of the young milk-avoiders had broken a bone before they were eight years old, frequently from slight trauma such as a minor trip or fall. "Forearm fractures were especially common," said the researchers, concluding that "young children avoiding milk are prone to fracture."

Dairy companies have made innovative strides to increase dairy consumption among children. Flavored milks, carbonated milk beverages, and flavored and colored cheese are among the newest dairy products that make dairy fun for kids. For example, *Raging Cow*™, from Dr Pepper/Seven Up Inc., Plano, Tex., is a five-flavor line of single-serve milk drinks. Chocolate Insanity, Pina Colada

Chaos, Chocolate Caramel Craze, Berry Mixed Up, and Jamocha Frenzy are the five flavors that make milk more exciting. The company's Web site states, "Boring milk needed a kick in the shorts, and with *Raging Cow*, that's just what boring milk got."

• **Calcium.** Because of insufficient dairy consumption, children's diets are lacking in calcium. "Children under 10 need about 900 mg of calcium," said Tanner. "Once they get to the age of 10, they need 1,300 mg of calcium per day."

Information from the *3-A-Day* program states that about 30% of kids ages 1-5 do not get the recommended amount of calcium in their diets; 70% of preteen girls and 60% of preteen boys (ages 6-11) do not meet current calcium recommendations; and nearly 90% of teenage girls and 70% of teenage boys (ages 12-19) do not meet daily calcium recommendations.

Not only is lack of calcium detrimental to children's bone and teeth health, but also recent studies have shown that calcium may play a role in children's weight. Research presented at the Experimental Biology Meeting in April 2003 (FASEB, 2003) suggested that girls who consume more calcium tend to weigh less and have lower body fat than those with low calcium consumption. Researchers at the University of Hawaii at Manoa and Kaiser Permanente Clinical Research Center in Honolulu studied 321 white, Asian, and mixed-ethnicity girls ages 9-14. They found that girls who consumed more calcium on average weighed less than similar girls who consumed less calcium. An increase of one serving of dairy—a cup of milk or a thumb-sized piece of cheese, about 300 mg of calcium—was associated with a 0.9 mm lower skin fold (about half an inch) and 1.9 lb lower weight.

Rachel Novotny, Professor in the Dept. of Human Nutrition, Food, and Animal Sciences at the University of Hawaii, explained that as calcium intake increases, the body increases its ability to break down fat and decreases fat synthesis.

Another study (Skinner et al., 2003) found that higher intake of dietary calcium was associated with lower body fat in young children. The study looked at 52 children ages 2-8 and their mothers. Results showed that dietary calcium and polyunsaturated fat intake were associated with a lower percentage of body fat. Milk and other dairy products were the main sources of dietary calcium in the study, with milk alone accounting for 50% of the total calcium intake.

• **Vitamin D.** This vitamin also is essential for bone health because it helps the body absorb calcium. Vitamin D deficiency largely is to blame for a rise of bone-deforming rickets in recent years among U.S. infants and toddlers, according to the Centers for Disease Control and Prevention.

Research at the University of Maine showed that during the winter, Maine girls are not getting enough vitamin D (Anonymous, 2004). Insufficient levels of vitamin D were detected in nearly half of 24 Bangor-area girls during a three-year study funded by the Maine Dairy and Nutrition Council. The findings worried Susan Sullivan, Assistant Professor of Human Nutrition at the university, because a history of persistent deficiencies of vitamin D could set the stage for osteoporosis later in life.

Infant Nutrition

Newborns and infants have different nutritional requirements than children. If not breastfed, infants' main source of food is formula. Docosahexaenoic acid (DHA), arachidonic acid (ARA), probiotics, and fiber, show promise in benefiting infant health. DHA and ARA are currently used in infant formulas in the U.S., probiotics enhance some formulas in Europe and Japan, and prebiotic fibers are used in some European formulas as well.

• **DHA and ARA.** These two fatty acids are used in infant formulas to improve the visual and brain development of infants. Researchers at the Retina Foundation of the Southwest in Dallas, Tex. (Hoffman et al., 2003), showed that infant formula supplemented with DHA and ARA significantly improved the visual development of infants compared to non-supplemented formula. They studied babies who were breastfed from birth to 4-6 months of age and then randomly weaned. The babies fed the supplemented formula had improved visual acuity at one year of age, compared to the babies fed the nonsupplemented formula after weaning.

"This study demonstrates the continued need for DHA and ARA in the infant diet beyond four months of age to optimize visual development during the first year of life," said lead researcher Dennis R. Hoffman.

• **Probiotics.** Research has shown that probiotics in infant formula may boost the immune system. Scientists at the Pediatric Gastroenterology and Nutrition Unit of Ben-Gurion University in Israel used a double-blind placebo-controlled trial with full term healthy infants between 4-10 months of age (Asli et al., 2003). They randomly received formulas supplemented with either *Bifidobacterium lactis* or *Lactobacillus reuteri*, or the same diet with no probiotics for 12 weeks. Infants fed a probiotics supplemented formula exhibited fewer febrile episodes and fewer gastrointestinal illnesses. They noted that this effect was more prominent in the *L. reuteri* group.

• **Fiber.** Research at the University of Illinois indicated that adding fiber to milk formula may be beneficial on bowel health of infants (Correa-Matos et al., 2003). The study showed that piglets that consumed formula with moderate levels of fermentable fiber tolerated an induced infection by *Salmonella typhimurium* much better than those fed a plain control formula or one with a nonfermentable fiber.

According to the study, diarrhea is a leading cause of morbidity and mortality in infants. The addition of fiber to infant formulas reduces recovery time following pathogenic infection in infants older than six months, but effects on neonates are unknown. The researchers concluded that because fermentable fiber enhanced intestinal function and reduced the severity of symptoms associated with *S. typhimurium* infection, it may be a cost-effective way in which to reduce the severity of pathogenic infection-associated symptoms in infants.

Vitamin D deficiency is most common in post-menopausal women and older Americans. However, Sullivan said, vitamin D intake is critical for children because they add calcium to their bones at a fast pace, maintain those levels into adulthood, then start to lose calcium as they grow elderly.

• **Iron.** "Iron is a part of blood's hemoglobin, which carries oxygen to the cells," Tanner said. "The oxygen helps cells produce energy, without which the body can become fatigued."

Infants need 6-10 mg of iron each day, and children need 10-15 mg. After age 10, children should be getting 15 mg of iron each day. Iron deficiency can be a problem, particularly for girls who experience very heavy periods. In fact, many teenage girls are at risk for iron deficiency because their diets may not contain enough iron to offset the blood loss. Also, teens can lose significant amounts of iron through sweating during intense exercise.

Iron deficiency can lead to fatigue, irritability, headaches, lack of energy, and tingling in the hands and feet. Significant iron deficiency can lead to iron-deficiency anemia.

- **Fiber.** Because children are not consuming five daily servings of fruits and vegetables, their fiber intakes are low as well. To determine how many grams of fiber a child should be consuming each day, it is recommended to add 5 to a child's age in years, said Tanner.

Fiber, especially in cereals, has been linked to the prevention of childhood obesity. A study by Albertson et al. (2003) showed that children who frequently consume cereal are less likely to be overweight. Cereal eaters were found to have a lower body mass index (BMI) and a higher nutrient intake than infrequent or non-cereal eaters.

The study, which included 603 children ages 4-12 years, examined the relationship between cereal consumption habits and BMI of school-aged children. The investigators concluded that children who consumed eight or more servings of cereal within a period of two weeks had significantly lower BMIs compared to the children who consumed fewer servings during that same time. Statistically, nearly 80% of the children who frequently consumed cereal boasted an appropriate body weight for their age and gender.

"For an average 10-year-old boy, the decision to eat cereal or not can equate to about a 12-pound difference," said G. Harvey Anderson, Professor of Nutrition at the University of Toronto and coauthor of the study. The authors also found that cereal consumption benefited the children in the study who were at risk of being overweight. Children of this age group who ate cereal lowered their risk to 21.3%.

Another study (Quaker Oats, 2003) showed that the risk of obesity is lower for children who eat oatmeal regularly compared to those who do not. The percentage of children 2-18 years old who are overweight or at risk of becoming overweight is almost 50% lower in oatmeal eaters than in children who do not consume the fiber, according to the study, which was funded by Quaker Oats.

In addition, the study found that children who eat oatmeal are about twice as likely to meet fiber intake recommendations—fiber intakes were 17% higher than for those who do not eat oatmeal.

The findings of the study were presented by researchers from Columbia University and Quaker Oats at Experimental Biology 2003.

"This study found that children and teens who consumed higher intakes of dietary fiber had lower BMI levels or less body fat," said Christine Williams, Professor of Clinical Pediatrics and Director of the Children's Cardiovascular Health Center at Columbia University. "Our data further suggests children who have diets rich in high-fiber foods, such as oatmeal, as early as age two could help them prevent obesity throughout their lives."

Suggestions for Food Manufacturers

When it comes to formulating food for children, Tanner stressed the importance of portion sizes, in addition to important nutrients, in her suggestions for food manufacturers:

- **Reduce portion size.** "Sell items in smaller packages. For example, lose the "grab bag" and go back to the 25-¢ ½-oz bag," she said. "Also consider smaller beverage containers."

- **Replace candy with fruit.** "A prepackaged lunch does not need candy to sell," she said. "Replace the goop with fruit. There are healthy options—the challenge is to keep them preserved so they are tasty and the fruit is fresh."

- **Add vegetables.** "Help make veggies cool. They have a great taste and are good for you, but for some reason the "not so cool" connection is there. Advertising speaks volumes!

- **Provide lower-fat, yet tasty options.** "The bottom line is that kids will not eat anything if it does not taste good."

REFERENCES

Albertson, A.M., Anderson, G.H., Crockett, S.J., and Goebel, M.T. 2003. Ready-to-eat cereal consumption: Its relationship with BMI and nutrient intake of children aged 4 to 12 years. J. Am. Dietetic Assn. 103: 1613-1619.

Anonymous, 2004. Umaine study: Teenage girls lacking in vitamin D. Univ. of Maine News press release, Jan. 29. www.umaine.edu/news/020204/GirlsVitaminD.htm.

Asli, G., Alsheikh, A., and Weizman, Z. 2003. Infant formula supplemented with probiotics reduces gastrointestinal infections' rate in day care infants. Presented at Ann. Mtg., Am. Pediatric Soc., May. www.reuteri.com/eng/sidor/studies/scientific_posters/stage2.pdf.

Correa-Matos, N.J., Donovan, S.M., Isaacson, R.E., Gaskins, H.R., White, B.A., and Tappenden, K.A. 2003. Fermentable fiber reduces recovery time and improves intestinal function in piglets following Salmonella typhimurium infection. J. Nutr. 133: 1845-1852.

FASEB 2003. Adolescent girls who consume more calcium weigh less. Press release. Fed. of Am. Socs. for Exp. Biol., www.eurekalert.org/pub_releases/2003-04/foasagw033003.php.

Goulding, A., Rockell, J.E.P., Black, R.E., Grant, A.M., Jones, I.E., and Williams, S.M. 2004. Children who avoid drinking cow's milk are at increased risk for prepubertal bone fractures. J. Am. Dietetic Assn. 104: 250-253.

Hoffman, D.R., Birch, E.E., Castaneda, Y.S., Fawcett, S.L., Wheaton, D.H., Birch, D.G., and Uauy, R. 2003. Visual function in breastfed term infants weaned to formula with or without long-chain polyunsaturates at 4 to 6 months: A randomized clinical trial. J. Pediatrics. 142: 669-677.

Quaker Oats. 2003. Study reveals oatmeal can play role in preventing childhood obesity. Press release, www.quakeroats.com/qfb_News/PressRelease.cfm?ID=201.

Skinner, J.D., Bounds, W., Carruth, B.R., and Ziegler, P. 2003. Longitudinal calcium intake is negatively related to children's body fat indexes. J. Am. Dietetic Assn. 103: 1626-1631.

From Food Technology, April 2004, pp. 65-69. Copyright © 2004 by Institute of Food Technologists. Reprinted by permission.

NO ONE TO BLAME

The age of their youngest patients has slipped to 9 years old, and doctors have begun to research the roots of this disease. Anorexia is probably hard-wired, the new thinking goes, and the best treatment is a family affair.

Peg Tyre

EMILY KRUDYS CAN PINPOINT the moment her life fell apart. It was a fall afternoon in the Virginia suburbs, and she was watching her daughter Katherine perform in the school play. Katherine had always been a happy girl, a slim beauty with a megawatt smile, but recently, her mother noticed, she'd been losing weight. "She's battling a virus," Emily kept on telling herself, but there, in the darkened auditorium, she could no longer deny the truth. Under the floodlights, Katherine looked frail, hollow-eyed and gaunt. At that moment, Emily had to admit to herself that her daughter had a serious eating disorder. Katherine was 10 years old.

Who could help their daughter get better? It was a question Emily and her husband, Mark, would ask themselves repeatedly over the next five weeks, growing increasingly frantic as Katherine's weight slid from 48 to 45 pounds. In the weeks after the school play, Katherine put herself on a brutal starvation diet, and no one—not the school psychologist, the private therapist, the family pediatrician or the high-powered internist—could stop her. Emily and Mark tried everything. They were firm. Then they begged their daughter to eat. Then they bribed her. We'll buy you a pony, they told her. But nothing worked. At dinnertime, Katherine ate portions that could be measured in tablespoons. "When I demanded that she eat some food—any food—she'd just shut down," Emily recalls. By Christmas, the girl was so weak she could barely leave the couch. A few days after New Year's, Emily bundled her eldest child into the car and rushed her to the emergency room, where she was immediately put on IV. Home again the following week, Katherine resumed her death march. It took one more hospitalization for the Krudyses to finally make the de-

cision they now believe saved their daughter's life. Last February, they enrolled her in a residential clinic halfway across the country in Omaha, Neb.—one of the few facilities nationwide that specialize in young children with eating disorders. Emily still blames herself for not acting sooner. "It was right in front of me," she says, "but I just didn't realize that children could get an eating disorder this young."

Most parents would forgive Emily Krudys for not believing her own eyes. Anorexia nervosa, a mental illness defined by an obsession with food and acute anxiety over gaining weight, has long been thought to strike teens and young women on the verge of growing up—not kids performing in the fourth-grade production of "The Pig's Picnic." But recently researchers, clinicians and mental-health specialists say they're seeing the age of their youngest anorexia patients decline to 9 from 13. Administrators at Arizona's Remuda Ranch, a residential treatment program for anorexics, received so many calls from parents of young children that last year, they launched a program for kids 13 years old and under; so far, they've treated 69 of them. Six months ago the eating-disorder program at Penn State began to treat the youngest ones, too—20 of them so far, some as young as 8. Elementary schools in Boston, Manhattan and Los Angeles are holding seminars for parents to help them identify eating disorders in their kids, and the parents, who have watched Mary-Kate Olsen morph from a child star into a rail-thin young woman, are all too ready to listen.

At a National Institute of Mental Health conference last spring, anorexia's youngest victims were a small part of the official agenda—but they were the only thing anyone talked about in the hallways, says David S. Rosen, a clinical faculty member at the University of Michigan and an eating-disorder specialist. Seven years ago "the idea of seeing a 9- or 10-year-old anorexic would have been shocking and prompted frantic calls to my colleagues. Now we're seeing kids this age all the time," Rosen says. There's no single explanation for the declining age of onset, although greater awareness on the part of parents certainly plays a role. Whatever the reason, these littlest patients, combined with new scientific research on the causes of anorexia, are pushing the clinical community—and families, and victims—to come up with new ways of thinking about and treating this devastating disease.

Not many years ago, the conventional wisdom held that adolescent girls "got" anorexia from the culture they lived in. Intense young women, mostly from white, wealthy families, were overwhelmed by pressure to be perfect from their suffocating parents, their demanding schools, their exacting coaches. And so they chose extreme dieting as a way to control their lives, to act out their frustration at never being perfect enough. In the past decade, though, psychiatrists have begun to see surprising diversity among their anorexic patients. Not only are anorexia's victims younger, they're also more likely to be black, Hispanic or Asian, more likely to be boys, more likely to be middle-aged. All of which caused doctors to question their core assumption: if anorexia isn't a disease of type-A girls from privileged backgrounds, then what is it?

Although no one can yet say for certain, new science is offering tantalizing clues. Doctors now compare anorexia to alcoholism and depression, potentially fatal diseases that may be set off by environmental factors such as stress or trauma, but have their roots in a complex combination of genes and brain chemistry. In other words, many kids are affected by pressure-cooker school environments and a culture of thinness promoted by magazines and music videos, but most of them don't secretly scrape their dinner into the garbage. The environment "pulls the trigger," says Cynthia Bulik, director of the eating-disorder program at the University of North Carolina at Chapel Hill. But it's a child's latent vulnerabilities that "load the gun."

ANOREXIA, WHICH AFFECTS 2.5 MILLION AMERICANS, HAS THE HIGHEST MORTALITY RATE OF ANY MENTAL ILLNESS. ABOUT HALF OF ANOREXICS RECOVER.

Parents do play a role, but most often it's a genetic one. In the last 10 years, studies of anorexics have shown that the disease often runs in families. In a 2000 study published in The American Journal of Psychiatry, researchers at Virginia Commonwealth University studied 2,163 female twins and found that 77 of them suffered from symptoms of anorexia. By com-

paring the number of identical twins who had anorexia with the significantly smaller number of fraternal twins who had it, scientists concluded that more than 50 percent of the risk for developing the disorder could be attributed to an individual's genetic makeup. A few small studies have even isolated a specific area on the human genome where some of the mutations that may influence anorexia exist, and now a five-year, $10 million NIMH study is underway to further pinpoint the locations of those genes.

AMY NELSON, 14, A NINTH grader from a Chicago suburb, thinks that genes played a role in her disease. Last year Amy's weight dropped from 105 to a skeletal 77 pounds, and her parents enrolled her in the day program at the Alexian Brothers Behavioral Health Hospital outside Chicago. Over the summer, as Amy was getting better, her father found the diary of his younger sister, who died at 18 of "unknown causes." In it, the teenager had calculated that she could lose 13 pounds in less than a month by restricting herself to less than 600 calories a day. No salt, no butter, no sugar, "not too many bananas," she wrote in 1980. "Depression can run in families," says Amy, "and an eating disorder is like depression. It's something wrong with your brain." These days, Amy is healthier and, though she doesn't weigh herself, thinks she's around 100. She has a part in the school play and is more casual about what she eats, even to the point of enjoying ice cream with friends.

Scientists are tracking important differences in the brain chemistry of anorexics. Using brain scans, researchers at the University of Pittsburgh, led by professor of psychiatry Dr. Walter Kaye, discovered that the level of serotonin activity in the brains of anorexics is abnormally high. Although normal levels of serotonin are believed to be associated with feelings of well-being, these pumped-up levels of hormones may be linked to feelings of anxiety and obsessional thinking, classic traits of anorexia. Kaye hypothesizes that anorexics use starvation as a mode of self-medication. How? Starvation prevents tryptophane, an essential amino acid that produces serotonin, from getting into the brain. By eating less, anorexics reduce the serotonin activity in their brains, says Kaye, "creating a sense of calm," even as they are about to die of malnutrition.

Almost everyone knows someone who has trouble with food: extremely picky eating, obsessive dieting, body-image problems, even voluntary vomiting are well known. But in the spectrum of eating disorders, anorexia, which affects about 2.5 million Americans, stands apart. For one thing, anorexics are often delusional. They can be weak with hunger while they describe physical sensations of overfullness that make it physically uncomfortable for them to swallow. They hear admonishing voices in their heads when they do manage to choke down a few morsels. They exercise compulsively, and even when they can count their ribs, their image in the mirror tells them to lose more.

When 12-year-old Erin Phillips, who lives outside Baltimore, was in her downward spiral, she stopped eating butter, then started eating with chopsticks, then refused solid food altogether, says her mother, Joann. Within two months, Erin's weight had slipped from 70 to 50 pounds. "Every day, I'd watch her melt away," Joann says. Before it struck her daughter, Joann had been dismissive about the disease. "I used to think the person should just eat something and get over it. But when you see it up close, you can't believe your eyes. They just can't." (Her confusion is natural: the term anorexia comes from a Greek word meaning "loss of appetite.")

Anorexia is a killer—it has the highest mortality rate of any mental illness, including depression. About half of anorexics get better. About 10 percent of them die. The rest remain chronically ill—exhausting, then bankrupting, parents, retreating from jobs and school, alienating friends as they struggle to manage the symptoms of their condition. Hannah Hartney of Tulsa, Okla., was first hospitalized with anorexia when she was 10. After eight weeks, she was returned to her watchful parents. For the last few years, she was able to maintain a normal weight but now, at 16, she's been battling her old demons again. "She's not out of the woods," says her mother, Kathryn.

While adults can drift along in a state of semi-starvation for years, the health risks for children under the age of 13 are dire. In their preteen years, kids should be gaining weight. During that critical period, their bones are thickening and lengthening, their hearts are getting stronger in order to pump blood to their growing bodies and their brains are adding mass, laying down new neurological pathways and pruning others—part of the explosion of mental and emotional development that occurs in those years. When children with eating disorders stop consuming sufficient calories, their bodies begin to conserve energy: heart function slows, blood pressure drops; they have trouble staying warm. Whatever estrogen or testosterone they have in their bodies drops. The stress hormone cortisol becomes elevated, preventing their bones from hardening. Their hair becomes brittle and falls out in patches. Their bodies begin to consume muscle tissue. The brain, which depends at least in part on dietary fat to grow, begins to atrophy. Unlike adult anorexics, children with eating disorders can develop these debilitating symptoms within months.

Lori Cornwell says her son's descent was horrifyingly fast. In the summer of 2004, 9-year-old Matthew Cornwell of Quincy, Ill., weighed a healthy 49 pounds. Always a picky eater, he began restricting his food intake until all he would eat was a carrot smeared with a tablespoon of peanut butter. Within three months, he was down to 39 pounds. When the Cornwells and their doctor finally located a clinic that would accept a 10-year-old boy, Lori tucked his limp body under blankets in the back seat of her car and drove all night across the country. Matthew was barely conscious when he arrived at the Children's Hospital in Omaha. "I knew that I had to get there before he slipped away," she says.

With stakes this high, how do you treat a malnourished third grader who is so ill she insists five Cheerios make a meal? First, say a growing number of doctors and patients, you have to let par-

FIGHTING ANOREXIA
THE PRICE OF PERFECTION

Because patients literally starve themselves, anorexia has one of the highest fatality rates of any emotional disorder. Its effects are particularly troubling in young people, whose developing bodies are more susceptible to deprivation.

Wasting Away

Deprived of food, the body cannibalizes itself for energy, first burning its fat stores, then turning to muscle and eventually its own organs.

Heart: Starved of energy, it can't pump properly. Patients of all ages feel weak, and have trouble keeping warm. Electrolyte shortages can cause palpitations.

Digestion: The GI tract slows, leaving patients feeling constipated and full. This can exacerbate their already strong aversion to eating.

Hormones: Extreme weight loss disrupts sex-hormone production. This can delay puberty in both girls and boys. Girls who remain anorexic into adulthood can suffer from infertility.

Nails turn brittle.

Hair becomes thin, dry and brittle from protein deficiences.

Skin dries out and it easily bruised; may sprout a fine layer of hair as insulation.

Brain

Kids can become lightheaded and unable to think straight; graddes often suffer. Brain scans show heightened levels of the chemical serotonin in patients. This imbalance may be linkded to feelings of anxiety and obsessional thinking.

Bones: Robbed of essential nutrients like calcium, anorexic children lack the basic building blocks for a strong skeletal system. If kids don't lay down enough bone during puberty, they're at increased risk for fractures later life.

Muscles: Atrophy sets in sapping strength and mass.

Kidneys: A severe lack of fluids can lead to organ failure.

1 in 100 females develops anorexia

10% of these patients could die of it*

*ESTIMATE

ents back into the treatment process. For more than a hundred years, parents have been regarded as an anorexic's biggest problem, and in 1978, in her book "Golden Cage," psychoanalyst Hilde Bruch suggested that narcissistic, cold and unloving parents (or, alternatively, hypercritical, overambitious and overinvolved ones) actually caused the disease by discouraging their children's natural maturation to adulthood. Thirty years ago stan-

THE SIGNS

A person with anorexia may show any or all of these symptoms. Parents should talk about their concerns to kids and consult a doctor or counselor for treatment options.

1. Loses weight dramatically
2. Refuses to eat certain foods
3. Obsesses over body weight, calories, food or dieting
4. Has bizarre eating rituals, such as rearranging food on the plate, excessive chewing or eating food in a certain order
5. Makes excuses to avoid mealtimes and eating
6. Complains frequently about feeling fat
7. Exercises obsessively, even during bad weather or illness; feels the need to burn off any calories taken in
8. Frequently weighs herself
9. Won't eat in front of others
10. Denies being hungry
11. Wears baggy clothes to hide appearance
12. Moody, depressed, withdrawn

dard treatment involved helping the starving and often delusional adolescents or young women to separate psychologically—and sometimes physically—from their toxic parents. "We used to talk about performing a parental-ectomy," says Dr. Ellen Rome, head of adolescent medicine at the Cleveland Clinic.

Too often these days, parents aren't so much banished from the treatment process as sidelined, watching powerlessly as doctors take what can be extreme measures to make their children well. In hospitals, severely malnourished anorexics are treated with IV drips and nasogastric tubes. In long-term residential treatment centers, an anorexic's food intake is weighed and measured, bite by bite. In individual therapy, an anorexic tries to uncover the roots of her obsession and her resistance to treatment. Most doctors use a combination of these approaches to help their patients get better. Although parents are no longer overtly blamed for their child's condition, says Marlene Schwartz, codirector of the Yale eating-disorder clinic, doctors and therapists "give parents the impression that eating disorders are something the parents did that the doctors are now going to fix."

Worse, the state-of-the-art protocols don't work for many young children. A prolonged stay in a hospital or treatment center can be traumatic. Talk therapy can help some kids, but many others are too young for it to be effective. Back at home, family mealtimes become a nightmare. Parents, advised not to badger their child about food, say nothing—and then they watch helpless and heartbroken as their child pushes the food away.

In the last three years, some prominent hospitals and clinics around the country have begun adopting a new treatment model in which families help anorexics get better. The most popular of the home-based models, the Maudsley approach, was developed in the 1980s at the Maudsley Hospital in London. Two doctors there noticed that when severely malnourished, treatment-resistant anorexics were put in the hospital and fed by nurses, they gradually gained weight and began to participate in their own recovery. They decided that given the right support, family members could get anorexics to eat in the same way the nurses did. These days, family-centered therapy works like this: A team of doctors, therapists and nutritionists meets with parents and the child. The team explains that while the causes of anorexia are unclear, it is a severe, life-threatening disease like cancer or diabetes. Food, the family is told, is the medicine that will help the child get better. Like oncologists prescribing chemotherapy, the team provides parents with a schedule of calories, lipids, carbohydrates and fiber that the patient must eat every day and instructs them on how to monitor the child's intake. It coaches siblings and other family members on how to become a sympathetic support team. After a few practice meals in the hospital or doctor's office, the whole family is sent home for a meal.

'I TELL THEM IT'S A BRAIN DISORDER,' SAYS DR. JULIE O'TOOLE. 'CHILDREN DON'T CHOOSE TO HAVE IT AND PARENTS DON'T CAUSE IT.'

"I told my daughter, 'You're going to hate this'," says Mitzi Miles, whose daughter Kaleigh began struggling with anorexia at 10. "She said, 'I could never hate you, Mom.' And I said, 'We'll see'." The first dinner at the Miles home outside Harrisburg, Pa., was a battle—but Mitzi, convinced by Kaleigh's doctor she was doing the right thing, didn't back down. After 45 minutes of yelling and crying, Kaleigh began to eat. Over the next 20 weeks, Kaleigh attended weekly therapy sessions, and Mitzi got support from the medical team, which instructed her to allow Kaleigh to make more food choices on her own. Eleven months later, Kaleigh is able to maintain a normal weight. Mitzi no longer measures out food portions or keeps a written log of her daily food intake.

CRITICS POINT OUT THAT THE Maudsley approach won't work well for adults who won't submit to other people's making their food choices. And they charge that in some children, parental oversight can do more harm than good. Young anorexics and their parents are already locked in a battle for control, says Dr. Alexander Lucas, an eating-disorder specialist and professor emeritus at the Mayo Clinic in Minnesota. The Maudsley approach, he says, "may backfire" by making meals into a battleground. "The focus on weight gain," he says, "has to be between the physician and the child." Even proponents say that family-centered treatment isn't right for everyone: families where there is violence, sexual abuse, alcoholism or drug addiction aren't good candidates. But several studies both in clinics at the Maudsley Hospital and at the University of Chicago show promising results: five years after treatment, more than 70 percent of patients recover using the family-centered method, compared with 50 percent who recover by themselves or using the old approaches. Currently, a large-scale NIH study of the Maudsley approach is underway.

Mental-health specialists say the success of the family-centered approach is finally putting the old stigmas to rest. "An 8-year-old with anorexia isn't in a flight from maturity," says Dr. Julie O'Toole, medical director of the Kartini Clinic in Portland, Ore., a family-friendly eating-disorder clinic. "These young patients are fully in childhood." Most young anorexics, O'Toole says, have wonderful, thoughtful, terribly worried parents. These days, when a desperately sick child enters the Kartini Clinic, O'Toole tries to set parents straight. "I tell them it's a brain disorder. Children don't choose to have it and parents don't cause it." Then she gives the parents a little pep talk. She reminds them that mothers were once blamed for causing schizophrenia and autism until that so-called science was debunked. And that the same will soon be true for anorexia. At the conclusion of O'Toole's speech, she says, parents often weep.

GETTING HELP

TREATMENT: The first step is restoring healthy body weight. Then:

1. **Psychotherapy** can address the underlying emotional issues of anorexia, such as obsessiveness-compulsiveness, profound mental rigidity and perfectionism
2. **Medications** help treat the depression and anxiety that often accompany anorexia
3. **Family therapy** can help young patients confront stresses in the home that may be exacerbating their conditions.

FOR MORE INFORMATION:

1. **National Eating Disorders Association** (tips for teachers and parents, specialist referrals): nationaleatingdisorders.org
2. **Something Fishy** (chat rooms offer online support for families and patients): www.something-fishy.org
3. **National Institute of Mental Health** (research news, treatment strategies, statistics); www.nimh.gov/publicat/eatingdisorders.cfm

—JOSH ULICK

THEY'RE NOT JUST YOUNGER. ANOREXICS ARE MORE LIKELY TO BE BLACK OR ASIAN, MORE LIKELY TO BE BOYS, MORE LIKELY TO BE MIDDLE-AGED.

Ironically, family dinners are one of the best ways to prevent a vulnerable child from becoming anorexic. Too often, dinner is eaten in the back seat of an SUV on the way to soccer practice. Parents who eat regular, balanced meals with their children model good eating practices. Family dinners also help parents spot any changes in their child's eating habits. Dieting, says Dr. Craig Johnson, director of the eating-disorder program at Laureate Psychiatric Hospital in Tulsa, triggers complex neurobiological reactions. If you have anorexia in the family and your 11-year-old tells you she's about to go on a diet and is thinking about joining the track team, says Johnson, "you want to be very careful about how you approach her request." For some kids, innocent-seeming behavior carries enormous risks.

Children predisposed to eating disorders are uniquely sensitive to media messages about dieting and health. And their interpretation can be starkly literal. When Ignatius Lau of Portland, Ore., was 11 years old, he decided that 140 pounds was too much for his 5-foot-2 frame. He had heard that oils and carbohydrates were fattening, so he became obsessed with food labels, cutting out all fats and almost all carbs. He lost 32 pounds in six months and ended up in a local hospital. "I told myself I was eating healthier," Ignatius says. He recovered, but for the next three years suffered frequent relapses. "I'd lose weight again and it would trigger some of my old behaviors, like reading food labels," he says. These days he knows what healthy feels like. Ignatius, now 17, is 5 feet 11, 180 pounds, and plays basketball.

Back in Richmond, Va., Emily Krudys says her family has changed. For two months Katherine stayed at the Omaha Children's Hospital, and slowly gained weight. Emily stayed nearby—attending the weekly therapy sessions designed to help integrate her into Katherine's treatment. After Katherine returned home, Emily home-schooled her while she regained her strength. This fall, Katherine entered sixth grade. She's got the pony, and she's become an avid horsewoman, sometimes riding five or six times a week. She's still slight, but she's gaining weight normally by eating three meals and three or four snacks a day. But the anxiety still lingers. When Katherine says she's hungry, Emily has been known to drop everything and whip up a three-course meal. The other day she was startled to see her daughter spreading sour cream on her potato. "I thought, 'My God, that's how regular kids eat all the time'," she recalls. Then she realized that her daughter was well on the way to becoming one of those kids.

The Role of the School Nutrition Environment for Promoting the Health of Young Adolescents

In spite of obesity and other nutrition-related health problems of young adolescents, middle schools have not put student health or the school nutrition environment very high on the priority list.

By Mary Kay Meyer, John Marshak, & Martha T. Conklin

While there is a growing emphasis on increasing middle grades students' achievement, nutrition has long been recognized for its impact on student success. What is really going on nutritionally at the middle level that is affecting the well being of students? To help answer this question, school superintendents and principals were asked to describe the practices they observed on a daily basis. Though some exceptional practices were found, overall the picture painted by the participants was bleak.

Participants confirmed the students' frequent consumption of foods such as pizza, chicken nuggets, hamburgers, French fries, tacos/burritos, chips, candy, and carbonated beverages during the school day. All of these foods would be classified as high fat or high sugar. It has been said that choices lead to behaviors, behaviors lead to habits, and habits lead to a way of life. Today, the health of adolescents and the adults they will become is critically linked to the health related behaviors they choose to adopt. The nutritional adequacy of students' diets does affect students' learning and performance today and will affect the health of the adults they will become.

A close relationship between nutrition and learning has been well established (Galler, Ramsey, Solimano, & Lowell, 1983; Murphy, Wheler, Pagano, Kleinman, & Jellinek, 1998; Pollitt, Leibel, & Greenfield, 1981; Pollitt, Lewis, Garza, & Shulman 1982; Scanlon,1989; Simeon, & Granthom-McGregor, 1989; Wahlstrom & Begalle, 1999). Chronically undernourished children are more likely to become sick, miss classes, and score lower on tests (Centers for Disease Control, 1997). Recent statistics show that the percentage of children meeting the recommended number of food group servings was 14% for fruit, 17% for meat/meat substitutes, 20% for vegetables, 23% for breads/grains, and 30% for milk. Girls ages 14 to 18 have especially low intakes of fruits and dairy products. More than two-thirds of females ages 14 to 18 exceed the recommendations for intake of total fat and saturated fat, but even greater percentages of children exceed these recommendations than among other age/gender groups. Children's diets are high in added sugars. For all children, sugars contribute an average of 20% of total food energy. Children are heavy consumers of regular or diet soda. Overall, 56% to 85% of children consume soda on any given day. Teenage males were especially heavy consumers of soda, with more than one-third consuming more than three servings a day (United States Department of Agriculture, 2001).

These trends have contributed to several serious diet-related concerns. The percentage of young people who are overweight has more than doubled in the past 30 years (Centers for Disease Control, 1997; United States Department of Agriculture, 2001). One of the most serious aspects of overweight and obesity in children is Type II diabetes. Type II diabetes accounted for 16% of the diabetes in children in 1994, up from 4% in 1992. Overweight adolescents are more likely to become overweight adults, with increased risk of developing heart disease; stroke; gallbladder disease; arthritis; and endometrial, breast, prostate, and colon cancer (U.S. Dept. of Health and Human Services, 1988).

Middle school students spend up to one-third of their days in the school environment and are greatly influenced by what they experience during these hours.

Adolescents' eating behavior is influenced by personal characteristics and environmental factors in the home, school, and the community (Bandura, 1986; Gillespie, 1981). These factors are composed of the objective and subjective culture of their behavior settings (Klepp, Wilhemsen, & Andrews, 1991). The objective cultures are the tangible effects of the environment and subjective cultures are the norms, attitudes, and learned values from family and peers (Triandis, 1972). Middle school students spend up to one-third of their days in the school environment and are greatly influenced by what they experience during these hours.

In today's school environment many tangible elements such as a la carte foods, vending machines, and snack bars compete with creating a nutrition environment that encourages healthy eating behaviors (Story & Neumark-Sztainer, 1999). Cullen, Eagen, Baranowski, Owens, and de Moore (2000) found that fifth-grade students who ate only meals from a snack bar consumed significantly less total fruits, juices, and vegetables than fifth-grade students who ate school meals. Wildey, Pampalone, Pelletier, Zive, Elder, and Sallis (2000) reported that in middle schools where school stores were available, 88.5% of inventory items were high in fat and/or sugar. Because of the limited research in assessing the nutrition environment in schools, coupled with the concern for the growth and development of children in middle grades, a research study was conducted throughout the country to identify the nature of the nutrition environment in the middle grades from the principals' and superintendents' points of view and to determine which elements of a school's nutrition environment these school administrators considered most relevant to students' health and well-being.

Method

Focus groups were used to explore the context for promoting healthy eating behaviors among students within the middle school environment. Focus groups allowed researchers to explore the socio-environmental, behavioral, and attitudinal dimensions of this issue without imposing predetermined boundaries. The *Focus Group Kit* developed by Morgan and Krueger (1998) was used as the basis for developing the research design. Dr. Richard Krueger, University of Minnesota, served as a consultant on the project.

The focus group sessions were held at three sites throughout the United States: Kansas City, Missouri; Las Vegas, Nevada; and Reston, Virginia. Participants included principals and superintendents from a nine-state radius around each location.

They included 17 school principals and 9 superintendents. Of the 26 participants, 17 had more than 17 years of experience and only three had less than five years of experience. The school system size of participating districts ranged from 267 to more than 131,000 students in middle grades. The percentage of students receiving meal assistance ranged from 6% to 69% free and from 3% to 22% reduced.

Figure 1

School District Characteristics of Participants in the Middle Grade Nutrition Environment Study (N=25)

Characteristic	Number of Participants
Schools participating in the federally funded breakfast program	23
School districts in which food service personnel are involved in nutrition education in the middle grades	8
School districts in which nutrition is included in the curriculum in middle grades	25
School districts in which a comprehensive health curriculum that includes nutrition is offered in middle grades	18
School districts which the school board had a policy concerning contracts with vendors for food/drink items	19

School districts serving middle grades with vending machines
  All buildings
  Some buildings
  No buildings
	13
	10
	3

School districts serving middle grades with school sponsored stores
  All buildings
  Some buildings
  No buildings
	5
	7
	14

Results

A la carte items were sold in 17 of the participating school districts. The most frequently sold a la carte items were pizza, French fries, and chips. The most frequently identified items sold in vending machines and school-sponsored stores were soda, candy, sports drinks, chips, cookies, and flavored water. This is consistent with Wildey and associates (2000) who reported that items sold in middle school stores were high in fat and sugar. Figure 1 shows additional school district characteristics.

Most school administrators did not think the environments in middle grades schools were conducive to healthy eating habits. Vending machines and a la carte sales of unhealthy food items received much discussion. One of the first questions asked participants was, "When you think of a school environment that promotes healthy eating behaviors, what comes to mind?" Participants mentioned healthful food choices, friendly staff, time to eat, low-fat foods, absence of vending machines, and a relaxed cafeteria environment as important. Several responses from participants concerned whose responsibility providing such an environment should be.

"It is the responsibility of the school to make sure what they do serve the children is healthy."

"School food service directors to superintendents and everyone between should be involved."

Participants were asked to identify five qualities they thought were essential to a school's nutritional environment. The most often given responses were an attractive dining environment, time to eat, friendly staff, taste of the food, and menu choices.

Another question posed to participants was, "When you consider all of the things that you have to contend with (administration, management, security, serving meals, day-to-day operations), where do you place the school's nutritional environment in your list of priorities? The average score for this question for all groups was 2.9 on a scale of 1= low to 7= high. When asked, "What would it take to move this rating to a higher priority?" numerous participants answered "time." Other responses included awareness, administrative support, vision for the school, and "When it becomes my responsibility."

The major barriers to having a good nutrition environment in middle grades identified by school administrators were:

- **Funding**

    Funding in various forms was the most frequently mentioned barrier in each focus group: "time, long lines, and the physical plant itself ... when you have an environment that is very inviting and conducive for students to come in, it helps with participation. If you had enough money to do this, it would be a dream cafeteria." Another participant's expression of the need to improve capital funding for the cafeteria: "I think it's the money. ... I really do, it's the simple matter of where are you going to put your priorities." This quotation addresses the importance of other issues, such as improving test scores, over building healthy eating habits in setting the budget priorities. "We have a 1965 budget with 2000 needs." Many participants expressed the need for the revenue generated by the sales of the less nutritious products to supplement the budget. No longer did they think it was just nice to have extra funds from vending and snack bar sales, but it has become a necessity to fund any number of essential needs.

- **Attitudes of parents and students**

    "It is the parents' attitudes that spill over to students' attitudes." "Eat junk at home; eat junk at school."

- **Outside influences**

    One of the greatest outside influences discussed was the media. "We have Channel 1 News every morning and between the news segments, soft drink and fast food hypes are on."

- **Peer pressure**

    "We had the best food going, but the kids would not eat it because it wasn't cool. ... We had to work to make it cool."

- **Lack of vision**

    "I think you have to have a vision of what you want for your nutritional program for your kids in your school and you use the same process that you use with everything else to get it done."

- **Lack of knowledge**

    "Major barriers are people based ... from a knowledge position ... because if I think, or the board thinks, or the community thinks that it is extremely important, the money will come from somewhere."

- **Inequity among free, reduced, and paying students**

    In some locations there is a social stigma associated with having to eat in the "regular" lunch line. Not all schools have been able to overcome the difficulties of differentiating between those students on free and reduced priced meals and those who are not. Therefore, students who qualify for free and reduced meals often choose not to eat.

- **Food preparation and limited choices**

    Limited choices were a concern. Participants frequently characterized the food as poor quality, greasy, tasting artificial, and lacking visual appeal.

- **Lack of commitment**

    Participants did not think that school districts acknowledged the importance of nutrition.

The topic of mixed messages generated great discussion in all groups. Included in the mixed messages being sent in the schools concerning nutrition were, vending machines and what is stocked in them, what is sold at concession stands, candy sales being used for fund raisers, teachers giving candy as classroom incentives, and serving hamburgers, corn dogs, and French fries in the cafeteria. "We are doing it. I am just as guilty. After a state exam we give all our kids chocolate chip cookies and donuts."

One of the two closing questions asked participants was, "Of all the things we have discussed, what is the most important?" Three themes consistently arose: involvement, funding, and vision.

"It was nice to hear that we all believe that all kids need to eat."

"We need more impact, communication, involvement at all levels from the superintendent down."

"You have to be a change agent in your school because no one else is going to do it."

"Money dictates what we do or don't do for kids, and I think that is a really sad scenario."

Conclusion and Application

Recently legislation has been introduced to regulate the sale of foods of minimal nutritional value in our nation's schools. Legislation will not solve the problem. Many states currently have such laws that are ignored by school administrators. Local school districts, communities, parents, educators, and school administrators must work together to eliminate the barriers to a healthy nutrition environment in our middle grades. School administrators can lead the challenge by ensuring that financial decisions do not undermine nutrition goals. This will not be easy and may necessitate making hard decisions about funding.

School administrators also can initiate the organization of a school health or nutrition advisory committee that includes teachers, parents, students, as well as the community. These stakeholders should also be involved in developing food and nutrition policy. These policies may involve questioning a decision to allow exclusive contracts with the large beverage companies.

Greater efforts should be made to ensure students have enough time to eat. It is critical for the health and well-being of our adolescents to receive proper nutrition. They cannot be expected to accomplish this when cafeterias are over crowded and it takes as much as 20 minutes of a 25 minute lunch period to be served. The physical environments of the cafeteria should allow students a pleasant and stress free environment for consuming the nutritious meals they need to nourish their bodies to allow them to better assimilate the knowledge gained through their classroom experiences.

Vending machines should be stocked with healthful snacks and beverages and the sale of high-fat and high-sugar snacks should be eliminated totally from middle school campuses. More healthful snack items such as baked chips, trail mix, dried fruit, low fat cookies, and 100% fruit juices should replace the high-fat and high-sugar items. Fund raisers should focus on non-food items. Raffles and silent auctions could replace the sale of candy and cookies as fund raisers for school organizations.

A comprehensive health education program with nutrition as a major component should be the national standard for middle school curriculum. Classroom and physical education teachers, food service managers, and other staff should work together to ensure the flow of nutrition throughout the curriculum.

Schools are in a unique position to promote healthful food choices and help assure appropriate nutrient intake of our young adolescents, as well as reinforce nutrition education and provide opportunities for students to practice healthful food choices. School administrators hold the keys to success. They must initiate and support efforts to provide a number of elements necessary to create a healthy environment for our young adolescents. But, it will take all involved parties working together to make this happen. One participant in the focus group research stated it best when he said, "When it becomes a priority, it will get done."

Acknowledgment

This article was written by the National Food Service Management Institute-Applied Research Division, located at The University of Southern Mississippi with headquarters at The University of Mississippi. Funding for the Institute has been provided with Federal funds from the U.S. Department of Agriculture, Food and Nutrition Services, The University of Mississippi. The contents of this publication do not necessarily reflect the views or policies of The University of Mississippi or the U.S. Department of Agriculture, nor does mention of trade names, commercial products, or organizations imply endorsement by the U.S. Government.

References

Bandura, A. (1986). *Social functions of thought and action: A social cognitive theory.* Englewood Cliffs, NJ: Prentice Hall.

Centers for Disease Control and Prevention. (1997). *CDC's guidelines for school health programs: Promoting lifelong healthy eating.* Atlanta, GA: Author.

Cullen, K. W., Eagen, J., Baranowski, T., Owens, E., & de Moore, C. (2000). Effect of a la carte and snack bar foods at school on children's lunchtime intake of fruits and vegetables. *Journal of the American Dietetic Association, 100,* 1482–1486.

Galler, J. R., Ramsey, F, Solimano, G., & Lowell, W. E. (1983). The influence of early malnutrition on subsequent behavioral development: Degree of impairment in intellectual performance. *Journal of the American Academy of Child Adolescent Psychiatry, 22,* 8–18.

Gillespie, A. (1981). A theoretical framework for studying school nutrition education programs. *Journal of Nutrition Education, 13,* 150–152.

Klepp, K., Wilhemsen, B. U., & Andrews, T. (1991) Promoting healthy eating patterns among Norwegian school children. In D. Nutbeam, B. Haglund, P. Farley, & P. Tillgren (Eds.), *Youth health promotion from theory to practice in school and community* (pp. 137–156). London: Forbes Publishers.

Morgan, D. L., & Krueger, R. A. (1998). *The focus group kit.* Thousand Oaks, CA: Sage Publications.

Murphy, J. M., Wheler, C. A., Pagano, M., Kleinman, R. K., & Jellinek, M. S. (1998). The relationship between hunger and psychological functioning in low-income American children. *Journal of the American Academy of Child Adolescent Psychiatry, 37,* 163–170.

Pollitt, E., Leibel, R., & Greenfield, D. (1981). Brief fasting, stress, and cognition in children. *American Journal of Clinical Nutrition, 34,* 1526–1533.

Pollitt, E., Lewis, N., Garza, C., & Shulman, R., (1982). Fasting and cognition. *Journal of Pediatric Research, 17,* 169–174.

Scanlon, K. S. (1989). *Activity and behavioral changes of marginally malnourished Mexican pre-schoolers.* Unpublished master's thesis, University of Connecticut, Storrs Connecticut.

Simeon, D. T., & Granthom-McGregor, S. (1989). Effects of missing breakfast on the cognitive functions of school children of different nutritional status. *American Journal of Clinical Nutrition, 49,* 646–653.

Story, M., &. Neumark-Sztainer, D. (1999). Competitive foods in schools: Issues, trends, and future directions. *Topics in Clinical Nutrition*, 15(1), 37–46.

Triandis, H. (1972). *The analysis of subjective culture*. New York: Wiley-interscience.

U.S. Department of Agriculture. (2001). *Foods sold in competition with USDA school meal programs. A report to Congress*. Washington, DC: Author. Retrieved June 2001 from `www.fns.usda.gov/cnd/Lunch/Competi.../competitive.foods.report.to.congress.html`

U.S. Department of Health and Human Services. (1988). *The Surgeon General's report on nutrition and health* (HHS Publication 88-50210). Washington, DC: U.S. Government Printing Office.

Wahlstrom, K. L., & Begalle, M. S. (1999). More than test scores: Results of the universal school breakfast pilot in Minnesota. *Topics in Clinical Nutrition*, 15, 17–29.

Wildey, M. B., Pampalone, S. Z., Pelletier, R. L., Zive, M. M., Elder, J. P., & Sallis, J. F. (2000). Fat and sugar levels are high in snacks purchased from student stores in middle schools. *Journal of the American Dietetic Association, 100*, 319–322.

Mary Kay Meyer is a research scientist at the National Food Service Management Institute, Division of Applied Research at the University of Southern Mississippi, Hattiesburg. E-mail: mk.meyer@usm.edu

John Marshak is an assistant professor of educational leadership at the State University of New York at Cortland.

Martha T. Conklin, formerly of Southern Mississippi University, is an associate professor at Pennsylvania State University, University Park.

UNIT 4

Obesity and Weight Control

Unit Selections

Key Points to Consider

- What are some of the causes behind a person becoming obese?

- As the incidence of obesity increases, how can it be prevented?

- What are some of the reasons that people have differential responses to weight loss and maintenance?

- Describe the role schools can play in preventing obesity in childhood and adolescence.

- Design a menu that would be in accordance with the new science of Volumetrics.

Student Website

www.mhcls.com/online

Internet References

Further information regarding these websites may be found in this book's preface or online.

American Anorexia Bulimia Association/National Eating Disorders Association (AABA)
http://www.nationaleatingdisorders.org/

American Society of Exercise Physiologists (ASEP)
http://www.asep.org/

Calorie Control Council
http://www.caloriecontrol.org

Eating Disorders: Body Image Betrayal
http://www.bibri.com/home/index.htm

Shape Up America!
http://www.shapeup.org

O verweight and obesity have become epidemic in the United States during the last century and are rising at a dangerous rate worldwide. Approximately 5 million adults are overweight or obese according to the new standards set by the US government using a body mass index (BMI) range of 30 to 39.9. Reports suggest that by the year 2050, half of the US population would be considered obese. This problem is prevalent in both genders and all ages, races, and ethnic groups. Twenty-five percent of US children and adolescents are overweight or at risk, which emphasizes the need for prevention, as obese children become obese adults. The catastrophic health consequences of obesity are heart disease, diabetes, gallbladder disease, osteoarthritis, and some cancers. The cost for treating this degenerative disease in the United States is approximately $100 billion per year.

Even though professionals have tried hard to prevent and combat obesity with behavior modification, a healthy diet, and exercise, it seems that these traditional ways have not proven effective. In a society where fast-food eateries are the mainstay of meals, where "big," including food servings, is better, where there is a universal reliance on automobiles, and where the food industry is more interested in profit than in the health of the population, we should not be surprised that obesity has become an epidemic. Dr. J. Tillotson examines the powerful influence of a few mega food companies on the food choices of Americans. They spend millions of dollars in advertising fast foods loaded with simple sugars and saturated fat. Their aggressive advertising coupled with food accessibility and large portion size has created the "obesigenic" characteristics of our environment whose interaction with genes resulted in the obesity pandemic. Other obstacles to maintaining a healthy diet are the lack of promoting healthy food and its low accessibility and high cost.

More recently, scientists have reported that fat is a dynamically active endocrine organ that releases hormones and inflammatory proteins that may predispose a person to chronic diseases including heart disease. Additionally, research has discovered the role of the "hunger hormone" and how individual differences in its levels affects our ability to lose weight. Thus, there is a great need for a multifaceted public health approach that would involve mobilization of private and public sectors and focus on building better coping skills and increasing activity. Inclusion of health officials, researchers, educators, legislators, transportation experts, urban planners, and businesses that would cooperate in formulating ways to combat obesity is crucial. A sound public-health policy would require that weight-loss

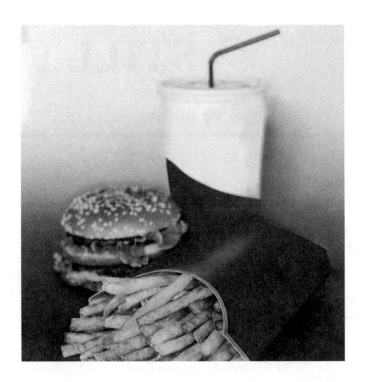

therapies have long-term maintenance and relapse-prevention measures built into them.

Healthy people 2010, is the US government's prevention agenda designed to ensure high quality of life and to reduce health risks. One of the 28 areas it focuses on is overweight and obesity. Its main objectives are to reduce the proportion of overweight and obese children, teens, and adults to 15 percent and to increase the proportion of adults who are at a healthy weight. Twice as many teens from poor households are overweight in comparison to those from middle to high income. Women with less education and lower incomes have high rates of obesity and the rates of obesity are higher among African American women than Caucasian. Gender differences in the incidence of obesity have been observed in Hispanics and African Americans with 80 percent greater in women than men.

The last three articles describe how childhood obesity is on the rise and suggest ways to prevent it—from changes in school-food quality and availability to home-based strategies in incorporating activity and addressing parent-child feeding relations.

STILL HUNGRY?

Fattening revelations—and new mysteries—about the hunger hormone

Janet Raloff

Too busy to cook, you drop by the neighborhood café and treat yourself to fried chicken with a side of macaroni and cheese. You wash it all down with a bottle of apple juice—to balance the high-fat entrees with something healthy. Although you've put away far more calories than usual, you still don't feel really full, so you select a slice of chocolate torte from the dessert case.

Recent studies have begun pointing to a wide variety of factors, including body weight, food choices, and lack of sleep, by which we can unwittingly alter not only when we experience hunger but also what items appear appetizing and how much food it takes to trigger a feeling that we've had enough.

Our bodies rely on a host of involuntary cues to regulate food consumption. In 1999, researchers discovered a hormone that contributes to strong feelings of hunger. Throughout the day, its concentration in our bodies rises and falls. Although we're not aware of these ups and downs, they drive our behavior, either moving us toward the table or letting us get on with the rest of our lives.

Cycles of this powerful hormone—dubbed ghrelin, after a Hindu word for "growth"—reflect a complex interplay of chemical signals that scientists are now beginning to untangle. In the last 2 years, research has also begun pointing to an array of diet and lifestyle factors that modify the body's production of ghrelin and other eating-related signals.

Such findings are not just curiosities. As the complex picture of ghrelin and its allies has been getting clearer, the medical community has begun considering new drugs, lifestyle changes, and other interventions to counter people's penchant for overeating. On the table are billions of dollars and the health of millions of people.

GUT REACTIONS Although many endocrinologists glibly refer to ghrelin as the "hunger hormone," it's got plenty of accomplices when it comes to making people eat—and stop eating—notes Aart Jan van der Lely of Erasmus University in Rotterdam, the Netherlands. Some 2 dozen chemical agents—many of them hormones—stimulate food intake, and a similar number suppress appetite, he says. But only a few of these substances appear to hold feature roles in dinner theater, while the rest serve as understudies or the chorus.

According to recent studies, ghrelin stars as a trigger of appetite (*SN: 2/16/02, p. 107*). The featured players in appetite suppression include insulin, which is made in the pancreas, and leptin, which fat cells manufacture. These two hormones turn down the dial on ghrelin production. Another appetite suppressor is PYY, a gut hormone that also appears to curb ghrelin manufacture.

All these hormones travel through the body, carrying their eat or don't-eat messages. They also trigger nerve signals running from the gut to the brain and are influenced, in turn, by messages returning from the brain.

As in a great theater production, there's depth in the cast of appetite regulators. When top-billed performers, such as ghrelin, are no-shows, the body turns to understudies to figure out when to eat and, somewhat less effectively, when to stop.

For instance, David E. Cummings of the University of Washington in Seattle and his coworkers reported in the October 2004 *Endocrinology* that the spike in insulin secretion that occurs after eating usually correlates with a dip in ghrelin production. The researchers found that when they killed rats' insulin-producing cells to model uncontrolled diabetes, food intake still suppressed ghrelin concentrations in the blood, but only about half as effectively as when insulin was present. One or more understudies must take a portion of ghrelin's role, the team concludes.

This study also showed that lack of insulin increased a rodent's sensitivity to ghrelin's call to eat. When Cummings and his coworkers infused a small amount of ghrelin into the diabetic rats, the animals more than tripled their food intake compared with that of healthy rats given the same treatment.

Related studies are homing in on other factors that perturb the normal checks and balances on ghrelin—changes that might keep the hunger bell ringing long after people would otherwise feel full. People may overeat not just when there's a problem with the ghrelin signal but also when something goes amiss in other parts of the control system.

With this new conceptual framework, scientists are looking for means to confront what many have characterized as a worldwide epidemic of obesity (*http://www.sciencesnews.org/articles/20020803/food.asp*).

ALL CALORIES AREN'T ALIKE Although most health guides recommend that we eat less fat, people have a hard time complying. The late Walter Mertz, when he was head of the Department of Agriculture's Human Nutrition Research Center in Beltsville, Md., used to sympathize: "The trouble with fat is that it tastes so good."

Cummings' new research points to a related problem: Calorie for calorie, fat is less effective than other nutrients at suppressing ghrelin's hunger call. During one recent study, his team on different days infused into rats' gastrointestinal tracts equal-calorie quantities of pure sugar, protein, or fat. In the February *Endocrinology*, the group reports that sugar and protein each prompted a rapid, 70-percent drop in the concentration of ghrelin circulating in the rodents' blood. When rats instead received fat, ghrelin concentrations fell far more slowly and by only about 50 percent.

"We've now found the same thing with humans," Cummings told *Science News.*

These results are consistent with earlier work by his team. For example, the researchers observed in 2003 that prebreakfast, or background, ghrelin concentrations rise as most people lose weight—as if the body is attempting to regain the pounds. However, when people trimmed their waistlines over several months via a low-fat diet, their prebreakfast ghrelin levels remained unchanged.

This "leads us to hypothesize," Cummings says, "that one of the mechanisms behind weight gain typically associated with high-fat diets is that they don't suppress the hunger hormone as well [as low-fat fare does]."

When it comes to sugars, different types can have different effects on ghrelin. For example, Peter J. Havel of the University of California, Davis and his coworkers gave 12 women standardized meals served with custom-prepared drinks sweetened with either of the two table sugar components: glucose, the sugar that cells use for energy, or fructose, the primary sugar in fruits and many soft drinks.

The meals silenced participants' ghrelin signals only about half as much on the days when the accompanying drinks had been sweetened with fructose compared with the days of glucose drinks, Havel's group reported in the June 2004 *Journal of Clinical Endocrinology & Metabolism* (*JCE&M*).

Even more interesting is what happened after each day of test drinks, when the women were permitted to eat anything from a buffet. The six women who had reported being careful about their food choices before the study chose fattier fare on the day after imbibing fructose drinks than they did on the day after drinking glucose-sweetened beverages. Moreover, these diners described themselves as being hungrier before meals on the day after getting fructose-sweetened drinks.

The sugar consumed the previous day didn't influence food choice or appetite of the other six women, Havel's team observed.

Though preliminary, these data suggest that even though fewer calories of fructose than calories of other sugars are required to sweeten a food, a high-fructose diet might boost calorie consumption in some people by fostering overeating, Havel notes.

WEIGHTY PROBLEMS One might expect that people with the highest background ghrelin concentrations in their blood would be the hungriest, eat the most, and end up fattest. It's just the opposite. This observation suggests that many people's bodies are misreading or ignoring hunger and satiety signals.

Obese individuals tend to have the lowest background ghrelin production, as if their bodies are encouraging them to fast (*SN: 7/6/02, p. 14*). Meanwhile, unhealthily lean people, such as those with anorexia nervosa, can have sky-high background ghrelin concentrations.

> "No wonder these poor people can't lose weight."
>
> — STEPHEN BLOOM, HAMMERSMITH HOSPITAL

Ian M. Chapman of the University of Adelaide in Australia is examining elderly individuals who are healthy except for their poor appetites and inordinately lean physiques. People with this "anorexia of aging" tend to produce twice as much ghrelin as do well-nourished seniors yet claim that they're never hungry, he says.

A similarly perplexing trend appears among 30 nondiabetic but overweight adults whom Arline D. Salbe has studied at a National Institutes of Health center in Phoenix. After being on a weight-maintenance diet for 3 days, the recruits got to eat all they wanted, whenever they wanted, for another 3 days. Each volunteer stayed in a hotel like hospital suite, and dieticians recorded every calorie consumed.

In the June 2004 *JCE&M*, Salbe's group reported that the higher a volunteer's prebreakfast concentration of ghrelin, the less he or she tended to eat.

Endocrinologist Stephen Bloom of Hammersmith Hospital in London isn't surprised.

Research by Cummings' group last year showed that in normal-weight volunteers, the more calories in a meal, the more it suppressed ghrelin production. But Bloom and his coworkers have found that hunger and satiety signals don't function well in heavy people.

Bloom's team fed 20 normal-weight and 20 heavy adults milkshakelike meals packed with anywhere from 250 to 3,000 calories. In the February *JCE&M*, the London researchers reported that ghrelin concentrations fell with increasing calories only among the normal-weight men and women. In the obese volunteers, the hormone showed the same drop after all meals, regardless of their milkshake's calorie content. The decline was similar to that in normal-weight people eating a meal with 1,000 calories.

In earlier work, Bloom's team had shown that after a meal the satiety-signaling gut hormone PYY rose less in obese volunteers than in people with normal weight (*http://www.sciencenews.org/articles/20030906/food.asp*).

"So now, you've got a double whammy," Bloom told *Science News*. Compared with other people, the obese remain hungry longer and don't feel full as quickly. "No wonder these poor people can't lose weight," he adds.

HUNGRY FOR SLEEP Since the mid-1960s, the rate of obesity in the United States has nearly tripled to one in three adults. Over the same period, U.S. citizens have deducted, on average, about 2 hours from their nightly slumber. Is there a connection?

Endocrinologist Eve Van Cauter strongly suspects that there is. She points to seven studies that have linked body weight to how long people sleep.

In her lab at the University of Chicago, Van Cauter has also been showing that blood concentrations of hunger and satiety hormones—as well as food preferences—depend on how well-rested people are. For instance, in the November 2004 *JCE&M*, her research team reported that prebreakfast concentrations of the satiety hormone leptin were roughly 20 percent lower in 11 healthy men who had slept only 4 hours a night for nearly a week than when they had slept 9 hours nightly.

In the December 2004 *Annals of Internal Medicine*, the researchers reported similar leptin differences in 12 healthy men after just 2 nights of each sleep regimen. Moreover, daytime concentrations of ghrelin climbed 28 percent during the sleep-deprived cycle.

After the second night of sleep deprivation, the recruits' appetites and food intake increased by 24 percent, compared with those after a good night's sleep. Moreover, when sleep deprived, the volunteers chose to consume a larger proportion of their food as high-calorie, carbohydrate-rich items, such as crackers and sweets. Those foods represented 33 to 45 percent more of the caloric intake than they did when the participants were well rested.

Van Cauter has also found that sleep loss increases the activity of the vagus nerve, the trunk line for signals between the gut and the brain. During stress, the brain signals the gut to alter its release of appetite-controlling hormones, which might be the mechanism by which sleep loss changes eating behavior. People are the only animals to voluntarily ignore their sleep needs, according to Van Cauter. They stay up to play, work, socialize, or watch television. However, she adds, "We're overstepping the boundaries of our biology because we are not wired for sleep deprivation."

HUNGER THERAPY Despite the complexity of appetite control, several large pharmaceutical companies have started developing ghrelin-blocking agents intended to blunt hunger in overweight individuals. Researchers are currently testing these substances on lab animals. From his own work, Cummings notes, ghrelin blockers "look pretty promising."

Currently, Bloom is probing dietary maneuvers to suppress ghrelin peaks and to increase the body's natural production of some of the understudy appetite-quenching hormones. He found that when he injected PYY into people, it suppressed appetite by 30 percent.

> With sleep deprivation, "we're overstepping the boundaries of our biology."
>
> —EVE VAN CAUTER, UNIVERSITY OF CHICAGO

The stomach hormone called oxyntomodulin also reduces ghrelin concentration and appetite in people. Indeed, "if we give a fair amount of oxyntomodulin to animals, they don't eat at all," Bloom notes.

In its search for appetite suppressors, van der Lely's team is focusing strictly on ghrelin, which comes in two forms. The type generally described as active is bound to a fatty acid and is called the acylated form. Although the unacylated form "used to be called inactive," van der Lely says, his team has found evidence that it has its own role in eating behavior.

In the February *JCE&M*, van der Lely and an international group of researchers report that unacylated ghrelin acts as a spoiler to the acylated form. "We have observed that if you experimentally co-administer both [ghrelins]—one in the left arm, and the other in the right arm of people—the unacylated ghrelin can completely abolish all of the effects of the other ghrelin on metabolism," he says. The finding suggests yet another means to silence the call to eat.

Ghrelin is emerging as a hunger hormone with multiple personalities.

EAT MORE WEIGH LESS

THE ANSWER MAY LIE IN THE NEW SCIENCE OF 'VOLUMETRICS'

Amanda Spake

Three young women scurry back and forth from the stainless steel counters to the big walk-in refrigerator, loading plates, written instructions, and questionnaires on trays in this commercial-style kitchen. But this is not like any other restaurant kitchen. The staff members not only prepare the food; they carefully weigh, measure, and record the food before it's served. They also weigh and measure what diners leave on their plates.

BARBARA ROLLS

Her "kitchen" at Pennsylvania State University also serves as her Volumetrics laboratory.

The adjoining dining room is also not typical. There are 16 individual cubicles separated by short walls and long, blue curtains, rather like the instant-photo booths once found in variety stores. Buffet tables are set up where dishes are kept hot. Small, unobtrusive video cameras record food selections at the buffet and the eating habits of diners inside the booths, all of it broadcast to monitors in the kitchen and in some of the offices surrounding the dining room.

Welcome to Pennsylvania State University's Laboratory for the Study of Human Ingestive Behavior, one of the world's most sophisticated centers for the study of what and how humans eat. The queen of this quirky culinary empire is Barbara Rolls, professor and Guthrie chair in nutrition at the university. For nearly three decades, Rolls, 60, has researched food choices, portion sizes, the caloric or energy density of foods, and myriad other factors that influence the human appetite and what satisfies it.

Most recently, the lab has been studying the impact of energy or calorie density—that is, the number of calories in a given weight of food—on satiety and weight control. Rolls calls this research "Volumetrics," and her new book, *The Volumetrics Eating Plan,* arrives in bookstores this week. Part weight-control program, part cookbook, it is an effort to put into practical form a lifetime of study on why people eat what they do and

how to satisfy the human biological drive for abundant food while achieving a healthy weight.

IN MANY WAYS, THE THEORY REPRESENTS THE ULTIMATE "VALUE MEAL": EAT MORE FOR LESS.

It was Rolls who realized that satiety, or the sensation of fullness, is "food specific." That is, when people are full of one food, they can still eat another—an explanation, says Rolls, "for why you always have room for dessert." She was among the first to notice that humans eat about the same weight or volume of food every day but not the same calories, a notion now accepted by nutrition scientists.

Supersize. Yet she also discovered an apparent contradiction: When food portions are "supersized," people eat more. Adults offered four different portions of macaroni and cheese at her lab ate 30 percent more calories when given the largest portion, compared with the smallest. Fewer than half noticed any difference in the serving sizes. Likewise, in Rolls's sandwich experiments, men and women were served 6-, 8-, 10-, and 12-inch submarine sandwiches. When given the 12-inch sub, women ate 31 percent more calories and men 56 percent more—compared with those given the 6-inch sub. Asked to rate their fullness after lunch, diners reported little difference whether they had eaten the larger or smaller sub. In a two-day study, portion sizes were increased for some dishes by as much as 100 percent, and people continued to eat more over both days. "As to why people respond this way, I don't know, but that is part of what we're working on," Rolls says. "Clearly, visual and cognitive cues are important."

What has become clear from her Volumetrics studies is that the key to weight management lies in "food choices that help you feel full with fewer calories." The absence of satiety is one reason most "diets" don't work very well or for very long. "Satiety is the missing ingredient in weight management," Rolls writes, and she's impatient with those who say the nation's obesity epidemic can be reversed by "telling people to eat less. People need to eat *more* low-energy-dense food, such as fruits and vegetables, so they get a satisfying amount of food and enough calories." This view is echoed in the 2005 Dietary Guidelines for Americans. And studies show that encouraging overweight families, for example, to eat more fruits and vegetables results in greater weight loss than telling them not to eat foods high in fat and sugar. "Emphasizing what people *can* eat rather than what they should not eat seems more sustainable," says Rolls.

In her lab, she tested these theories recently in the first year-long clinical trial of Volumetrics, involving 97 obese women. One group was given Volumetrics ideas and encouraged to eat more fruits, vegetables, soups, whole grains, and legumes. The other group received more traditional and negative messages about restricting fat and portion sizes. Neither group counted calories or fat grams, yet both groups showed a similar reduction in fat intake, and both groups lost weight. "The low-energy-density diet group ate a greater weight of food over a year but lost more body weight—about 20 pounds," says Rolls. The group given negative messages, to eat less fat and smaller portions, lost about 15 pounds. While the 33 percent greater amount of weight lost by the Volumetrics group may not have made anybody skinny, the group also ate more fruits and vegetables—five servings a day compared with 3.5—and a diet lower in energy density and richer in important nutrients.

While the trial is encouraging, Rolls is the first to say that it's small. Volumetrics needs to be tested at a number of medical centers, among more participants, and over a longer time. "There is so much research money going into diets that change the proportion of macronutrients [fat, protein, and carbohydrates]," says Rolls. "Yet what we're advocating will lead people to follow the new dietary guidelines and optimize not only weight but nutritional status as well."

In many ways, the theory represents the ultimate "value meal": Eat more for less. The secret ingredients that make foods less energy dense are water and fiber, which explains why most vegetables are among the lowest-energy-dense foods available, while vegetable oils, with all the water and fiber removed, are the highest. The principle becomes obvious when thinking of fruit: One hundred calories of grapes represents a great deal more food in terms of weight and volume, and is more filling, than 100 calories of raisins, or dried grapes. The same is true for nearly any dish. The drier the food, the higher its energy density. Potato chips (dry and cooked in vegetable oil) are five times as energy dense as a baked potato. Pasta, which absorbs water as it cooks, is about half as energy dense as Italian bread, even though the ingredients are similar. Adding water or water-rich foods, like vegetables, and using oils and energy-dense ingredients sparingly lower the density of most dishes, allowing larger portions and increasing satiety.

VEGGIES OR JUNK?

Nothing wrong with a few chips now and then, but the fiber and water in veggies will leave you far more satisfied.

The formula. Energy density is easy to calculate from a food label. Just divide the calories in one serving by its weight in grams, and you have the energy density of the food. To use Volumetrics for weight control, Rolls recommends making up a large portion of the diet with foods that have fewer calories in a serving than their weight in grams, resulting in energy densities below 1 (most fruits, vegetables, and low-fat dairy products). Also good are foods with calories equal to or slightly greater than their weight, or an energy density of 1 to 2 (beans, fish, chicken without fat or skin, potatoes, pasta, rice, low-fat salad dressings). Foods that have two or more times as many calories as their weight (ice cream, beef, french fries, cheese, pretzels, full-fat salad dressings, chips, cookies, bacon, oils) need to be controlled.

The Volumetrics principles are also useful for lowering the caloric density of whole meals. Rolls demonstrated the concept in her salad studies. Different groups of diners ate different sizes of salads with different energy densities. High-density salads had full-fat dressing and cheese, for example, while low-density salads were vegetables with fat-free dressing. She found that the diners who ate the large, low-density salads before a pasta entree ate about 100 fewer calories of pasta and 12 percent fewer calories for the meal. By contrast, the high-density salads increased the total calories by 17 percent. In a similar study of 200 overweight individuals on a weight-loss diet, those who ate soup as a snack twice a day lost 50 percent more weight than dieters snacking on dry, low-fat, calorie-dense foods, like pretzels or baked chips.

"We're being urged to manage calories," says Rolls. "So Volumetrics gives people a way to do that without having to count calories. If people understand where the calories are in foods, they can go for lower calories, lower density, and bigger portions of foods." Portion size and energy density independently contribute to the total calories of a meal, says Rolls, which is why restaurant eating is such a waist-expanding experience—energy density is high, and portions are large. "When people really get the energy-density message, they can accommodate in their diet some high-energy-dense foods in moderation," says Rolls. "But it's all trade-offs: You can eat a lot more apples than apple pie, but if you really want that piece of apple pie, it's better to accommodate it."

Food family. Rolls comes from a family fascinated by food. Her great-grandparents were farmers. Her grandfather, a professor at Cornell University, helped establish the New York agricultural extension program. Rolls grew up in Adelphi, Md., outside Washington, D.C., where her father spent most of his career at the U.S. Department of Agriculture. Her mother was a teacher and homemaker who struggled with food choices and weight control. "She was obese," Rolls says, "and she died of obesity-related illnesses—diabetes and cardiovascular disease."

A premed student at the University of Pennsylvania, Rolls graduated in biology and secured a fellowship to Cambridge University in England. She stayed in England, became a research fellow in experimental psychology and nutrition, and married Edmund Rolls, a professor of experimental psychology at Oxford. Her first studies of satiety were in the early 1980s. "My ex-husband was doing some neurophysiology experiments and found that cells in the brain stopped firing when we reached satiety with a certain kind of food but started firing again when we eat another food. This was fascinating because it meant that satiety is not global. It can be specific to the food or type of food you have been eating. People tire of salty or spicy foods and like the change to the sweet taste. So, when we have a variety of foods, we eat more."

Spice of life. In a series of experiments, Rolls looked at how variety influences the amount of food people eat. Students fed four courses at a meal ate 60 percent more than when they were served just one of the foods. When student nurses were offered sandwiches for lunch with either one filling or four different fillings, they ate 33 percent more food when offered the variety. Even the shape of food affects how much people eat: Volunteers ate 15 percent more pasta when served three different shapes than when served only one. "This is why it's important to have on hand a variety of low-energy-dense foods [oranges, pears, apples, carrots, celery, salad greens, soup, stew]. Otherwise, we eat high-density foods that are all too readily available [chips, crackers, cookies, pizza, fast-food burgers, and fries] because we want variety."

Rolls divorced and came back to the United States in 1984 with her two daughters, Juliet and Melissa, to an associate professorship in psychiatry at Johns Hopkins School of Medicine. "Members of the department were interested in the role gut hormones play in satiety," she says. She became a full professor in 1991 and made the move to Pennsylvania State in 1992 when the university offered her the directorship of the school's new Laboratory for the Study of Human Ingestive Behavior.

> ## SALAD SOLUTION
>
> **A large, low-fat salad before the main course reduces the amount of calories people eat during the entire meal.**

"I spent the 1990s comparing proportions of carbohydrate and fat because that's where the action was," she says, meaning the research money. "But we really weren't finding much difference in the effect of fat or carbohydrates on the total calories people ate. So, I noticed that people were eating the same weight or volume of food. I remember going to meetings where everybody was talking about the right proportion of fat or protein in the diet, and I'd say, 'Look at the weight of the food people are eating! It's the same, whether it's high in fat or carbohydrates.' See, we all thought people were eating for calories, the same number of calories per day. But they weren't. They were eating for the same weight or volume of food." The idea of Volumetrics was born.

Much nutritional research still focuses on macronutrients, or the ratio of fat, protein, and carbohydrate in the diet. Clinical studies on the effectiveness of low-carbohydrate versus low-fat diets for weight loss are still underway, but so far most show similar outcomes and modest long-term results. In fact, much of the public remains confused about these seemingly contradic-

tory diet strategies, in part, as Rolls puts it, "because there has really been a lot of controversy in the field over fat. Understanding energy density resolves a lot of these issues." Both high-fat foods and foods high in refined carbohydrates are energy dense and make weight control difficult.

One of the first studies on this subject was done not by Rolls but by researchers at the University of Alabama in 1983, who found that people on a low-energy-dense diet reached satiety with about half the calories of those on a high-density diet. Rolls uses the study in her presentations and laments that the researchers didn't continue it. But that article and Rolls's subsequent studies began to influence those working in the weight-loss trenches. "I was in private practice at that time," says James J. Kenney, nutritionist at the Pritikin Longevity Center. "I had this one woman who wasn't losing weight on a low-fat diet. I started looking at what she was eating, and everything was dry: dried fruit, dried cereal, dry crackers, energy-dense foods." When she switched to soups, salads, fresh fruit, and vegetables, her weight dropped.

Once at Pritikin, Kenney suggested the center change its emphasis from the low-fat regimen that the program had been founded upon to one emphasizing a lower-caloric-density approach. Kenney was fearful that the wave of low-fat but high-energy-dense cookies, crackers, and snack foods hitting the market would lead to more obesity and confuse the public about the usefulness of reducing fat calories. "And that's just what happened," he says. "In the 1990s, we saw Americans gaining weight like never before. … The public has been oblivious to the very important role calorie density plays in how full people feel when they eat a set amount of calories."

Of course, a small group of elite dieters who attend some of the premier weight-control centers have been schooled in energy density. At the Duke Diet and Fitness Center, as at Pritikin, nutrition manager Elisabetta Politi has been using an energy-density approach for a few years. "I think Barbara Rolls has a great theory, and there is a lot of interest in it," says Politi. "We take advantage of what she's found in what we do here. We start with a big salad, soup, smaller servings of protein and higher-density foods; and our clients feel satisfied on 1,200 or 1,300 calories a day." Likewise, Brian Zehetner, the lead nutritionist at Canyon Ranch SpaClub at the Venetian in Las Vegas, says, "We promote foods that are high in fiber and water. They add bulk, but it's not calorie-containing bulk. So theoretically, you can decrease your calorie intake and eat more food while eating low-energy-dense foods compared to eating high-energy-dense foods." Rolls wants Volumetrics to be accepted by a wider audience, however. She's now on the board of the Jenny Craig weight-loss program, and she notes that Weight Watchers seems to be incorporating aspects of Volumetrics as well, though she quibbles with both of these programs.

Paradigm. If the majority of the public, outside of a few weight-control programs, has been oblivious to the role energy density could play in cleaning up the American diet, so have many nutritional scientists. "This is a paradigm shift," agrees Gary Foster, clinical director of the Weight and Eating Disorders Program at the University of Pennsylvania School of Medicine. Volumetrics is "an overarching concept, less based on macronutrients, though clearly, high-fat foods have higher energy density. It's a more unifying approach to diet, and there are data to support it." The downside, Foster says, is that energy density is not listed on food labels. Rolls hopes that will change: "If we had an energy-density number on food labels, it would give people an immediate way to compare foods and the calories in a portion."

"My sense is people are becoming disenchanted with a low-carbohydrate diet, which is a high-energy-dense diet," says Columbia University's Xavier Pi-Sunyer, a member of the dietary guidelines advisory committee and director of the Obesity Research Center at St. Luke's-Roosevelt Hospital Center. "So this would be a return to a lower-energy-density diet. And that is in line with the new guidelines."

THIS EXPLAINS WHY YOU ALWAYS HAVE ROOM FOR DESSERT.

The grocery bill for a week of Volumetrics meals may be higher, says Adam Drewnowski, director of the Nutritional Sciences Program at the University of Washington. "On a per-calorie basis, fruits, vegetables, fish, lean protein, and low-fat dairy products are more expensive sources of pure calories. But we spend so little on food and so much on our cellphones; it really should be the other way around." Drewnowski is an advocate of a diet based on its nutrient density. "But Barbara and I end up in the same place—eating more fruits, vegetables, whole grains, water, and fiber-rich foods, which are nutrient dense."

Foster, Drewnowski, and Pi-Sunyer, like Rolls herself, would like to see Volumetrics and the energy-density concept fully evaluated in long-term clinical trials. "Let's roll this out now to three or four different centers," says Foster, "and see how it works for 300 to 400 people."

A longtime practitioner of Volumetrics, Rolls herself is slim. She swims every day in a lap pool at her house on a mountaintop near the university, walks on campus, takes the stairs instead of the elevator, and encourages people to use step counters to monitor their activity. A past president of the North American Association for the Study of Obesity, Rolls is no ascetic, however. She loves good food, and as she puts it, "I save my juice calories for wine." She and her partner of seven years, Charles Brueggbors, an architect turned foodie, developed the recipes in the book. Brueggbors came to a Volumetrics diet before he met Rolls, after consulting a dietitian some 15 years ago when he developed hypertension and a spare tire. "I still want chips; I still want sausage," Brueggbors says. "But I've learned to like the fresh veggies and low-fat foods, too. And so now I have chips, but I get a bowl, put in a small amount, and when it's gone, I just don't go back."

It's lunchtime, and the first volunteer diner enters the laboratory and is seated in a curtained booth. He's told he may take his plate to the buffet, get as much as he wants, and go back as often as he wants for any of the four dishes: a chicken and noodle casserole; a creamy, green bean and fried onion dish; a broccoli salad; and whipped sweet potatoes. Most diet programs recommend using a small plate to reduce calories in a meal. "We're not finding it's true," says Rolls. "People just go back for more."

Rolls watches on a video monitor as the man makes his way to the buffet table for the third time, piling the noodle casserole and the green bean and onion rings concoction onto his small plate. "Look at that," Rolls laments. "He's not even touching the broccoli salad."

Clearly, we have a long way to go.

A Call to
ACTION

Seeking Answers to Childhood Weight Issues

To solve the current obesity dilemma, more attention should be focused on increasing children's activity levels.

BY CAROL M. MEERSCHAERT, RD, LDN

One morning, I grabbed a cup of consciousness (or espresso roast coffee) and headed to the computer. In my e-mail inbox was one of those "words of wisdom" letters titled "People Over 35 Should Be Dead." Being older than 35 myself, the heading quickly woke me from my morning stupor.

The e-mail read: "Those of us who were kids in the 1940s, 1950s, 1960s, or even maybe the early 1970s probably shouldn't have survived. We ate cupcakes, bread and butter, and drank soda pop and Kool-Aid with sugar in it, but we were never overweight because we were always outside playing. We would leave home in the morning and play all day, as long as we were back when the street lights came on. We did not have PlayStations, Nintendo 64, X-Boxes—no video games at all—no 99 channels on cable, videotape movies, personal computers, or Internet chat rooms. We had friends! We went outside and found them."

As a dietitian, parent, and lover of physical activity, this message struck home. We have struggled to find the answers to the complex issues of childhood overweight prevention and treatment, and there, suddenly, the answer seemed to be staring at me from my inbox.

You all know the statistics on overweight: Currently, 64% of the adult population—or 123 million people—is either overweight or obese. The rate has doubled in children and tripled in adolescents since 1980. Approximately 15% of children and teens are overweight. The problem of overweight/obesity in America costs $117 billion annually and accounts for at least 14% of deaths in the United States, or some 300,000 premature deaths each year. As professional nutritionists, you also know that weight control is the time-honored balance of caloric intake and expenditure. So how do we help overweight children deal with this problem? How do we help prevent other children from becoming overweight?

> ## Could it be that a large decrease in physical activity, not changes in caloric intake, is responsible for increases in childhood obesity rates since 1980?

While everyone agrees that children should be encouraged to eat a healthful diet, weight-loss diets are not the answer. The National Institutes of Health-funded Growing Up Today Study examined a cohort of children who are offspring of the Nurses' Health Study II participants. These children were followed for three years, and those who were on weight-loss diets gained more weight relative to predicted body weight than the nondieters. Binge eating was also associated with dieting to control weight.[1] The authors concluded that for many adolescents, chronic dieting is not only ineffective, but it also may promote weight gain.

In an earlier study, Field and colleagues found that dieting among teens did not necessarily lead to lower caloric intake, nor was dieting restricted to girls who were overweight. Sadly, 50% of the girls who were below the national age-standardized 15th percentile for body mass index (BMI) reported their ideal weight as less than their current weight.[2] Emphasis on thinness and dieting seems to backfire.

A prospective, three-year study of female students in grades 7 to 10 found that restrained eating, body dissatisfaction, drive for thinness, self-induced vomiting, laxative use, diet pill use, and alcohol use significantly increased, while attitudes about physical appearance and self-concept significantly decreased among frequent dieters compared with nondieters.[3]

What about the energy expenditure side of the energy balance equation? A group at Brigham and Women's Hospital in Boston examined a nationwide cohort of 6,149 girls and 4,620 boys aged 9 to 14. They found that in both boys and girls, a one-year increase in BMI was larger in those who reported more time with TV and videos. Larger increases in BMI were also seen among girls who reported higher caloric intakes and less physical activity.[4]

Lisa Sutherland, PhD, RD, research assistant professor of nutrition at the University of North Carolina at Chapel Hill, studied national health data on adolescent obesity, calorie intake, and physical activity from 1980 to 2000. To determine overweight in children, she used National Health and Nutrition Examination Survey II and III and 1999 Centers for Disease Control and Prevention (CDC) data on BMI. Calorie intake was determined using the Nationwide Food Consumption Survey (NFCS) and the Continuing Survey of Food Intake by Individuals from the U.S. Department of Agriculture. Physical activity was determined by examining data from the Youth Risk Behavior Survey, CDC.[5] The result was that in people aged 12 to 19, obesity rose 10% during that time frame; calorie intake rose a mere 1%; and physical activity fell a substantial 13%.

Could it be that a large decrease in physical activity, not changes in caloric intake, is responsible for increases in childhood obesity rates since 1980? Decreased physical activity has an impact on adolescent overweight. Sutherland concluded that both sides of the energy equation need to be addressed when creating community, state, and federal programs and policy that address childhood obesity.

A National Bureau of Economic Research paper by Lakdawalla and Philipson gives compelling evidence that technological change has induced weight gain by making people more sedentary.[6] They argue that 60% of the weight gain seen in the U.S. population may be due to factors such as declining physical activity from technological changes. When was the last time your kids shoveled the driveway? Hung clothes on a clothesline? Chopped wood for the woodstove? Waxed the floor?

A National Association for Sport and Physical Education survey found that 81% of adults said they believe daily physical education should be mandatory in schools. Surprisingly, Illinois is the only state that requires daily physical education classes for students in grades kindergarten through 12. The California Education Code mandates physical education for all students in grades 1 through 9, but only one additional year in the four years of high school. In contrast, Colorado and South Dakota do not have any mandate for physical education at any grade level. The result is that grade school children are now 24% more active than high school students. Schools struggle to meet the demands of state education initiatives and federal initiatives such as "No Child Left Behind," so physical education and recess get squeezed out of the school day.

When trying to solve the puzzle of increasing childhood overweight, ponder this: In my elementary school, we had recess three times per day. In my son's school, they get one 15-minute recess after lunch. I walked to school; now my children take a bus. According to the CDC, 85% of children's trips to school are by car or school bus, and only 13% are on foot or by bike. Does your community have bike racks and sidewalks? Crossing guards? Sutherland suggests that nutrition professionals get active in community programs, creating links with parents to increase opportunities for children to be active. She is currently a coinvestigator in the National Evaluation of the Walk to School Project. This critical evaluation seeks to understand how and why the program works and to identify parent and child barriers that prevent walking or biking to school. (To learn more, check out the CDC Kids Walk to School Program at www.cdc.gov/nccdphp/dnpa/kidswalk.)

American children do not walk as much as others. Susan D. Vincent, PhD, from Brigham Young University used pedometers to measure walking and showed that Americans walked less than their Swedish or Australian counterparts. Swedish boys, for instance, took as many as 18,346 steps per day, Australians took 15,023, and Americans took 13,872 steps.[7]

Schools struggle to meet the demands of state education initiatives and federal initiatives such as "No Child Left Behind," so physical education and recess get squeezed out of the school day.

Often, tight budgets are the scapegoat for cutting physical education, sports, and other opportunities for kids to get active. However, a Harvard School of Public Health survey of 1,002 adults presented at their Spring Obesity conference found that 76% of adults would support measures such as offering more physical education classes and educating parents about healthful eating and exercise, even if it meant higher taxes. Further, 42% would pay $100 more per year in taxes to support these kinds of efforts.

Physically active children gain more than just weight control. A California Study matched scores from the spring 2001 administration of the Stanford Achievement Test, Ninth Edition (SAT-9), with results of the state-mandated physical fitness test, known as the Fitnessgram, given in 2001 to students in grades 5, 7, and 9. Reading and math scores were matched with fitness scores of 353,000 fifth-graders, 322,000 seventh-graders, and 279,000 ninth-graders. Higher achievement was associated with higher levels of fitness at each of the three grade levels measured. The relationship between academic achievement and fitness was greater in mathematics than in reading, particularly at higher fitness levels. Students who met minimum fitness levels in three or more physical fitness areas showed the greatest gains in academic achievement at all three grade levels.

How can nutrition professionals get more information to get more involved?

• Visit www.cdc.gov/mmwr to read a report on how your state measures up. The CDC, in the August 15, 2003, issue of MMWR, "New Physical Activity Measures include Lifestyle Activities, Behavioral Risk Factor Surveillance System 2001" provides baseline data nationally and for each state and U.S. territory based upon the measurements used for 2001.

• The California Department of Education (www.cde. ca.gov/cyfsbranch/lsp/health/pecommunications.htm) has recommendations on physical education for teachers, students, and their families.

• Check out www.presidentschallenge.org, a new interactive Web site to help all Americans build a regular physical activity routine. This Web site tracks progress toward earning presidential awards for active lifestyle and physical fitness.

• Download or order materials from the VERB Campaign (www.cdc.gov/youthcampaign/materials/index. htm) to increase physical activity. The materials feature campaign materials for use with 'tween audiences, including posters, stickers, and temporary tattoos that organizations can order free of charge.

• The CDC also has free brochures to help increase physical activity among elementary and middle school-aged children. The parents' brochure is available in English and Spanish versions at www.cdc.gov/healthyyouth/physicalactivity.

• Learn about the National School Fitness Foundation (www.cdc.gov/youthcampaign/materials/index.htm), a public, nonprofit organization, founded in March 2000 to fight childhood obesity and inactivity. Their Leadership in Fitness Training (LIFT) program offers aerobic and strength training equipment, computerized assessment kiosks, curriculum, and complete faculty training and certification to schools. As of September 2003, the LIFT Program was being utilized by students in more than 450 schools in 18 states (www.nsff.net).

• Use the tools found on www.kidnetic.com, a healthy eating and active living Web site designed for kids aged 9 to 12 and their families to inspire them to move toward healthier lifestyles. Kidnetic.com is also a resource for health professionals and educators to use when working with patients and students. Kidnetic.com is the initial program element of ACTIVATE, an educational outreach program of the International Food Information Council Foundation developed in partnership with the American Academy of Family Physicians, American College of Sports Medicine, American Dietetic Association, International Life Sciences Institute Center for Health Promotion, and National Recreation and Park Association.

References

1. Field AE, et al. *Pediatrics*. 2003;112(4):900-906.
2. Field, et al. *J Am Acad Child Adolesc Psychiatry*. 1993;32(6):1246-1252.
3. French SA. *J Adolesc Health*. 1995;16(6):438-447.
4. Berkey CS, et al. *Pediatrics*. 2000;105(4):E56.
5. Centers for Disease Control and Prevention. National Center for Chronic Disease Prevention and Health Promotion. Youth Risk Behavior Surveillance System, 2001.
6. Lakdawalla D, Philipson T. The Growth of Obesity and Technological Change: A Theoretical and Empirical Examination NBER Working Paper No. w8946. May 2002.
7. Medicine and Science in Sports and Exercise. August 2003. Available at: http://www.ms-se.com

—Carol M. Meerschaert, RD, LDN, is a freelance writer in Falmouth, Me.

Social Change and Obesity Prevention

Where Do We Begin?

Obesity in the United States has reached epidemic proportions in both adults and children. Multi-factorial causes are responsible, including social, economic, and other environmental forces acting on a susceptible genetic heritage. Halting and reversing the epidemic will require multi-factorial solutions, including implementing cognitive coping strategies and mounting an effective social change movement.

John C. Peters, PhD

Dramatic increases during the past 2 decades in the prevalence of overweight and obesity in the United States have prompted medical and public health officials to declare the situation epidemic. Rising obesity rates have also fueled alarming increases in type 2 diabetes in children and adults, projecting a tremendous toll on health and quality of life and an escalating financial burden to individuals and society.[1-5]

Historically, the first response to an epidemic is to find and isolate the causal agent, and then strategies can be put in place to stem the outbreak and prevent future incidents. What is the cause of the obesity epidemic? Can we isolate the offending agent(s) and eradicate the problem? Can we inoculate the population against further attack?

There is an emerging scientific consensus that the recent rise in obesity is a function of multi-factorial causes, reflecting an interaction between our susceptible genetic heritage and an environment that promotes excessive food consumption and a sedentary lifestyle.[6, 7] Our human ancestors developed multiple and redundant biologic systems that encouraged us to eat when food was available and conserve energy when expending it was not required to meet basic survival needs. It is no wonder that in our age of relative food abundance and accessible high-technology machines, people are eating more, moving less, and gaining weight.

Obesity and Our Environment

It is easy to identify characteristics of our everyday environment that promote eating ... from the ready accessibility of food in virtually every locale to large portions and aggressive advertising. Today, food is inexpensive and it takes little time or energy to prepare it for consumption. Thanks to technological advances in food production, stabilization, and preparation, "fast" food is available at home, at school, in the workplace, and in restaurants and other venues throughout our communities. Literally centuries of efforts to create a world in which food availability, cost, and convenience are no longer problems have finally paid off.

However, there are new problems. In addition to the seemingly constant pressure to eat, the temptation or even the requirement to be sedentary is a defining feature of our modern lifestyle—in schools, on the job, and at home. In the most sought-after high-paying jobs, people are essentially paid to be sedentary, spending hours in front of a computer screen managing and transacting business with the click of a mouse. Outside of work we can conduct most aspects of daily business without ever having to step out of our cars. Never has going to the bank, picking up a prescription, or getting dinner been easier or taken less physical exertion. Leisure time entertainment has become increasingly sedentary and ever more attractive, with hundreds of television channels to watch, movies to rent, and electronic games to play. We have engineered the need for physical activity out of our lives to a large extent. Just a few decades ago, physically active jobs were typically low paying and less desirable. Ironically, more and more of us now pay to be physically active, as evidenced by the dramatic growth of the health club market.[8]

As our technological prowess grew and our lifestyle priorities changed, we built our communities to reflect these evolving preferences. Land use and community design changed dramatically in ways that now make it difficult to adopt a more physically active lifestyle, even if this became a priority.[9] For example, traditional early 20th-century neighborhood design followed a characteristic grid pattern in which there were many intersections and few major thoroughfares.[9] It was easy to walk to school; the park, the grocery store, or the beauty salon. Doing business on foot was as safe and convenient as relying on the automobile.

Contemporary neighborhoods are characterized by a more amorphous design, with few intersections and large multilane thoroughfares.[9] Because of land costs in suburban America, new schools are often built miles from population centers so that walking or riding a bike is not an option. Sidewalks are absent from many neighborhoods, making even casual physical activity a safety risk. We have constructed the modern world to best suit conducting our lives from the comfort and safety of our chairs, couches, and automobiles. Inadvertently, we have nearly eliminated the single largest source of physical activity (energy expenditure involved in moving our bodies) from our traditional human existence—walking.

It is easy to find what appear to be important factors in the causal chain leading to obesity. Are these features of our food and physical activity environment the root causes of obesity, or are they merely symptoms of deeper sociocultural issues? Clearly, no one set out to make the American public obese. The myriad businesses that promote food consumption and physical inactivity are not purposefully targeted at making people gain weight. So what is driving the epidemic?

Sociocultural Drivers of Obesity

One could argue that these "obesigenic" features of our environment arose and evolved to meet the demands of a population that was seeking the proverbial American dream. Who *wouldn't* want abundant food that was convenient, tasted great, and was inexpensive? Who *wouldn't* want a subsistence that didn't require hard physical exertion? Who *wouldn't* want wide access to affordable and enjoyable entertainment?

In the tradition of our ancestors, most of us toil to make a better life for our children, to make life easier in every way, so future generations can be as happy and productive as possible. Individuals and society have benefited enormously from the technological advances that have transformed the food supply, the workplace,

and our community and home environments. Standards of living for most people have never been higher. The food is less expensive, more convenient, and tastes better than ever. We don't have to do hard physical labor on the job, but there have been unintended consequences of achieving this once only-imagined American dream.

Prominent among them is the ever-accelerating pace of our modern globally connected "electronic" lives. "Keeping up" not only eliminates the time we would otherwise spend preparing wholesome nutritious meals and enjoying physical activity but also adds stress to our lives, reducing sleep and making us vulnerable to eating as a way to medicate the stress. To top it off, a multitude of sedentary entertainment options help us cope with the strain brought about by life in the fast lane.

All of these environmental features and adaptive behaviors provide immediate gratification and are strong drivers of the choices we make every day about what and how much to eat and how much physical activity in which to engage. However, in our quest for the American dream, we haven't taken time to examine the long-term health consequences on body weight and chronic disease of these short-term benefits. The question is: now that we are beginning to recognize these unintended consequences and confront the problem … what do we do about it?

The underlying cultural, economic, and social drivers that shaped our current environment are so complex and interrelated that changing the environment will be a long-term process—but it is one that can begin today. Although there is a natural tendency to search for the single cause or "villain" in the obesity epidemic, this will be essentially impossible to do retrospectively, and finding someone or something to blame will not solve the obesity crisis. Rather, we must embark on two parallel efforts: First, we need to mount a concerted social change movement to create a future state in which healthy lifestyle behaviors are socially normative behavior. Second, we need to provide people with better tools to support cognitive management of body weight within the prevailing environment—before the future state becomes a reality.

The solution: two parallel efforts—a social change movement to create socially normative healthy lifestyle behaviors and tools to help in cognitive management of body weight.

Building for Social Change

What will this take? There are numerous examples of previous successful social change campaigns, including the recycling movement, smoking cessation campaigns, and the move toward routine seat belt use.[10] These movements shared many common features, including a definition of the crisis in immediate terms relevant to individuals, eg, "how will this affect me personally" a strong science base, and the importance of a solution that was economically feasible and sensible. Although there is currently much media attention on the obesity epidemic, recent surveys show the average consumer does not place this at the top of his or her list of personal concerns.[11]

Perhaps one way to highlight the immediacy and personally threatening nature of the crisis is to highlight the externality of this issue. That is, to show how unhealthy lifestyle choices by one individual may have a negative effect on others—without their consent. The turning point in the movement to provide wide availability of smoke-free environments was driven by the release of the secondhand smoke report in the mid-1980s, which showed that one person's decision to smoke can have a negative health effect on nonsmokers via secondhand smoke.[10] This was seen as a violation of personal liberty, one of the strongest values in America. One could apply the same logic to eating and physical activity health behaviors. For example, among participants in a group health insurance plan, those making healthy lifestyle choices and consequently spending less on healthcare are effectively subsidizing other consumers who may not be making healthy choices and consequently cost the insured group more money. If this situation were made clear to those in the group making healthy lifestyle choices, they might be inspired to drive a campaign for change—tied to our American values of personal liberty and fairness/justice.

Build in immediate benefits for healthy choices to reinforce them

---

In the end, a successful social change movement will require cooperation among all sectors of society—public and private. Creating and sustaining a future state in which the prevailing environment supports healthy eating and physical activity behaviors will require institutionalizing incentive systems that provide people with immediate benefits for "doing the right thing." Years of public health and behavioral research has shown that few people will change these immediately rewarding behaviors based solely on the long-term promise of better "health."[12–14] In our current environment and social system, there are essentially no short-term incentives to maintain healthful eating and physical activity patterns. Instead, health behaviors must come from within the individual—supported by a level of self-actualization that is likely present in only a minority of the population. Because the immediate benefits of eating too much and moving too little are strongly reinforced by our biologic predisposition (eat when food is available and rest when

you can), the incentives (and possibly disincentives) for alternative behaviors will have to be strong and compelling.

Building Better Coping Skills

Comprehensive social change will take time, yet the obesity epidemic is worsening rapidly. We need to provide people now with better tools to use in their day-to-day lives to combat weight gain. In the current environment, we can no longer rely on our body's inherent physiology to manage body weight—we will need to exert cognitive control over the current environmental pressures to eat and be sedentary.[15] Current diet and physical activity guidelines are difficult to implement for many people. For example, although the current guidelines recommend a certain number of servings of specific food types and so many minutes of physical activity per day, how many people can or do keep cumulative track of their progress toward these goals during the day. Most of us don't carry food diaries to log our servings of fruits and vegetables or stop watches to log the number of minutes we spend in various activities. Furthermore, most people don't know how to equate the energy value of food and physical activity, so they do not have the knowledge or skills to balance energy intake and energy expenditure. Finally, the diet and physical activity goals set by public health authorities may be scientifically sound and appropriate, but for many people, starting from where they are, these targets may seem too high and too far out of reach to even begin contemplating change.

As a nation, we need to set more realistic goals for combating obesity. *Healthy People 2010* set as a goal to reduce obesity prevalence to 15%[16]—we are now at more than 30%[17] and rising! A more realistic goal might be to simply stop any further excess weight gain in the population—among adults and children. Over time, this would lead to reductions in population obesity prevalence as our youth would not join the ranks of the overweight when they became adults—but what about adults who are already overweight and obese? Stopping further weight gain alone could have tremendously positive benefits for health and healthcare costs.[18] Furthermore, even if we were to focus on reversing established obesity, we have had little success in doing so with individually focused treatments thus far,[19, 20] and there are no proven effective population-based solutions.

Better coping skills and more realistic targets for decreasing overweight are needed

---

To stop weight gain, we need to provide people with simple tools to better cope within the current environment—actionable solutions that can help them balance energy in and energy out. Increasing lifestyle physical activity would seem to be a promising approach to helping manage energy balance, because it is easy to monitor using readily available technology and can be related to the energy value of food. A recent report shows that the median weight gain of the US population is approximately 2 lb per year.[7] A positive energy balance of 100 kcal/day can explain the weight gain of 90% of the population. Simply eating less and moving more in some combination adding up to 100 kcal/day could stop weight gain in 90% of the population.[7] On the physical activity side of the equation, walking 2,000 additional steps (almost a mile) each day would burn the entire 100 kcal. In addition, taking 100 calories out of daily food intake would be equally accessible using simple strategies such as like food substitution (eg, using a reduced-fat or reduced-calorie option) and portion "right-sizing."

Cutting back a little on eating or increasing energy output by 100 calories a day would help a lot

---

Using a combination of both strategies would offer consumers the most flexibility and choice—as long as we can keep it simple and consumers can easily keep track. Monitoring the extra steps (walking) is easy using inexpensive electronic pedometers and can be an easy first step toward implementing a strategy to stop weight gain.[21] Framing the problem and the solution in these terms—small steps can have a big impact—might seem less daunting for individuals and the population as a whole, and it offers hope that making progress in combating obesity may be surprisingly within our reach.

As an example of this approach—simple steps to better health—is a new national initiative called America on the Move (**www.americaonthemove.org**). Sponsored by a nonprofit public-private organization, the Partnership to Promote Healthy Eating and Active Living, America on the Move (AOM) promotes a simple and fun way for people to begin the process of adopting a healthier lifestyle. Based on the analysis showing that weight gain could be prevented by a reduction in positive energy balance of only 100 calories per day,[7] AOM emphasizes making small daily changes in eating and walking that can fit with peoples' hectic lives. As a start, the initiative encourages people to take 2,000 more steps per day than they take currently (monitored by a pedometer) and to reduce food intake by 100 calories. The program was successfully pilot tested in Colorado, showing that these goals are easily achievable by the majority of participants.[21] AOM was launched nationally on the Internet in July 2003 and is currently being implemented into communities via a network of state affiliates. Ongoing research (J.O. Hill, personal communication) is

showing that once people reach these initial goals, their confidence and self-efficacy increase and they often go beyond to achieve more challenging health behavior goals. Importantly, AOM is working with both the public and private sectors, including the retail and food industries, to provide incentives and other support in work sites, schools, restaurants, businesses, and communities for people to engage in these healthy behaviors.

Solving the obesity crisis facing the nation today will likely take generations. Obesity is a multifaceted problem that will require multifaceted and comprehensive solutions. It will take time to generate the political will to begin changing the systems and institutions and social values that support the current environment and that, in effect, reward people for practicing behaviors that promote obesity. It will take time before we find affordable and sustainable ways of engaging and rewarding people to "do the right thing" from a purely personal health perspective. It will take time for society to evolve so that leading a healthy active lifestyle becomes "normative behavior" and, thus, becomes self-sustaining. As a society, we will succeed in bringing about these changes because we must—we can't afford not to. In the meantime, we should all be working to inspire our families, friends, and communities to take those first small steps that can have a big effect. After all, you have to start somewhere.

Notes

1. McGinnis JM, Foege WH, Actual causes of death in the United States. *JAMA*. 1993;270:2207–2212.
2. Allison DB, Fontaine KR, Manson JE, Stevens J, VanItallie TB. Annual deaths attributable to obesity in the United States. *JAMA*. 1999;282: 1530–1538.
3. Sturm R, Wells KB. Does obesity contribute as much to morbidity as poverty or smoking? *Public Health*. 2001;115:229–235.
4. Ford ES, Williamson DF, Liu S. Weight change and diabetes incidence: findings from a national cohort of U.S. adults. *Am J Epidemiol*. 1997;146:214–222.
5. Wolf AM, Colditz GA. Current estimates of the economic cost of obesity in the United States. *Obes Res*. 1998;6:97–106.
6. Hill JO, Peters JC. Environmental contributions to the obesity epidemic, *Science*. 1998;280:1371–1374.
7. Hill JO, Wyatt HR, Reed GW, Peters JC. Obesity and the environment: where do we go from here? *Science*. 2003;299:853–855.
8. Sturm R. The economics of physical activity: societal trends and rationales for interventions. *Am J Prev Med*. 2004. In press.
9. Saelens BE, Sallis JF, Frank LD. Environmental correlates of walking and cycling: findings from the transportation, urban design, and planning literatures. *Ann Behav Med*. 2003;25:80–91.

10. Economos CD, Brownson RC, DeAngelis, MA, et al. What lessons have been learned from other attempts to guide social change? *Nutrition Reviews.* 2001;59:S40–S56.

11. Lee T and Oliver JE. Public opinion and the politics of America's obesity epidemic. Available at: `http://ksgnotesl.harvard.edu/Research/wpaper.nsf/rwp/RW PO2-017?OpenDocumen.` Accessed March 3, 2003.

12. Hill JO, Goldberg GP, Pate RR, Peters JC. Summit on promoting healthy eating and active living: developing a framework for progress. *Nutr Rev.* 2001;59:S4–S6.

13. Wetter AC, Goldberg GP, King AC, et al. How and why do individuals make food and physical activity choices? *Nutr Rev.* 2001;59:S11–S20.

14. Booth SL, Sallis JF, Ritenbaugh C, et al. Environmental and societal factors affect food choice and physical activity: rationale, influences and leverage points. *Nutr Rev.* 2001;59:S21–S39.

15. Peters JC, Wyatt HR, Donahoo WT, Hill JO. From instinct to intellect: The challenge of maintaining health weight in the modern world. *Obesity Reviews.* 2002;3:69–74.

16. U.S. Department of Health and Human Services. *Healthy People 2010: Understanding and Improving Health and Objectives for Improving Health.* Washington, DC: Government Printing Office; 2000.

17. Flegal KM, Carroll MD, Ogden CL, Johnson CL. Prevalence and trends in obesity among US adults, 1999–2000. *JAMA.* 2002;288: 1723–1727.

18. Willett WC, Manson JE, Stampfer MJ, et al. Weight, weight change, and coronary heart disease in women. Risk within the "normal" weight range. *JAMA.* 1995;273:461–465.

19. Wing RR. Behavioral interventions for obesity: recognizing our progress and future challenges. *Obesity Res.* 2003; 11:3S–6S.

20. Lowe MR. Self-regulation of energy intake in the prevention and treatment of obesity: Is it feasible? *Obesity Res.* 2003;11:44S–59S.

21. Wyatt HR, Peters JC, Reed GW, et al. Using electronic step counters to increase lifestyle physical activity: Colorado on the move. *J Physical Activity Health.* 2004. In press.

John C. Peters, PhD, is the Head, Nutrition Science Institute, and Associate Director of Food and Beverage Technology, Procter and Gamble, Cincinnati, Ohio.

Correspondence: John Peters, PhD, Procter and Gamble, 11810 Miami River Rd, Room 1D32A, Box 742, Cincinnati, OH 45252 (e-mail: Peters.jc.1@pg.com).

UNIT 5

Health Claims

Unit Selections

Key Points to Consider

- How can consumers protect themselves from misinformation in the nutrition field?

- Discuss advantages and disadvantages of the Food Industry developing functional foods?

- Research the interactions among the two most popular herbal supplements, Echinacea Purpurea and St. John's wort combined with antidepressant medications.

- What is your opinion of assessing your own risk for degenerative disease and self-prescribing supplements?

- What should the role of the FDA be in monitoring and regulating use of supplements?

Student Website

www.mhcls.com/online

Internet References

Further information regarding these websites may be found in this book's preface or online.

Federal Trade Commission (FTC): Diet, Health & Fitness
http://www.ftc.gov/bcp/menu-health.htm

Food and Drug Administration (FDA)
http://www.fda.gov/default.htm

National Council Against Health Fraud (NCAHF)
http://www.ncahf.org

QuackWatch
http://www.quackwatch.com

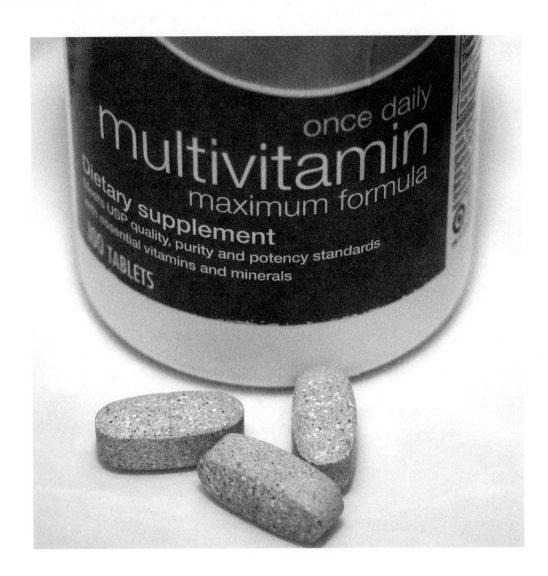

Americans spend approximately $25 billion on alternative treatments. According to an American Dietetic Association (ADA) Survey, ninety percent of consumers polled get their nutrition information from television, magazines, and newspapers.

It is very discouraging that Americans are confused and overwhelmed about the controversies surrounding food and health and that they have stopped paying attention to the contradictory claims reported by news media. The media very frequently misinterpret results, simplify them, and take them out of context. Additionally the media is too eager to publish sensational information and not solid science. A new source of information is the Internet, which allows distribution and promotion of just about anything. About 29 percent of Americans turn to the Internet for information. We need to be vigilant as to the type of information we get from different Web sites.

Functional foods are foods that may provide a health benefit beyond basic nutrition and are becoming one of the fastest growing segments of the food industry especially among affluent baby boomers. The US government has no regulatory category of functional foods. Despite their popularity, their efficacy and safety is questionable due to lack of scientific evidence. So we are far from declaring them "magic bullets" to improve health and prevent disease. Omega-3 fatty acids and omega-6 fatty acids, referred to as functional fatty acids are very popular supplements nowadays because of their benefits on heart disease, cancer prevention and treatment, and brain and eye development. The consumer though, should be advised to eat a variety of foods that contain the above fatty acids as part of an overall healthful diet. The same applies to soy and soy products that the food industry is developing because of their beneficial role on bone health, cancer, and cardiovascular disease among others. Scientists are also developing new lines of crops with intense antioxidant pigments that alter the color, flavor, and antioxidant content of the plant. Questions about enriching the food supply with megadoses of a single nutrient without studying the health risks on the population are some of the questions addressed by one of the articles.

Herbal supplements have become very popular in the US but what the consumer does not know is that manufacturers have problems with quality control. Activity of the herbal product components depends on many factors and what the label describes is not usually what is in the bottle. Safety of herbal supplements and their interactions with other herbs and medications are generally unknown. It is unsettling to discover the adverse health problems through cases of people who died due to the above interactions.

Using Nutrition-Related Claims to Build a Healthful Diet

The newly released *Dietary Guidelines for Americans, 2005* provides the latest scientific consensus about the role that diet plays in living a healthful lifestyle. It also points to the importance of providing consumers with the necessary tools so that they can be successful in meeting that goal. The role of nutrition communicators, dietitians, and other health professionals in helping Americans learn how to implement the new *Dietary Guidelines* cannot be overemphasized. Various educational tools exist, and as the new *Dietary Guidelines* points out, "the food label and the Nutrition Facts panel provide information that is useful for implementing the key recommendations in the *Dietary Guidelines* and should be integrated into educational and communication messages."

Consumers indicate that they are looking at labels to make food choices. According to the *2004 Food Marketing Institute (FMI)/Prevention Magazine: Shopping for Health* consumer trends survey, shoppers are buying products that claim to reduce the risk of disease. Forty-two percent of respondents said that they have purchased foods claiming to reduce their risk of developing heart disease, and 26 percent said that they

had purchased foods claiming to reduce the risk of cancer. We also know that consumers are interested in seeking out foods on the basis of the health-related benefits that they provide. In fact, consumers state that they want to learn more about such foods.

Today, the food label offers more complete, useful, and accurate information than ever before. Fifteen years have passed since the enactment of the Nutrition Labeling and Education Act (NLEA)—and as the scientific community continues to learn more about the emerging research on diet and health—more and more foods bear nutrition-related claims to inform consumers of the special nutritional properties that certain foods and dietary supplements may deliver. NLEA was designed to give consumers scientifically valid information about the foods that they eat, including the use of "truthful, non-misleading, and useful" label statements that describe the relationship between a food and health-related conditions. With oversight from the US Food and Drug Administration (FDA) and the US Department of Agriculture (USDA), food labels provide a wealth of information that consum-

ers can use. In fact, FDA has been increasing its efforts to expand opportunities for food manufacturers to provide meaningful, up-to-date information to consumers about the health effects of their dietary choices, through additional health claims based on emerging science ("qualified" health claims).

With more emphasis on the recommendation/advice to *"get the most nutrition out of our calories"* in the words of the recently released *Dietary Guidelines for Americans, 2005*, there is an even greater need for consumers to understand how to put this information into practice. The Nutrition Facts Panel and label claims on the food package can be used to identify the amount of key nutrients a serving provides to help ensure consumption of essential nutrients for good health. Rather than using the food label to determine only those nutrients that should potentially be decreased in the diet, consumers can also use the food label to learn which foods provide important nutrients that should be increased in the diet. Further, nutrition-related claims also provide consumers with the opportunity to learn about the positive health benefits of various nutrients and food components not included on the Nutrition Facts panel.

What's in a Claim? Making Sense of Nutrition-Related Claims

Claims on food labels are made to identify the nutrition-related attribute of a food. Regulated claims that can be used on food and dietary supplement labels fall into the following categories: (1) health claims, (2) nutrient content claims, (3) structure-function claims, and (4) dietary guidance statements. For the first two, health and nutrient content claims, a food must meet criteria pre-approved by the FDA.

1) Health claims confirm a relationship between a food or a component in a food—such as calcium, fat, soluble fiber, soy protein, or plant sterols—and risk of a health-related condition or disease, like heart disease or cancer. Health claims can be authorized in three ways:

- NLEA-Authorized Health Claims. These claims are based on a rigorous review of scientific literature, using a *significant scientific agreement (SSA)* standard. They are sometimes called unqualified health claims because they meet the SSA standard and do not require a qualifying statement to explain the state of the science (see Qualified Health Claims below). *"Diets low in saturated fat and cholesterol that include 25 grams of soy protein a day may reduce the risk of heart disease. One serving of [name of food] provides X grams of soy protein"* is an example of an unqualified health claim.
- Authoritative Statements Based on the Food and Drug Administration Modernization Act of 1997 (FDAMA). This Act allows a health claim to be used on the basis of an authoritative statement by a scientific body of the US government or the National Acad-

emy of Sciences. They still must be approved by FDA. An example of a FDAMA-authorized health claim is *"Diets containing foods that are a good source of potassium and that are low in sodium may reduce the risk of high blood pressure and stroke."*

- Qualified Health Claims. The launch in March 2003 of FDA's Consumer Health Information for Better Nutrition Initiative provided for the use of qualified health claims to communicate emerging evidence for a relationship between a food, food component, or a dietary supplement and the reduced risk of a disease or health-related condition. Therefore, qualified health claims convey a developing relationship between components in the diet and risk of disease on the basis of the *weight of the credible scientific evidence available.* "Qualifying" language is included as part of the claim to indicate that the evidence supporting the claim has not yet reached the standard of SSA. An example of a qualified health claim is, *"Scientific evidence suggests but does not prove that eating 1.5 ounces per day of most nuts [such as name of specific nut] as part of a diet low in saturated fat and cholesterol may reduce the risk of heart disease."*

2) Nutrient content claims
on a food label characterize the level of a nutrient in a serving of the food. This type of claim is authorized under NLEA. To make this type of claim, a food product must contain a FDA-designated amount of the nutrient per reference amount (or standard serving size). Example phrases used for nutrient content claims include excellent source of [nutrient], good source of [nutrient], fat-free, rich in [nutrient], low cholesterol, reduced saturated fat, less sugar, more fiber, light, and many more.

3) Structure-function claims
describe the role of a nutrient or di-

etary ingredient that affects or maintains the normal structure or function of the body. For example, "calcium builds strong bones," "fiber maintains bowel regularity," or "lycopene maintains cell integrity."

4) Dietary Guidance Statements are statements on a label that describe the health effects of a broad category of foods. FDA, as part of a cooperative effort with the National Cancer Institute (NCI), offers this dietary guidance message for consumers: *"Diets rich in fruits and vegetables may reduce the risk of some types of cancer and other chronic diseases."*

Consumers can use nutrition labels to make informed food choices for improved health. However, the food label is only one way to guide consumers to make healthful dietary choices; the food label is a tool and does not, in and of itself, provide education to consumers. Research shows time and again that consumers continue to be confused by nutrition information; they often state that they hear conflicting advice from a variety of sources—family, friends, professional colleagues, journalists, and the Internet, among others. This can result in information overload. Thus, the context that can help put the information into perspective and therefore, practice, is often lacking.

Consumer-based communications and education are essential to the success and effectiveness of any dietary guidance or food labeling system. Additional consumer research is needed to better understand how and to what extent labeling information is used and understood by consumers. This will ensure that the information effectively promotes consumer awareness and is helpful in making purchase decisions, allowing consumers the opportunity to better implement the *Dietary Guidelines for Americans, 2005.* In the meantime, health professionals, in coordination with other health communicators such as the government, media, and industry, have the opportunity to provide the context that consumers need to interpret labels so that they can translate the information into a set of actionable choices that will lead to achieving the goal of an overall healthful diet and lifestyle.

Reprinted from the International Food Information Council Foundation, 2005, pp. 2-3.

Nutraceuticals
& Functional Foods

LINDA MILO OHR
Contributing Editor, Chicago, Ill.
l_milo@yahoo.com

Functional Fatty Acids

News about fatty acids has evolved from the negative to the positive. Media focus on the evils of *trans* fatty acids is shifting to the benefits of specific fatty acids, mostly the omega-3 fatty acids. Not only do these ingredients provide benefits across a span of health conditions, they also provide these benefits to people across a range of ages, from infants to the elderly.

Omega-3s received a recent boost in consumer awareness with both the Food and Drug Administration's 2004 qualified heart-health claim and the newly revised *2005 Dietary Guidelines for Americans*. The Dietary Guidelines recognize that "limited evidence suggests an association between consumption of fatty acids in fish and reduced risks of mortality from cardiovascular disease for the general population." In addition, they recognize that there are other sources of docosahexaenoic acid (DHA) and eicosapentaenoic acid (EPA) that may provide similar cardiovascular benefits, but state that "more research is needed."

"The market for omega-3s is growing at a double-digit rate in the U.S., as well as in the EU," says Beth Way, Market Development Specialist, Encapsulation, National Starch Food Innovation, Bridgewater, N.J., citing information from Frost & Sullivan. "Industry observers note that market opportunities for omega-3 fatty acids in the global nutrition and food fortification markets could reach a conservative value of $500 million. Current estimated North American consumption for fish-oil-based omega-3 fatty acids in dietary supplements, excluding infant formula, is 6–10 times higher compared to the food sector. Supplement sales grew from $103 million in 1999 to $230 million in 2004."

> Naturlinea products are fortified with safflower-derived conjugated linoleic acid, a fatty acid that has shown to help reduce body fat.

DHA and EPA are the two omega-3 fatty acids currently in the media spotlight. The qualified heart-health claim specifically mentions them. Although omega-3 fatty acids are the most widely reported on and most commonly known, other fatty acids, both polyunsaturated and monounsaturated, show promise for health benefits as well. They include alphalinolenic acid, oleic acid, and conjugated linoleic acid.

Benefits of Omega-3

"Awareness of the positive health benefits of omega-3 is high, with most consumer studies suggesting 60% have heard of omega-3 and believe it is positive," says Ian Lucas, Vice President of Marketing and New Product Development, Ocean Nutrition Canada. "We have conducted our own qualitative primary research with over 250 individual consumers, and every market research project was consistent with the trends published in the syndicated reports. Our studies suggested that 60% of people have heard of omega-3 and believe it is important for health; 80% associated it with fish. Most people we interviewed associated heart health and brain health with eating fish." Infant development and cancer prevention and treatment are other areas where omega-3 fatty acids show benefits.

• **Cardiovascular Health.** According to the American Heart Association (AHA) large-scale epidemiological studies suggest that individuals at risk for coronary heart disease (CHD) benefit from the consumption of plant- and marine-derived omega-3 fatty acids (AHA website).

"EPA prevents vascular inflammation, which can lead to plaque buildup that can ultimately lead to narrowing of the coronary vessels on the heart," explains Lucas. "At the same time, DHA is considered to be important in the electrical conduction in the heart and is associated with reducing ventricular arrhythmias. Strong scientific evidence has actually led to an EPA/DHA supplement product in Italy being indicated as a prescription for preventing a second heart attack."

In September 2004, the Food and Drug Administration announced the availability of a qualified health claim for reduced risk of CHD on conventional foods that contain EPA and DHA. PDA recommends that consumers not exceed more than a total of 3 g of EPA and DHA per day, with no more than 2 g/day from a dietary supplement.

"The heart-health benefits of EPA and DHA position products very well for the Baby Boomer generation," observes Lucas. "In addition, the anti-inflammatory effects of EPA are suited for middle age people with arthritis."

Ocean Nutrition's *MEG-3™ Omega-3 Powder* is currently used in several bread products in the United States and other countries, says Lucas. For example, in January 2005, Wegman's Food Markets, Rochester, N.Y., launched a line of breads fortified with *MEG-3* omega-3 fats: *100% Whole Wheat, 12 Grain and Very Low Sodium Bread*, two slices of which offers 80–90 mg of omega-3s.

"*MEG-3™ Omega-3 Powder* ingredient is really a breakthrough technology in that it provides the health benefits of fish, conveniently in food products people love, without the taste or smell of fish," states Lucas. "Our patented microencapsulation technology is very unique. It is a free-flowing powder with undetectable free oil, meaning the goodness of fish is kept inside the powder, so foods don't smell or taste fishy."

Another encapsulated omega-3 fatty acid ingredient will also help make it easier to produce fortified baked goods. Earlier this year, National Starch Innovation introduced *Novomega™* encapsulated omega-3. The powder ingredient is the result of a joint agreement by National Starch and Omega Protein, Houston, Tex., a producer of fish oil and protein products derived from menhaden. The ingredient is said to be easily added to baked goods without affecting their taste, texture, or aroma.

Independent sensory research has shown that *Novomega* can be incorporated into foods without affecting flavor, which is still the number one criteria for purchase, says Way. "We have found a way to protect this valuable ingredient from harsh processing, other ingredient interaction, and light and air, which contribute to rancidity."

• **Infant Nutrition.** Omega-3 fatty acids also fortify many infant formulas, such as Mead Johnson Nutritionals' *Enfamil*® *Lipil*® *with Iron*. It contains both DHA and arachidonic acid (ARA), an omega-6 fatty acid. The two fatty acids support a baby's brain and eye development.

A study using the product showed that it helped to significantly improve the visual development of infants compared to non-supplemented formula (Hoffman et al., 2003). Researchers at the Retina Foundation of the Southwest in Dallas, Tex., studied babies who were breastfed from birth to four to six months and then randomly weaned either to the formula supplemented with DHA and ARA or to a formula without them. The babies fed the supplemented formula had improved visual acuity at one year of age, compared to the babies fed the non-supplemented formula.

"The successful addition of DHA and ARA to infant formula has helped consumers become aware of the need for these important nutrients," observes Laura Coury, Director, Marketing Food & Beverage, Martek Biosciences, Columbia, Md. "This also has paved the way to reach consumers outside of the traditional infant formula market. Some infant formula companies are now offering DHA and ARA fortified formulas for toddlers up to 24 months old. Their moms understand the health benefits of DHA, creating a ready-made market for more DHA-fortified foods. Food manufacturers are looking at ways to take advantage of this opportunity by adding DHA to their food products."

In February of this year, for example, Martek signed a non-exclusive license agreement with Kellogg Co., under which it will supply DHA for use in a new line of fortified foods. Products containing microalgae-derived Martek DHA are expected to hit the shelves by mid-2006. The *Martek DHA* logo will appear on packaging, in print advertisements, and on other promotional materials.

• **Brain and Eye Development.** Infants are not the only ones who benefit from omega-3 fatty acids' role in brain and eye development. "EPA's effect on triglyceride lowering, inflammation, and plaque formation can maintain a healthy blood flow to the brain, while DHA is an important structural component of the brain," says Lucas. "Research suggests 60% of the brain is made up of fat, and half the fat is DHA. EPA and DHA are therefore important for normal brain and nervous system growth and development." Research indicates that omega-3 deficiencies may be linked to attention deficit/hyperactivity disorder (ADHD), dyslexia, depression and aggression, Alzheimer's disease, and dementia.

"Since there is a strong association with brain health and development, we expect to see many products in the future with EPA and DHA associated with foods for people who are in school or are learning" says Lucas.

• **Cancer Prevention and Treatment.** The American Institute for Cancer Research (AICR) states that omega-3 fatty acids have displayed a range of anti-cancer activities in the laboratory and have been repeatedly associated with lower cancer risks in population studies (American Institute for Cancer Research, 2004).

Research funded by AICR has shown that adding omega-3 fatty acids to the diet of mice can actually reduce the occurrence of tumors and slow tumor growth. W. Elaine Hardman, a researcher at the Pennington Biomedical Research Center of Louisiana State University, has received several AICR grants to study the cancer-fighting potential of omega-3 fatty acids.

Her previous AICR-funded research has demonstrated that omega-3s also have a potential role in helping chemotherapy drugs work more effectively and in reducing side effects from cancer treatment.

Another AICR grantee is investigating another possible protective mechanism. Researchers Robert Chapkin and Joanne Lupton of Texas A&M University are investigating how DHA interferes with a specific protein that is critical for tumor formation in the colon.

Studies on Other Fatty Acids

Studies have been conducted on various other fatty acids, as well:

• **Alpha-Linolenic Acid** (ALA) is found in a variety of green leafy vegetables, some types of nuts, canola oil, flaxseed oil, and flaxseed supplements and can be converted to omega-3 fatty acids in the body. Two recent studies showed ALA's benefits in cardiovascular disease

(CVD). At the November 2004 AHA Scientific Sessions, researchers reported that protection from sudden cardiac death in women may be linked with a diet rich in ALA (Albert et al., 2004). Women who reported eating diets rich in oils containing ALA seemed to have a lower risk of dying from heart disease and sudden cardiac death than women whose diets were low in the plant-derived fatty acid.

Researchers at Pennsylvania State University reported last year that a diet rich in ALA reduced CVD risk, possibly by favorably changing vascular inflammation and endothelial dysfunction (Zhao et al., 2004). Inflammatory markers and lipids and lipoproteins were assessed in hypercholesterolemic subjects fed two diets low in saturated fat and cholesterol and high in polyunsaturated fatty acids varying in ALA and linoleic acid compared to those fed an average American diet.

- **Oleic acid** is a monounsaturated fatty acid, most commonly associated with olive oil. Recent experiments using breast cancer cell lines showed that the fatty acid dramatically cut the levels of an oncogene called Her-2/neu (also known as erb B-2) (Menendez et al., 2005). High levels of Her-2/neu occur in more than a fifth of breast cancer patients and are associated with highly aggressive tumors that have a poor prognosis.

A team of researchers in both the U.S. and Spain reported not only that oleic acid suppressed over-expression of the gene but also that other tests on the cell lines showed that it also boosted the effectiveness of trastuzumab (Herceptin), the monoclonal antibody treatment that targets the Her-2/neu gene and has helped to prolong the lives of many breast cancer patients.

- **Conjugated Linoleic Acid** (CLA), derived from both dairy and safflower sources, has reported benefits in cancer and body composition or body shaping. The majority of research to date has focused on the biological effects of the *cis*-9, *trans*-11 and *trans*-10, *cis*-12 CLA isomers. Dairy-derived CLA, for example, has been shown to inhibit carcinogenesis in experimental animals (Ip et al., 1999).

A group headed by Dale Bauman at Cornell University works with dairy-derived CLA, looking at the effects of CLA in cancer models. Some of the group's earlier work determined that the CLA in milk fat can function as an anti-carcinogen. They designed a diet that enhanced the *cis*-9, *trans*-11 CLA content of milk fat in milk collected from cows. Workers in Cornell's Food Science Dept. used the milk to produce a butter that had a CLA content eightfold greater than control butter. Researchers at Roswell Park Cancer Institute, Buffalo, N.Y., used the butter in a study of chemically induced mammary carcinogenesis in rats. The CLA-enhanced butter was shown to be effective in reducing tumor formation (The Bauman Group).

Bauman Group is continuing research on the effects of CLA in cancer models and is looking at the effects of a high-CLA butter in an atherosclerosis model. The group is also involved in on-going research to find feeding/management practices that will elevate and maintain *cis*-9, *trans*-11 CLA levels in milk fat (Lock and Bauman, 2004).

Commercial forms of CLA currently available in the marketplace are derived from safflower oil. These have shown benefits in weight control. A brand of CLA called *Tonalin CLA*®, supplied by Cognis Nutrition and Health, Cincinnati, Ohio, was shown to help reduce body fat mass in healthy overweight humans when taken as a dietary supplement for one year (Gaullier et al, 2004). The study concluded that that the CLA safely reduced body fat mass by as much as 9%. According to the company, the randomized; double-blind, placebo-controlled study is the first to document the long-term safety and efficacy of CLA supplementation over a 12-month period without additional lifestyle or dietary restrictions.

Study participants who took 3.4 g of CLA/day experienced a significant reduction in their body fat mass compared to those in the placebo group, said Jean-Michel Gaullier, project manager of the study.

A panel of independent experts has found that *Tonalin* is safe for use in yogurt, meal-replacement bars and drinks, fruit juices, chocolate, milk-based beverages, and coffee cream substitutes. The ingredient was introduced for the first time in food products last year from the Spanish dairy Corporacion Alimentaria Penasanta (CAPSA) (Fig 1.). Called *Naturlinea*, the line includes a milk and orange juice-milk blend. The *Tonalin* logo is featured on the milk carton, which features a claim for helping to reduce body fat.

Cognis produces the ingredient through a proprietary process that converts linoleic acid from safflower into CLA. The company will soon be publishing a study showing that the ingredient can keep fat cells from refilling with fat, protecting dieters from regaining lost weight, potentially preventing the yo-yo diet effect.

Another commercial form of safflower oil-derived CLA, *Clarinol*™, has also been shown to have benefits on body composition. Last year, its manufacturer, Lipid Nutrition, Channahon, Ill., announced that *Clarinol* CLA may use four structure function claims: it reduces weight gain, increases lean muscle mass, reduces the amount of body fat, and maintains body weight level. According to the company, its unique manufacturing method suppresses the inclusion of isomers other than *cis*-9, *trans*-11 and *trans*-10, *cis*-12, yielding the highest available concentration for these two active CLA isomers, which have been identified as being helpful in reducing the amount of body fat and increasing lean muscle mass.

REFERENCES

Albert, C., Oh, K., Whang, W., Manson, J.E., Chae, C.U., Stampfer, M.J., Willett, W.C., and Hu, F.B. 2004. American Heart Association meeting report: Protection from sudden cardiac death in women may be linked with a diet rich in alpha-linolenic acid. News release Nov. 8, Am. Heart Assn., Dallas, Tex, http://scientificsessions.american-heart.org/portal/scientificsessions/ss/newsrelease11.08.04b.

American Heart Association. Fish and Omega-3 Fatty Acids, http://www.americanheart.org/presenter.jhtml?identifier=4632.

American Institute for Cancer Research. 2004. Experts Concerned Over Unhealthy "Fat Ratio" in American Diets. Press Release, May 13.

The Bauman Group, http://www.ansci.cornell.edu/bauman/

Gaullier, J.M., Halse, J., Hoye, K., Kristiansen, K., Fagertun, H., Vik, H., and Gudmundsen, O. 2004. Conjugated linoieic acid supplementation for 1 year reduces body fat mass in healthy overweight humans. Am. J. Clin. Nutr. 79: 1118-1125.

Hoffman, D.R., Birch, E.E., Castaneda, Y.S., Fawcett, S.L., Wheaton, D.H., Birch, D.G., and Uauy, R. 2003. Visual function in breast-fed term infants weaned to formula with or without long-chain polyunsaturates at 4 to 6 months: A randomized clinical trial. J. Pediatrics 142: 669-677.

Ip, C., Banni, S., Angioni, E., Carta, G., McGinley, J., Thompson, H.J., Barbano, D., and Bauman, D.E. 1999. Conjugated linoleic acid-enriched butter fat alters mammary gland morphogenesis and reduces cancer risk in rats. J. Nutr. 129: 2135-2142.

Lock, A.L. and Bauman, D.E. 2004. Modifying milk fat composition of dairy cows to enhance fatty acids beneficial to human health. Lipids 39:1197-1206.

Menendez, J.A., Vellon, L., Colomer, R., and Lupu, R. 2005. Oleic acid, the main monounsaturated fatty acid of olive oil, suppresses Her-2/neu (erbB-2) expression and synergistically enhances the growth inhibitory effects of trastuzumab (Herceptin™) in breast cancer cells with Her-2/neu oncogene amplification, Annals Oncology 16: 359-371.

Zhao, G., Etherton, T.D., Martin, K.R., West, S.G., Gillies, P.J., and Kris-Etherton, P.M. 2004. Dietary-linolenic acid reduces inflammatory and lipid cardiovascular risk factors in hypercholesterolemic men and women. J. Nutr. 134: 2991-2997.

Herbal foods:

Are They Efficacious and Safe?

In recent years, a new market has developed for food products designed to reduce the risk or effect of disease on consumers. Some of these so-called functional foods contain plant-derived bioactives, yet there is a lack of knowledge about their use, efficacy, and safety in foods. Some of these plant-derived substances are not normally consumed in the diet as concentrated extracts, and others have only previously been used as herbal medicines. The implications of the food-as-medicine concept when using plant-derived bioactives are discussed.

Karen M. Silvers, PhD; Emmeline L. R. Taptiklis, MSc

In recent years, a new market has developed for food products designed to reduce the risk or effect of disease. Research has shown a generally positive consumer response to the concept of foods as medicine, which has led to health claims being approved for some products. Recent estimates indicate that the value of this functional food market is $56 billion. Annual growth is forecast at 8-9%, and it is predicted that this market will eventually account for 5% of total food expenditure. Despite this, the evidence that functional foods contribute to short-term or long-term health and well-being is unsubstantiated.

The terms used to describe food products based on the food-as-medicine concept include nutraceuticals, pharmafoods, phytofoods, designer foods, nutritional foods, pharmafoodicals, medifoods, superfoods, therapeutic foods, prescriptive foods, fitness foods, longevity foods, and foodiceuticals.[1] However, nutraceuticals and functional foods are the terms most commonly used.

A functional food can be defined in a variety of ways: "A natural food, a food to which a component has been added, or a food from which a component has been removed by technological or biotechnological means. It can also be a food where the nature of one or more components has been modified, or any combination of these possibilities."[2] The functional food concept is one that goes beyond that of basic nutrition and fits with the perceived ideology of modern medicine, which aims to treat disease with a single therapeutic modality. Indeed, the growing popularity and projected sales of functional foods can be considered to be an extension of our desire to find a magic bullet to cure disease. Because plant-derived bioactives are perceived as natural, it may be appealing to consume them in a food, but this raises serious concerns about their safety and efficacy.

Herbs in foods are increasingly common.

Herbal Foods

Many so-called functional foods contain plant-derived bioactive ingredients, such as herbs. Plant-derived bioactives include whole plants, roots, stems, leaves, fruits, seeds, extracts, and purified compounds that provide health-promoting or health-protecting functions. The usual approach when producing a functional food containing a plant-derived bioactive is to add the bioactive with a known health benefit to a food or beverage base. Examples include muesli bars containing Spirulina, acidophilus yogurt containing echinacea, aloe vera herbal tonics, herbal soft drinks, and yogurt smoothies.

Medicinal Uses of Plant-Derived Bioactives

There has been a dramatic increase in the use of plants for medicinal purposes in the last 10 years. This is not without rationale because there is now increasing evidence substantiating the therapeutic effects of numerous natural plant products. These include many commonly found in the diet, such as garlic and ginger but also include herbal medicines, St John's wort, and valerian.

The modern use of herbs, or herbalism, in Western cultures is part of a holistic philosophy. Plant extracts are used in the belief that they help the body make the physiologic and biochemical adjustments necessary to maintain homeostasis and support the body's own healing processes. This belief relies on the concept of synergy in the bioactive properties of herbs. Prescriptions of herbal medicines may include using a single herb with more than one bioactivity to treat more than one ailment or the synergistic use of herbs with similar or complementary bioactivities to treat a single ailment. Many herbal treatments offer the benefit of lower toxicity and reduced side effects compared with modern pharmaceuticals.[3] However, little is known about contraindications, potential adverse effects, and herb-drug interactions.

Both safety and efficacy of herbal ingredients needs to be assessed.

Although several drugs used in conventional medicine are extracted from plants (e.g., digitoxin from foxglove and morphine from the opium poppy), the systematic and scientific study of herbs and their medicinal uses has only recently begun to lose its association with quack medicine. It has been shown that many of the beliefs of the old herb physicians were indeed true; for example, plants do possess different properties if harvested at different times of the day or year, and certain combinations of plants are more active than the individual herbs used separately.[4]

Botanicals and their extracts can be divided into 3 broad categories: (1) those already frequently consumed as foods, such as garlic and rosemary (leaf); (2) those derived from culinary botanicals/herbs but not normally consumed as concentrated extracts, e.g., rosemary oil; and (3) those that previously have been used only as herbal medicines, e.g., valerian.

Efficacy of Botanicals/Herbs or Their Extracts in Functional Foods

Few traditionally used herbs or plant extracts that do not normally occur in the diet have been rigorously assessed for clinical efficacy. Furthermore, standardized methods for extracting the bioactive ingredients and measuring their activity have often not been established. Where there is some scientific evidence of a therapeutic effect, the evidence has often come from in vitro cell-culture experiments or in vivo animal studies, both of which are a long way from testing the effectiveness of botanicals in human clinical trials. Even when some bioactivity has been established for an herb or extract, it is not always clear which components are biologically active. Indeed, the efficacy of an herbal remedy is usually attributed to many compounds, typically approximately 600 in the whole plant, compared with a single active compound in a pharmaceutical. The proportions of these compounds can vary depending on a range of factors, including location, climate, and time of harvest.

To ensure consumer satisfaction and prevent disillusionment with the product, the efficacy of the plant-derived bioactive must be assessed in its new matrix. This may not be straightforward because the product must contain the ingredient in a form and amount that will provide a therapeutic effect even after processing, storage, consumption, and digestion.

Safety Related to the Use of Plant Bioactives in Functional Foods

Although interest in the use of herbs or their extracts as ingredients in functional foods is based on their known or suspected therapeutic effects, safety must also be considered if the amount of plant material or extract exceeds levels normally achieved in the diet, the form of plant material is different from that usually ingested, or the substance has only previously been used as an herbal medicine. Even though adequate information about safety and toxicity of many of the botanicals or their extracts is not currently available for the majority of botanicals/herbs or their extracts, our knowledge is continuing to develop. The exceptions to this are those botanicals more commonly used, such as garlic, St John's wort, and echinacea.

The safety of such functional foods will relate directly to the dose of bioactive consumed. Unlike conventional medicines, there are few, if any, regulations governing the use of botanicals and their extracts in foods and whereas the dosage of a conventional medicine is controlled by the amount of active ingredient contained in each capsule, pill, or spoonful, the dose of a plant-derived bioactive ingredient in functional food is much more difficult to control and regulate. This is because the proportions of the many compounds associated with efficacy in a herb/botanical or extract may vary according to a range of factors, including location, climate, and time of harvest and because people eat according to their appetite and desire for a particular food. Generally, the more therapeutically active the material, the more likely it is that high and/or frequent dosages will lead to adverse effects, including skin allergies, gastrointestinal upsets, drug interactions, genetic mutation, tachycardia, peripheral paralysis, and intoxication or psychoses.[5] It is, therefore, imperative that the dose-response-toxicity relationship is considered when selecting a suitable botanical, sourcing extracts with consistent levels of active ingredients, and developing the product in relation to dose per product unit.

As the physiologic effect of many plant-derived bioacrive ingredients increases with increasing dose, so will any associated adverse effects. Although some whole plants/compounds are considered to be nontoxic, it is always necessary to consider dose, particularly when botanicals are incorporated into food staples in the diet. Adverse reactions after consumption of such a food need to be systematically assessed, as well as the implications of frequent and long-term use of such functional food products. This may involve modeling intakes for a range of dietary patterns and consumption levels, as is done before fortification of a food with a nutrient.

Herb-Drug Interactions

It has been found that up to 31% of consumers use herbal supplements with prescription drugs and 48% with over-the-counter drugs,[6] and recent evidence suggests that this will continue to increase.[7] In addition, many patients are not reporting the use of dietary supplements to their physicians, increasing the likelihood that adverse effects resulting from herb-drug interactions are not recorded or are wrongly attributed to the drug being taken.[6] Indeed, little is known about herb-herb and herb-drug interactions for the majority of botanicals, and what is known is anecdotal or based only on case reports.

Herb-drug interactions may cause adverse or beneficial effects.[8] Herbs can be partially additive or additive, may potentiate the action of the drug, or may be directly antagonistic to a drug's action.[8] For instance, St John's wort has been reported to increase serotonin levels in patients using selective serotonin reuptake inhibitors.[9] It also appears to affect the hepatic cytochrome P450 by increasing the isoenzyme CYP3A4, therefore lowering the activity of drugs that are known to be substrates for this enzyme, including oral contraceptives, some antiretrovirals, nonse dating antihistamines, antiepileptics, cyclosporine, macrolide antibiotics, some antifungals, calcium channel blockers, and some chemotherapeutics.[10-11] Garlic has been found to increase bleeding times for patients taking warfarin.[12-13] Likewise, Ginkgo leaf extract may have an additive effect with other blood-thinning agents, such as aspirin,[14] and has been found to potentiate the action of a drug used for erectile dysfunction.[15]

A systematic assessment of contraindications and adverse reactions after the consumption of functional foods containing plant material or extracts, at levels or in forms not normally found in the diet, should be carried out if consumers are to be assured of their safety. Until more is known, consumers should be advised of possible interactions and the need to inform their physicians if using dietary supplements and functional foods containing herbs or other botanical material. In addition, there is a need for physicians and pharmacists to request information about the use of these products when prescribing medications.

Conclusion

Our desire for a quick fix from acute and chronic disease, combined with our growing interest in natural therapies, has led to the emergence of foods and beverages that contain botanical ingredients not previously found in our diet. Many of these botanicals have previously only been used as herbal medicines and are not normally consumed. However, the efficacy of such foods has not been proved, and, more importantly, their safety cannot be assured without a systematic assessment of contraindications and adverse reactions after their consumption.

REFERENCES

1. Jullestad A. Crafting appetizing nutraceuticals. *Food Product Design.* 1998;March:97-119.
2. Aggett PJ, Alexander J, Alles M, et al. Scientific concepts of functional foods in Europe: consensus document. *Br J Nutr.* 1999;91(Suppl 1):1-27.
3. Perry EK, Pickering AT, Wang WW, et al. Medicinal plants and Alzheimer's disease: from ethnobotany to phytotherapy. *J Pharm Pharmacol.* 1999;51:527-534.
4. Stuart M. *The Encyclopedia of Herbs and Herbalism.* London: Orbis; 1979.
5. Miller LG. Herbal medicinals: selected clinical considerations focusing on known or potential drug-herb interactions. *Arch Intern Med.* 1998;158:2200-2211.
6. Eisenberg DM, Davis RB, Ettner SL, et al. Trends in alternative medicine use in the United States, 1990-1997. *JAMA.* 1998;280:1569-1575.
7. Johnston BA. Prevention magazine assesses the use of dietary supplements. *Herbalgram.* 2000;48-65.
8. Blumenthal M, Goldberg A, Brinkmann J. *Herbal Medicine-Expanded Commission E Monographs.* Newton, Mass: Integrative Medicine Communications; 2000.
9. Lanz MS, Buchalter E, Giambanco V. St John's wort and antidepressant drug interactions in the elderly. *J Geriatr Psychiatry Neurol.* 1999;12:7-10.
10. Roby CA, Kantor E, Anderson GD, et al. St John's wort: effect on CYP3A4 activity. *Clin Phannacol Ther.* 2000;67:451-457.
11. Roby CA, Kantor E, Anderson GD, et al. St John's wort impact on CYP3A4 activity [poster presentation]. Boca Raton, FL: Presented at the 39th Annual Meeting of New Clinical Drug Evaluation Unit Program; June 1-4 1999.
12. World Health Organization. *WHO Monographs on Selected Medicinal Plants.* Vol 1. Geneva: World Health Organization; 1999.
13. Sunter WH. Warfarin and garlic [letter]. *Pharm J.* 1991; 246:722.
14. Rosenblatt M, Mindel J. Spontaneous hyphema associated with ingestion of Gingko biloba extract [letter]. *N Eng J Med.* 1997;336:1108.

15. Sikora R, Sohn M, Duetz FJ, et al. Gingko biloba extract in the therapy of erectile dysfunction [abstract]. *J Urol*. 1989; 141:188A.

She takes a multidisciplinary approach and has strong links with biochemists, psychologists, and other health researchers both in New Zealand and internationally.

Karen M. Silvers, PhD, is a human nutrition scientist with a background in clinical research, antioxidants, and health. Her current interests are related to maintenance and promotion of brain function, mental health, and well-being.

Emmeline L. R. Taptiklis, MSc, is a nutritionist at, Crop & Food Research, Palmerston North, New Zealand. Corresponding author: Karen M. Silvers, PhD, Crop & Food Research, Private Bag 11600, Palmerston North, New Zealand (e-mail: silversk@crop.cri.nz).

HERBAL LOTTERY

What's on a dietary supplement's label may not be what's in the bottle

JANET RALOFF

Echinacea is a commercial success. The dietary supplement—made from the flowers, stems, and leaves of the purple coneflower—has become a popular and lucrative over-the-counter cold remedy. It's also one of the few nutraceuticals—natural products with medicinal reputations—that have substantial scientific evidence to support its purported functions: Various studies suggest that echinacea supplements can boost immunity or shorten the duration of colds.

Several years ago, however, Christine M. Gilroy of the University of Colorado Health Sciences Center in Denver was unsure whether to trust data from those experiments because few reports included biochemical proof of which species of purple coneflower had been used. That's important, she notes, because three species—*Echinacea pallida, Echinacea purpurea,* and *Echinacea angustifolia*—turn up in supplements "and only the first two have data indicating they might make colds better."

Not Twins—*Echinacea pallida* and *Echinacea purpurea* look different, but manufacturers sometimes swap one for the other in dietary supplements—even though the plants contain different chemicals and may perform differently.

Curious about *E. pallida's* reputed power against colds, Gilroy designed a study and then ordered dried samples from three suppliers. She sent some of each delivery out for analysis of chemicals that were known to distinguish the species and that might even have therapeutic activity.

The data that came back put her study on hold. They showed no batch containing pure *E. pallida.* The one from a bulk wholesaler that supplies herbal-products companies contained almost no *Echinacea* from any species, and what little there was consisted solely of *E. purpurea.* The other batches, acquired directly from coneflower growers, did contain *E. pallida*—but also contaminating plants, including *E. angustifolia.*

Gilroy then turned to 59 commercial echinacea products from local stores. Her team's analyses, reported in the March 24 *Archives of Internal Medicine,* show that none offered con-

sumers what had been promised by its label. Six contained no evidence of any echinacea, and 28 failed to contain the specific species that was listed on the box. Some offered echinacea in quantities exceeding or, more often, falling below the quantity on the label, sometimes substantially.

These findings call into question the conclusions of the many earlier studies of echinacea's purported cure for the common cold, says Gilroy. At the least, they suggest that health effects seen with one sample of supplement might not hold for others.

This is just the latest in a string of studies revealing variability in the ingredients of dietary supplements on the market today. Uniform products require consistent ingredients and processes throughout every stage of manufacturing. The troubling findings suggest that many herbal-product makers aren't maintaining adequate quality control.

Several weeks ago, the Food and Drug Administration proposed rules designed to stem quality-control problems in dietary supplements, including nutraceuticals. The agency would mandate so-called good manufacturing practices, or GMPs, in the industry. Under GMPs like those now governing pharmaceuticals, all manufacturers of dietary supplements would have to chemically validate their ingredients and keep stringent records. These would include temperature readings from each batch as it's made and notes about any breakdowns of factory equipment.

However, representatives of the nutraceutical industry say they plan to call for amendments to the proposed FDA rules. They're currently analyzing the hundreds of pages of details before requesting changes. Moreover, any set of standard practices may be severely challenged by the complex makeup of herbal products, several scientists told *Science News.*

"For the most part, with [herbal] supplements, we still don't know what all the active ingredients are," so nobody knows the ideal formulation of most supplements, observes Bill J. Gurley of the University of Arkansas for Medical Sciences in Little Rock.

Says David J. Newman of the National Cancer Institute in Frederick, Md., "The bottom line remains *caveat emptor,*" or let the buyer beware.

Beyond Echinacea

There's evidence for poor quality control in the making of many dietary supplements, says Chien M. Wai of the University of Idaho in Moscow. His work focuses on those made from leaves of the maidenhair tree (*Ginkgo biloba L.*). Ginkgo supplements fight memory loss and reinvigorate blood flow in the brain, according to users of the herb.

Scientists have identified five purported active ingredients in ginkgo. In most cases, Wai finds, a product's label describes only how much bulk ginkgo tissue a tablet, powder, or tincture contains without quantifying the active agents. Concentrations of those agents can vary widely in plant tissue.

In 2001, Wai's group reported data showing that, for instance, supposedly equally potent ginkgo supplements could contain anywhere from 0 to almost 4 milligrams of active compounds. Brands varied in which active chemicals dominated them, and some brands exhibited large batch-to-batch variation.

His subsequent studies, Wai says, indicate "the situation is not getting better."

Consumers can't use his team's reports to avoid supplements with weak or erratic ingredients because the researchers haven't published any brand names. Companies challenge any implied criticism of their products, Wai explains, and "we can't afford the time to fight lawsuits."

Gurley has named brands in his published analyses of supplements containing the weight-loss stimulant ephedra and indeed "stirred up a hornet's nest," he notes. It started 3 years ago, when his team first surveyed 20 over-the-counter ephedra products. As Gilroy found with echinacea, the ingredients often didn't match label claims.

Tissues from the *Ephedra sinica* plant, like ginkgo, contain at least five purported active ingredients, which are in the chemical family named alkaloids. Each alkaloid has a different effectiveness as a stimulant, and its concentration varies among individual plants. Most supplements that are labeled with ingredient information claim only to have some specified quantity of mixed ephedra alkaloids—information too general to offer much gauge of potency, says Gurley.

Although one brand that his team tested contained none of the five stimulant alkaloids, most had several, but the amounts varied among brands. When the researchers tested several batches of a brand, some differed in concentration by up to tenfold. Only 13 of the 20 products listed a total quantity of alkaloids on the label; others just listed quantities of the raw source plant. In many cases, Gurley says, those values bore no relation to what was present. His group published its findings in 2000. Since then, the researchers' tests of 130 additional ephedra products found far fewer discrepancies between labels and contents, "although they do still occur," says Gurley.

His team has lately turned to St. John's wort (*Hypericum perforatum*), a possible antidepressant. The researchers are finding a wide range of concentrations of St. John's wort's purported active ingredient, which is called hyperforin. Batch-to-batch hyperforin differences in one supplement brand varied 15-fold.

Gurley acknowledges that some herbal-supplement companies reliably produce what their labels promise. The trick is identifying them, Gurley says, a task beyond the capability of most consumers.

Many Explanations

Quality-control problems in herbal supplements often start with the hundreds of chemicals that plants contain. The type and quantity of these compounds vary in response to the environment in which a plant grew: its soil type and nutrition, water availability, excessive heat or cold, exposure to toxic minerals, degree of shading, and any hybridization.

One team is studying horticulturally triggered variations in several citrus compounds that are regarded as potential nutraceuticals because they've inhibited cancers in laboratory animals. Data collected by Bhimanagouda S. Patil and his colleagues at Texas A&M University in Weslaco show that concentrations of one such chemical—limonin glycoside—peaks midway through the crop's harvest season. So, when it comes to this agent, Patil says, "you must eat two grapefruit in May to get what one picked around Christmas will give you."

He's also been quantifying lycopene, a potential anticancer carotenoid that turns plants red. When his group planted Florida-derived rootstock of Star Ruby grapefruit in Texas, the fruit produced some 50 percent more of this carotenoid than it had in Florida.

Researchers at the University of Newcastle in Ourimbah, Australia, are studying effects of manufacturing techniques on nutraceutical quality. For instance, Douglas L. Stuart and Ron B.H. Wills report that high temperatures reduce concentrations of one of the potential therapeutic agents derived from *E. purpurea*. The scientists report in the March 15 *Journal of Agricultural and Food Chemistry* that drying the plant at 40°C results in one-third more cichoric acid than drying it at 70°C does.

Moreover, Wai's team has shown that whether oil, alcohol, or water is used can effect which chemicals are extracted from a plant. These products can have different potencies.

Even if purported active ingredients make it into a supplement, poor manufacturing techniques can yield tablets that don't effectively release those chemicals, notes Larry L. Augsburger of the University of Maryland in Baltimore.

Working with a synthetic version of melatonin, a hormone that promotes sleep, seems to fight jet lag (*SN: 5/13/95, p. 300*), and maybe even battles cancer (*SN: 10/17/98, p. 252*: http://www.sciencenews.org/sn_arc98/10_17_98/19981017fob.asp), his team showed that tablets don't always release their contents in a timely fashion. Although industry standards for the breakdown of conventional drugs is generally 30 minutes or less, his test-tube studies showed that some commercial melatonin supplements didn't disintegrate or release their contents for periods of 4 hours to more than 20 hours, by which time an ingested tablet may well have been excreted.

Help on the Way?

In the early 1990s, nutraceutical manufacturers feared that FDA would challenge their label claims. Then, the 1994 Dietary Supplement Health and Education Act was passed, permitting the sale of nutraceuticals and other supplements that are nontoxic and make no curative claims.

Immediately following the act's passage, sales of herbal supplements skyrocketed, with many companies regularly reporting up to 11 percent annual growth. But by 2000, U.S. sales started flagging, observes Clare M. Hasler of the University of Illinois at Urbana-Champaign. Reports were emerging of health risks associated with some products, such as ephedra; uncertain efficacy of others; and quality-control problems in the industry.

Because that last item appears to be the easiest for manufacturers to fix, some nutraceutical makers have been voluntarily adopting GMPs of their own design, says Nancy Childs of St. Joseph's University in Philadelphia. These companies tend to be the large prescription-drug manufacturers that have entered the nutraceuticals market in the past half-decade, she adds.

Most nutraceutical makers are far smaller than those companies, notes Kim Smith, an attorney with the National Nutritional Food Association (NNFA) of Newport Beach, Calif. Since 1999, her trade group—which represents many nutraceutical makers with 20 to 500 employees—has provided guidance for developing voluntary GMPs. NNFA also officially supports FDA's March 28 proposal for mandatory GMPs. "It will go a long way toward improving credibility in the industry," Smith says.

However, she adds, small firms could have a hard time paying for stringent FDA-required monitoring and record keeping. The agency estimates that first-year costs for small firms will run about $100,000, with annual costs of $60,000 or so thereafter. In fact, Smith says, her group suspects FDA is substantially underestimating those costs.

Success in complying with mandatory GMPs, Hasler suspects, "is going to sort out the [nutraceutical industry's] major players from the fly-by-night companies and probably put some small players out of business." She adds, "I'm not sure that's a bad thing."

Allen Montgomery, executive director of the American Nutraceuticals Association in Birmingham, Ala., which represents pharmacists and other health professionals, agrees. He says, "I don't know of any other billion-dollar industry that makes ingested products for which [mandatory] GMPs are not in place."

Within the nutraceutical industry generally, Gurley charges, "there are so many bad actors right now, that it's giving the whole industry a bad name."

Fortunately, Montgomery notes, several independent groups—such as the U.S. Pharmacopoeia (USP) of Rockville, Md.—have already begun validating voluntary GMPs for several products. USP is the official standards-setting body for all U.S. medicines and dietary supplements.

Companies that want to carry the USP logo must submit products for a series of stringent tests of such features as a product's purity, potency, and consistency. Also, USP inspectors visit factories to confirm that GMPs are in place, notes Sherrie L. Borden, the organization's spokesperson. "Then we do postmarket surveillance [of a supplement] once a product is on the shelf. It's very rigorous," she notes, "because this mark carries a lot of credibility."

All this sounds comforting, Gurley says, except that pharmaceutical-grade uniformity in herbal products may be amazingly difficult to achieve, and FDA's new rules don't address the complexity of a plant's make-up. Synthetic drugs and vitamins tend to have only one or two well-characterized active ingredients, he explains, while herbal supplements "are a veritable pharmacological Pandora's box."

Indeed, the 48 nutraceuticals that USP recently vetted—all produced under the Nature Made or Kirkland Signature labels—contain only vitamins, minerals, or fish oil—not complex herbal products.

Since plant tissue may contain hundreds of compounds with perhaps dozens of active ingredients, Gurley asks, who knows which of these should be standardized in each product? This "truly daunting" problem would challenge the best pharmaceutical manufacturer, he says, let alone a 30-employee herbal-products company.

Wai and Newman say that they'd like to see the herbal-supplements market develop into a natural-products offshoot of the over-the-counter drug industry. They argue that the best route for making safe and effective nutraceuticals would be to identify each plant's active agents, isolate them for testing in the same kind of trials that conventional pharmaceuticals go through, and then package the proven chemicals in carefully measured doses.

An advantage to this approach for manufacturers, Newman argues, is that unlike an herb, the recipe for a cocktail of natural chemicals is patentable. Thus, it might be market forces after all that bring consistency to the nutraceutical marketplace.

Reprinted with permission from *Science News*, the weekly newsmagazine of science, June 7, 2003, copyright 2003 by Science Service.

The Latest Scoop on Soy

Twenty-eight percent of Americans consume soyfoods or soy beverages once a week or more, according to the United Soybean Board's 2003–04 annual study, "Consumer Attitudes about Nutrition." According to the survey, soymilk, tofu, and soy veggie burgers are the top soy products regularly consumed (see table).

The USB study found that significantly more consumers are aware of soymilk, soy ice cream or cheese, miso, and tempeh compared to 2002. In addition to becoming more aware of soy products, consumers are also learning more about soy's health benefits. The study found that 74% of U.S. consumers perceive soy as healthy. Heart health is the main benefit that consumers associate with soy. Other areas of awareness include menopause relief, obesity prevention/ weight loss, cancer prevention, and protein source.

As awareness grows and as research accumulates, so do the soy ingredients that companies offer. Ingredients such as soy protein isolates, soy protein concentrates, soy isoflavones, soy flour, and soy nuggets have evolved through the years to become more functional for manufacturers' needs. Solubility and flavor of soy ingredients are two areas that have vastly improved.

Here's a brief update on some of the latest soy news related to health and ingredient offerings.

The Healthy Side of Soy

Soy is most commonly known for its cardiovascular benefits, particularly soy protein. This is evident in the Food and Drug Administration's approved soy protein health claim linking it to a reduced risk for heart disease. The health claim is based on clinical trials showing that consumption of soy protein can lower total and low-density-lipoprotein (LDL) cholesterol levels.

Soy is most commonly known for its cardiovascular benefits [but] bone health, prostate cancer, and menopause are three main areas where consumers may soon be learning more about soy's benefits.

Additional research and clinical trials are pointing to other potential health benefits of soy protein and soy isoflavones. Bone health, prostate cancer, and menopause are three main areas where consumers may soon be learning more about soy's benefits.

Bone Health

"In my view, there is probably the most support for the skeletal benefits of soy protein and isoflavones," said Mark Messina, Adjunct Associate Professor at California's Loma Linda University and co-owner of Nutrition Matters Inc. "When soy protein is substituted for milk protein, several studies have found that urinary calcium excretion is decreased. The metabolism of the sulfur amino acids in protein leads to the production of acid, which requires buffering. The skeletal system is the largest source of buffering agent in the body. In response to acid, the bones are broken down, which leads to an increase in urinary calcium. Since soy protein contains lower amounts of sulfur amino acids than milk protein, it causes less calcium excretion."

In addition to soy protein, isoflavones may have possible skeletal benefits. Mes-sina discussed two studies that have drawn attention to this. "A recent one-year trial found that genistein, the main isoflavone in soybeans, was even more effective than conventional hormone replacement therapy (HRT) at reducing bone loss at the hip in postmenopausal women and was only slightly less effective than HRT at the spine," he said. "Another recently presented two-year trial found that isoflavone-rich soymilk reduced bone loss at the hip and spine in comparison to soymilk low in isoflavones."

He added that long-term studies are currently underway to firmly conclude that isoflavones have the same effect as HRT in reducing fracture risk. "Nevertheless, because soy protein is high quality, the current data justify recommending that isoflavone-rich soyfoods be part of an overall bone-healthy diet. When using soy in place of dairy products, calcium-fortified soy products should be used."

Breast and Prostate Cancer

"There is a large body of literature on the cancer prevention actions of a diet that includes soy. These data support a beneficial effect especially on breast cancer and prostate cancer risk," stated Debra Miller, Director, Nutrition Science Communications, The Solae Co., St. Louis, Mo.

For example, a recent Japanese study suggested that eating foods rich in isoflavones reduced the risk of breast cancer, especially in postmenopausal women. Frequent consumption of soy-rich miso soup was found to be particularly effective (Yamamoto et al., 2003).

Researchers from the National Cancer Center Research Institute in Japan evaluated the relationship between isoflavone consumption and breast cancer risk among women as part of the Ja-

What consumers say about soy foods, according to the United Soybean Board's 2003–04 annual study	
Soy products used regularly	**Soy products tried at least once during the year**
1. Soymilk (17%)	1. Tofu (48%)
2. Tofu (12%)	2. Soy veggie burgers (44%)
3. Soy veggie burgers (12%)	3. Soymilk (39%)
4. Soy protein bars (5%)	4. Soy nuts (26%)
5. Soy nuts (4%)	5. Soy protein bars (22%)

pan Public Health Center-based prospective study on cancer and cardiovascular diseases.

The JPHC study began in 1990, when nearly 22,000 Japanese female residents age 40–59 years from four public health center areas completed a questionnaire which included items about the frequency of soy consumption. Ten years later, 179 of these women had been diagnosed with breast cancer.

Researchers found that while soyfoods alone did not have a significant effect, both consumption of miso soup and overall isoflavone intake reduced the risk of breast cancer. In addition, the researchers reported that the association was found to be stronger in postmenopausal women.

Because of increasing evidence of the benefits of isoflavones, a European Union-funded project, called the Isoheart project, has recently been established to explore the physiological effects from eating foods with added soy-derived isoflavones. One of the project's aims is to establish the presumed health benefits of phytoestrogens in reducing the risk of heart disease in postmenopausal women, as well as to study the consumer acceptability of foods enriched with isoflavones.

In men, soy isoflavones are believed to help in preventing prostate cancer. "Personally, I am most excited about the role that soy may have in preventing and even treating prostate cancer," said Messina. "One key to preventing prostate cancer mortality is preventing the latent (small, clinically irrelevant) tumors from progressing to the larger tumors that can metastasize and which are life threatening," he said. "The International Prostate Health Council concluded that isoflavones stop this progression. Animal

studies are very supportive of this hypothesis, and a recent pilot study found that isoflavones were of benefit to prostate cancer patients resistant to conventional medical treatment. Still, all this remains speculative, although I strongly recommend that men consume soy."

Research presented at a recent American Urological Association meeting in Chicago showed that genistein reduced prostate-specific antigen (PSA) levels in men with untreated cancer, in some cases by almost two thirds.

PSA is a protein produced by the cells of the prostate gland. PSA levels tend to rise if the prostate gland is enlarged due to cancer. The researchers from the University of California Davis Cancer Center said their study suggested that genistein could help men at risk of developing prostate cancer.

The researchers studied 62 men known to have prostate cancer and elevated PSA levels. The men were given 5 g of a dietary supplement containing genistein every day for six months. Sixteen of the men had untreated prostate cancer—they were in the "watchful waiting" group, where the cancer is slow-growing and causing no symptoms. In this group, three had to stop the therapy because they suffered from diarrhea, but eight saw their PSA level fall between 3 and 61%. The remaining five (38%) saw their PSA levels rise, but the researchers say this is a far smaller proportion than in the remaining 46 men who had been treated for prostate cancer, 98% of whom saw a rise.

Ralph de Vere White, Director of the UC-Davis Cancer Center, said, "It must be interpreted cautiously because the numbers of men enrolled are small. He added, however, that "patients on watchful waiting may do better due to grade of

disease or distribution and concentration of genistein within the prostate."

Menopausal Symptoms

A number of studies have shown that consuming both soy protein and soy isoflavone extracts can help reduce the severity and frequency of hot flashes, said Miller. "It should be noted, however, that consuming soyfoods or supplements will not result in the powerful and quick results that HRT provides. However HRT has recently been associated with a number of long-term health risks such as heart attack, stroke, breast cancer, and Alzheimer's disease. In light of these risks, many women find consuming soyfoods a healthy option."

In an article in the *Journal of Medicinal Food*, Messina and Hughes (2003) reviewed the evidence to date on the impact of soyfoods and soy isoflavones on hot flush symptoms in women. They found a statistically significant relationship between initial hot flush frequency and treatment efficacy.

"Initial hot flush frequency explained about 46 percent of the treatment effects, and hot flush frequency decreased by about 5 percent (above placebo or control effects) for every additional initial hot flush per day in women whose initial hot flush frequency was five or more per day," the authors reported.

Soy has received attention as an alternative to HRT largely because it is a unique dietary source of isoflavones. However, there have been conflicting results from trials measuring the ability of isoflavones to reduce menopausal symptoms. In their review, Messina and Hughes eliminated trials on breast cancer patients. They also eliminated non-blinded trials.

Out of 11 studies on soyfoods, only one found that women showed a significant decrease in hot flush frequency. The researchers noted, however, that "the large placebo effect makes most of these trials underpowered to detect modest effects." In four out of six studies on isoflavone supplements, there was a positive link to reduced menopausal symptoms. But the baseline level of hot flush frequency was higher on average among participants in the supplement trials. This led the authors to the theory that efficacy increased with hot flush frequency, so that those women having around 10 hot flushes each day saw this frequency halved, while those experiencing only seven daily only saw a reduction of around three flushes, after taking isoflavones.

The researchers wrote that although conclusions based on the analysis should be considered tentative, "the available data justify the recommendation that patients with frequent hot flushes consider trying soyfoods or isoflavone supplements for the alleviation of their symptoms."

They added that future trials involving soyfoods and isoflavone supplements are warranted, "but should focus on women who have frequent hot flushes." The correlation between initial hot flush frequency and the extent of reduction of symptoms should also be studied, they said.

Weight Management/Diabetes Control

"Given the enormous problem with obesity and its secondary effects, such as type 2 diabetes in the Western world, many people are looking at alterations in diet. Many have opted for high protein/lower carbohydrate diets and found success with such diets," said Miller. "However, health professionals are concerned with long-term high animal protein consumption. Eating large amounts of meat, cheese, and eggs can cause calcium loss from bones and cause the kidneys to work harder than usual (a big risk factor for those who have type 2 diabetes already). Interestingly, soy protein, as a vegetable protein, does not cause calcium loss and is actually the protein recommended to many patients on dialysis to prevent protein malnutrition because

even patients with impaired renal function can tolerate soy protein."

Soy protein and its constituents have also been linked to enhancements in glucose tolerance and reductions in insulin resistance, added Miller. "This research is encouraging. Certainly adding soy protein to food in place of carbohydrates can help reduce the glycemic index of foods."

Soy proteins and isoflavones are becoming more versatile and functional for various products.

Cognitive Ability

"One of the most exciting areas of research regarding soy foods is the association with better recognition and recall ability in memory testing when people eat a diet high in soy compared to those on a low-soy diet," said Miller. Research is ongoing in this area.

Improvements in Soy Ingredients

"Who thought that soy protein would be used in cold cereal four or five years ago?" said Mian Riaz, Head of the Extrusion Technology Program and Research Scientist at the Food Protein Research and Development Center at Texas A&M University, College Station. "With improved ingredients, we will see more soy-cultured products with improved flavor and taste, real soy cheese and ice cream, which taste just like traditional cheese and ice cream products, soy water, soy tea, and soy candy."

He added that there is a lot of research going on to process a soy meat analog that is very close to real meat. "This meat texture will resemble fresh meat and have the same composition as real meat you buy from the butcher (with 70% moisture content)."

Novel soy products such as these would not have been possible if not for the continuous improvement of soy ingredients. From the following information from three soy suppliers, we can see that the ingredients are becoming more refined and tailored for specific food product applications. Both soy proteins and isofla-

vones are becoming more versatile and functional for various products.

New Soy Ingredient Developments

"What's happened overall with soy ingredients is that companies have figured out how to create better-tasting ingredients for different applications. That now has allowed us to put together food systems with better taste and texture," said Tony DeLio, Vice President, Marketing and External Affairs, Archer Daniels Midland Co., Natural Health and Nutrition Division, Decatur, Ill.

The company offers a range of soy products, from flours, to soy protein concentrates and isolates, to soy isoflavones. "It all depends on what your end product is. Our soy flours enable us to work in bread applications, for example. Utilizing our baking expertise, we can easily get 6.25 g of soy protein into two slices of sandwich bread without compromising texture and flavor," said DeLio.

A new addition to the company's *NutriSoy* line is *Wholebean Soy Powder*, an organic ingredient for soymilk and other dairy-like products. It offers the superior nutrition of whole soybeans—fiber and isoflavones—in a form that can be easily incorporated into virtually any dairy or dairy analog product, he said.

"We can also incorporate soy into chocolate coating systems and have worked with a number of companies to create soy rice crispies for nutrition bars," DeLio added. "On the meat analog side, we tend to use soy concentrates and isolates to get a higher level of protein. We are currently developing technology to simulate whole-muscle meat products. We hope to have this revolutionary new product on the market within the next six months."

Regarding isoflavones, approximately 125 different retail product labels carry the *NovaSoy* brand name. "Isoflavones have gone from being primarily in dietary supplements to functional foods such as beverages and snack bars," he said. "We provide all different concentration levels of isoflavones. We have recently licensed technology that allows the time release of isoflavones. For example, you could have a time-released steady stream of isoflavones in a product."

DeLio concluded that with the innovation in soy ingredients, there is no reason why the food industry can't have a line of branded soy products that cut across all food segments. This would be similar to the line of *Healthy Choice* products that cater to low salt and low fat demand. "The consumer interest is there and the time is right for somebody."

Concept Beverage with Soy Isoflavones.

A ready-to-drink raspberry tea that supports bone health was unveiled by Cargill Health & Food Technologies, Minneapolis, Minn., at the Institute of Food Technologists' Annual Meeting + Food Expo® last month. The prototype beverage, named *Bone Appetit*, contains Cargill's *AdvantaSoy™* Clear isoflavones, *Oliggo-Fiber™* inulin, and calcium. Proprietary processing technology results in beverages that retain their traditional flavor, color, and consistency. "*AdvantaSoy Clear* isoflavones allow us to meet the challenge of creating new functional beverages that promote health and retain the delicious flavor and aroma which made them popular in the first place," said Steve Snyder, Cargill's Director of Sales and Marketing, Nutraceuticals.

"What we try to do is look at the retail market and create a product solution based on consumer input," said Lee Knudson, *Advantasoy* Product Manager. "This will help our customers be more successful in key product launches. The ready-to-drink tea is one example."

The *AdvantaSoy line* is available in three different forms depending on the application, he explained. Produced using proprietary technology and available in isoflavone concentrations of up to 50%, *AdvantaSoy Clear* has improved solubility, a whiter appearance, and reduced undesirable taste and odor, ideal for beverages and more-attractive food product applications. The product is GRAS for beverages, nutrition bars, yogurt, meal replacement, and confections. *AdvantaSoy Complete Isoflavones* are created using a natural, solvent-free processing technique. The ingredient is a combination of soy protein and isoflavones, ideal for breads, cereals, and meal replacements. *AdvantaSoy Compress*, available in isoflavone concentrations of up to 50%, is formulated for dietary supplements.

"Our soy isoflavones are really next-generation ingredients in the sense that we concentrate ours in a proprietary process from the soy germ," said Snyder. "The first generation of isoflavones was concentrated from the soy protein isolate manufacturing process."

In the future, said Snyder, we'll see soy ingredients that are easier to formulate, with better taste attributes. "Ingredients will be tailored to individual food products."

Improved Flavor and Functional Performance

New soy developments center on improving the flavor and functional performance and developing new ingredient forms to allow use in a wider array of food products. "We have also focused on innovations that contribute unique textures in food products," said Jim Holbrook, Vice President, Food Science Research and Development, The Solae Co. For example, the company's *Supro® XT* proteins, based on soy isolate technology, provide flavor and functional improvements in beverages. The *Alpha®* proteins, based on a revolutionary new manufacturing process, provide improved flavor performance in beverages and a range of dairy alternative products.

Other new offerings include extruded soy nuggets, now delivering protein contents up to 80% protein and providing unique texture and crunch in nutritional food bars and other grain-based foods. "For meat alternatives, we have introduced a range of high-moisture extruded ingredients for use in this application, which provide consumers a more meat-like eating experience," Holbrook said. "We have also introduced a number of products that offer enhanced nutritional attributes, such as soy proteins co-processed with other ingredients, such as calcium phosphate, carbohydrates, and fibers to enhance the nutritional value and functional performance of our ingredients in various food products. We also offer products with guaranteed levels of isoflavones, important health-promoting components found in soy."

Applications that will benefit from Solae's innovations include beverages, nutrition bars, and meat alternatives. "We have recently introduced new technology that makes soy protein more functional in acidic beverages, a big growth area for soy protein today," Holbrook said. "We are looking at both powdered isolate and extruded soy nuggets as technologies we can employ to positively affect shelf life in bars. We are also continuing to innovate with new extruded products and forms for meat alternatives. Additionally, we are very excited about our new *Alpha* technology, based on an innovative new process that delivers very bland-flavored soy proteins. We believe this technology has tremendous potential for future development across a spectrum of new applications."

Better Soy Ingredients

So, in the future, we can expect soy ingredients with improved flavor, texture, color, and mouthfeel. "The food industry will be able to find soy ingredients with very specific functionality, like foaming, whipping, emulsification, solubility, and texturization for specific food applications," said Riaz. "Improved soy ingredients will be available for soy beverages without the chalky flavor. There will be improvement in soybean oil for taste, flavor, and overall quality without the hydrogenation. The food industry will also find soy flour with higher protein levels, through breeding and improved processing techniques."

Expect more great things to come from soy!

REFERENCES

1. Messina, M. and Hughes, C. 2003. Efficacy of soyfoods and soybean isoflavone supplements for alleviating menopausal symptoms is positively related to initial hot flush frequency. J. Medicinal Food 6(1): 1–11.
2. Yamamoto, S., Sobue, T., Kobayashi, M., Sasaki, S., and Tsugane, S. 2003. Soy, isoflavones, and breast cancer risk in Japan. J. Natl. Cancer Inst. 95: 906–913.

Q & A on Functional Foods

Q. What are "functional foods"?

"Functional foods" is simply a convenient way to describe foods or their components which may provide a health benefit beyond basic nutrition. In other words, functional foods do more than meet your minimum daily requirements of nutrients—they also can play a role in reducing risk of disease and promoting good health. While all foods are functional in that they provide nutrients, "functional foods" tend to be those with health-promoting ingredients or natural components that have been found to have potential benefit in the body. They can include whole foods as well as fortified, enriched or enhanced foods and dietary supplements that have a beneficial effect on health.

The concept of functional foods is not entirely new, although it has evolved considerably over the years. In the early 1900s, food manufacturers in the United States began adding iodine to salt in an effort to prevent goiter, representing one of the first attempts at creating a functional component through fortification. Today, researchers have identified hundreds of compounds with functional qualities, and they continue to make new discoveries surrounding the complex benefits of phytochemicals in foods.

Q. How does a food become "functional"?

Since many of these foods are just natural, whole foods with new information about their potential health qualities, they do not become "functional" except for the way we perceive them. On the other hand, functional foods can result from agricultural breeding or added nutrients/ingredients.

Many—if not most—fruits, vegetables, grains, fish, and dairy and meat products contain several natural components that deliver benefits beyond basic nutrition, such as lycopene in tomatoes, omega-3 fatty acids in salmon or saponins in soy. Even tea and chocolate have been noted in some studies as possessing functional attributes.

Agricultural scientists are able to boost the nutritional content of certain crops through the same breeding techniques that are used to bring out other beneficial traits in plants and animals—everything from beta-carotene-rich rice to vitamin-enhanced broccoli and soybeans, just to name a couple of examples. And research is under way to improve the nutritional quality of dozens of other crops.

Below is a sampling of a few functional foods, their components and their potential benefits for human health.

Functional Component	Source	Potential Health Benefit
Lutein	Green vegetables	Contributes to maintenance of healthy vision
Insoluble fiber	Wheat bran	May reduce risk of breast and/or colon cancer
Lactobacillus	Yogurt, other dairy	May improve gastrointestinal health
Soy protein	Soy-based foods	May reduce risk of cardiovascular disease
Omega-3 fatty acids	Salmon, tuna, fish/marine oils	May reduce risk of cardiovascular disease and improve mental, visual functions
Xylitol	Nutritional bars, beverages	Improves oral health; Does not promote tooth decay

Other foods may be specially formulated with nutrients or other ingredients. This is true of products such as orange juice fortified with calcium, cereals with added vitamins or minerals, or flour with added folic acid. In fact, more and more foods are being fortified with nutrients and other physiologically active components (such as plant stanols and sterols) as researchers uncover more evidence about their role in health and even disease risk reduction.

Q. What are some of the health benefits associated with functional foods?

The scientific community has only just begun to understand the complex interactions between nutritional components and the human body. However, there is already a large body of scientific evidence showing that eating foods with functional benefits on a regular basis as part of a varied diet can help reduce the risk of, or manage a number of health concerns, including cancer, heart and cardiovascular disease, gastrointestinal health, menopausal symptoms, osteoporosis and eye health, to name a few.

Q. How can I get more functional foods in my diet?

The most effective way to reap the health benefits from foods is to eat a balanced and varied diet, including fruits and vegetables as well as foods with added beneficial components. Watch labels and read articles for information about foods and health. Before you decide to make any major dietary changes, however, take the time to evaluate your personal health, or speak to your health care provider on ways to help reduce your risk of certain diseases. It is also important to remember that there is no single "magic bullet" food that can cure or prevent most health concerns, even when eaten in abundance. The best advice is to choose foods wisely from each level of the food guide pyramid in order to incorporate many potentially beneficial components into the diet.

Q. Where can I learn about scientific research related to the functional benefits of foods?

There are several universities and research institutions conducting scientific studies on various food components. You can find out more about current research by visiting the home page of the Functional Foods for Health program administered by the University of Illinois at Urbana-Champaign and Chicago. Information on functional foods research is also available from the U.S. Department of Agriculture's Agricultural Research Service, the Institute of Food Technologists, the American Dietetic Association, and the food science programs at Rutgers University and the University of California, Davis.

Q. Are functional foods regulated by the federal government?

Yes. "Functional foods" has no official meaning and do not constitute a distinctly separate category of foods. Most often they are simply natural whole foods we have been eating for thousands of years. Therefore, the Food and Drug Administration (FDA) regulates them in the same way they regulate all foods—safety of ingredients must be assured in advance, and all claims must be substantiated, truthful, and non-misleading.

A significant amount of credible scientific data is needed to confirm any "health claims"—messages pertaining to a relationship between dietary components and a disease or health condition, for example soy protein and heart disease. Foods also can bear another type of claim to convey their potential benefits, and those are called "structure/function claims." These statements describe or imply a relationship between the product itself, or its components, and normal bodily functions (for example, "may help support digestion"). All such claims must be adequately substantiated.

A 1994 law stipulates that dietary supplements-for example an herb, vitamin, mineral or other substance added to one's total diet—shall continue to be treated as foods for regulatory purposes, but with just a few differences in approach. Regardless of any differences in approach, like all other foods, supplements are regulated by FDA to assure safety and accuracy of label claims.

There has been some criticism of certain foods containing herbal ingredients—whether or not such ingredients are allowed in food and whether their label claims are substantiated. The FDA is looking into these allegations. While herb-containing foods may be considered "functional", it is important to keep in mind that they represent only a small number of the broad spectrum of foods that are thought of as "functional foods".

Consumers need to remember that functional foods represent an important breakthrough in understanding the connection between diet, health, and even disease risk reduction. With regard to all claims pertaining to diseases and health conditions, consumers may be reassured to know that they must be pre-approved by FDA and substantiated by a large body of credible scientific evidence. And, although structure/function claims do not require FDA pre-approval, they too must be adequately substantiated by the producers of the food.

Q. What health claims have been approved so far by FDA?

Since 1993, FDA has approved 14 health claims, eight of which are related to the functional benefits of food:

- Potassium and reduced risk of high blood pressure and stroke
- Plant sterol and plant stanol esters and coronary heart disease
- Soy protein and coronary heart disease
- Calcium and reduced risk of osteoporosis
- Fiber-containing grain products, fruits and vegetables and cancer

- Fruits, vegetables and grain products that contain fiber, particularly soluble fiber, and risk of coronary heart disease
- Fruits and vegetables and cancer
- Folate and neural tube birth defects
- Dietary soluble fiber, such as that found in whole oats and psyllium seed husk, and coronary heart disease
- Dietary sugar alcohol and dental caries (cavaties)

The remaining three are based on diets low in "negative" nutrients in food, such as sodium:

- Dietary fat and cancer
- Dietary saturated fat and cholesterol and risk of coronary heart disease
- Sodium and high blood pressure

Q. What is the relationship between biotechnology and functional foods?

While many of the nutritional compounds in functional foods are either naturally present or added during processing, some may be the result of agricultural breeding techniques, including conventional crossbreeding and biotechnology.

Crossbreeding a plant for a specific genetic trait, such as higher vitamin A content, can take as long as a decade or more. Modern biotechnology, however, makes it possible to select a specific genetic trait from any plant and move it into the genetic code of another plant in a much shorter time span, and with more precision than crossbreeding allows.

Researchers are working with farmers around the world to develop dozens of functional foods through the use of this promising technology.

From *International Food Information Council Foundation*, November 2002. © 2002 by International Food Information Council Foundation.

ARE YOUR SUPPLEMENTS SAFE?

**Which supplements are safe? Which aren't? Which should you avoid if
you're taking blood-thinners or antidepressants?**

**Don't bother asking the manufacturers...or the government, for that matter. When it comes
to herbs and other over-the-counter supplements, you're pretty much on your own.**

Seven out of every ten adults in the U.S take vitamins, minerals, herbs, or other supplements, according to a 2002 Harris Poll. Some—calcium, folic acid, glucosamine, and saw palmetto, for example—are beneficial. Others—soy isoflavones, ginseng, ginkgo—may or may not be. And still others—ephedra, usnic acid, kava—can be dangerous.

And *any* supplement can do damage if you take too much or take it in the wrong combinations.

"How many supplement takers suffer adverse reactions, no one really knows," says Christine Haller, a medical toxicologist at the University of California at San Francisco who has analyzed reports on the toxicity of ephedra for the Food and Drug Administration (FDA). (Ephedra, which has been called an "herbal fat burner," was linked to the death of Baltimore Orioles pitcher Steve Bechler last spring.)

"We really can't tell how serious the safety questions are for dietary supplements until we look at these products more carefully," says Mary Palmer, an emergency room physician and toxicologist in Alexandria, Virginia.

Palmer, Haller, and their colleagues recently analyzed nearly 500 calls about bad reactions to supplements that had been phoned in to 11 poison control centers in the U.S. in 1998.[1]

"When I started the study I thought that maybe the safety problems with supplements really were mild and that my worries were unfounded," says Palmer. "I was very surprised to see how serious the adverse reactions really were." A third of them included heart attacks, liver failure, bleeding, seizures, and death.

Prescription medications cause an estimated 100,000 deaths and 2.2 million adverse reactions each year. While the toll from supplements is nowhere near as great, it's far from trivial. For example, more than 20,000 complaints about weight-loss products containing ephedra, including scores of deaths, have been registered during the past decade.

Supplements are regulated so much more loosely than drugs that it's impossible to know how much harm they cause.

"Drugs can be sold only if companies have enough evidence to convince the FDA and panels of independent experts that they're safe and effective and that their benefits justify their risks," says Bruce Silverglade, director of legal affairs at the Center for Science in the Public Interest (publisher of *Nutrition Action Healthletter*).

In contrast, "The dietary supplement market is the Wild West," says Congressman Henry Waxman, a California Democrat and longtime champion of measures to protect consumers' health.

"There are no requirements that a company prove anything about either the safety or the effectiveness of its products before they go to market."

Most people don't realize that.

"About 60 percent of U.S. consumers believe that dietary supplements must be approved by a government agency like the Food and Drug Administration before they can be sold to the public," says Nancy Wong of the Harris Poll.

Not so. Congress made sure of that when it passed the Dietary Supplement Health and Education Act (DSHEA) in 1994. "DSHEA put manufacturers in the driver's seat when it comes to which supplements are sold and what claims can be made for them," notes Palmer.

Before DSHEA, if the FDA questioned a supplement's safety, the manufacturer had to prove that it was safe. "DSHEA shifted the burden of proof," says Silverglade. "With drugs, food additives, and pesticides, it's always up to the manufacturer to prove safety. But thanks to DSHEA, the FDA has to prove that supplements are dangerous."

"Because of DSHEA," says Silverglade, "the FDA has been reduced to regulating by press release."

When the agency considers a supplement unsafe, it typically issues a consumer advisory and then discourages—but doesn't prohibit—companies from continuing to sell the product. How many consumers hear about these FDA advisories? "We don't know," concedes FDA spokesperson Sebastian Cianci. "To find that out would require research we don't have the resources to do."

Bottom line: The FDA can only bark, not bite.

In late 2001, for example, the agency received reports of young adults who developed liver damage or failure soon after starting to use a weight-loss product called LipoKinetix. (It contained usnic acid, the same substance thought to have destroyed Jennifer Rosenthal's liver a year later.) In response, the agency put out a press release advising consumers to "immediately stop use of LipoKinetix."

But the FDA didn't ban or suspend its sale. "Given the serious hazard presented by the use of your product," the agency wrote in a letter to the manufacturer, "we strongly recommend that you take prompt action to remove LipoKinetix from the market." (As it happened, the company had already suspended production because it couldn't get a steady supply of one ingredient.) Two years later, anyone can still purchase supplements that contain usnic acid on the Internet.

Consumers are protected from unsafe *drugs* by at least three lines of defense: The law requires manufacturers to test drugs for safety before they're sold, the FDA removes drugs from the marketplace when serious problems become evident, and manufacturers must track and disclose adverse effects, drug interactions, and other safety problems.

But against potentially unsafe *dietary supplements,* consumers are left to fend for themselves. Among the obstacles they face:

No Safety Testing

Pharmaceutical companies have to test their drugs to make sure they don't cause cancer, interfere with reproduction, damage organs, or cause other problems greater than they solve. In contrast, "Supplement companies have no obligation to test their products for safety before they market them," points out Christine Haller of the University of California at San Francisco.

"Some companies do small studies, but certainly not of the magnitude you would need to detect adverse effects," adds toxicologist Mary Palmer. "In many cases, there will be no information at all about a product's safety. But that doesn't mean it's safe."

"The dietary supplement market is the Wild West."

"Supplement manufacturers like to say that their products are safe because they've been used for centuries in other cultures," says Haller. "But traditional use didn't mean taking capsules of herbs day after day, so it was really different from the way we use them now." Continual exposure to concentrated extracts "probably changes the body's response to the herbs," notes Haller. "So these products might become ineffective or even have a detrimental effect."

How can an herb that has been used for centuries still be dangerous? If it causes cancer in, say, one out of every 100 people 20 years after they take it, the increased risk would never be noticed. Yet the government calls some food additives pesticides, and drugs carcinogens if they cause cancer in one out of every *million* people. That's the level that animal studies on those substances are designed to detect.

Supplement manufacturers, on the other hand, don't even have to understand how the body metabolizes their products. If they did, physicians would have learned long ago that St. John's wort can be life-threatening. (It can interfere with HIV drugs and immunosuppressants for transplant patients.)

And if companies had been required to thoroughly research the safety of hydroxycitrate before putting it in weight-loss supplements, they would have learned that the pharmaceutical giant Hoffman-La Roche abandoned the compound in the 1980s because of toxicity problems.

"We dropped hydroxycitrate when we saw that it seemed to cause testicular atrophy and other toxicities in animals," said a Hoffmann-La Roche spokesperson. "We never got as far as testing it in humans."

When told about the potential problems, a spokesperson for the firm that produces one of the two most popular hydroxycitrate formulations sold in the U.S. said, "I'm really, really surprised."

"There's no incentive for supplement companies to study the safety of their products," says Palmer. "It would be nothing but trouble for them, because they have a good deal right now." If anything's going to hurt their sales, "it's going to be safety issues. So why would they go looking for trouble?"

Take usnic acid. It's produced by lichen plants, so it falls within the loose definition of a dietary supplement. You can buy it on the Internet in the form of Usnea Lichen liquid herbal extracts. (We found one company that sells bottles of usnic acid capsules "for experimental research use only and not for human consumption" to anyone who claims to be at least 18 years old.)

Yet usnic acid may have destroyed the livers of at least half a dozen people in the U.S. over the past few years. Apparently that's not enough to motivate the companies that sell it—or the FDA—to investigate its toxicity.

"I don't know anyone else who's working on the toxicity of usnic acid besides me," says Neil Kaplowitz, director of the University of Southern California Research Center for Liver Diseases in Los Angeles.

Underreported Reactions

"Mild symptoms are definitely underreported to physicians and health agencies, and, as a result, there are probably many problems with supplements that are not being described," says toxicologist Christine Haller. A 2001 report by the U.S. Department of Health and Human Services estimated that only about one out of every 100 adverse reactions is reported to the FDA.[2]

EIGHT TO AVOID

Despite evidence that these eight products can cause serious problems, most are still available, either over the counter or via the Internet.

- **Aristolochic acid.** The ingredient in some traditional Chinese medicines is toxic to the kidneys.
- **Chaparral.** In 1992, the FDA advised consumers to "stop taking chaparral immediately" because it can cause hepatitis.
- **Comfrey.** It can cause chronic liver disease.
- **Ephedra.** It has been linked to high blood pressure, strokes, and heart attacks and is 200 times more likely to cause an adverse reaction than all other herbs combined.
- **Kava.** It's a suspect in liver damage that has resulted in 11 liver transplants over the last several years.

- **PC SPES and SPES.** These supplements, which held promise as prostate-cancer fighters, turned out to be frauds. They worked like hormones only because they were spiked with hormones, a blood thinner, an anti-inflammatory, and several other drugs.
- **Tiratricol.** In 2000, the FDA warned consumers not to use weight-loss supplements containing this thyroid hormone, which can cause strokes and heart attacks.
- **Usnic acid.** This "natural" compound (it's found in lichen), which is used in some herbal mixtures, appears to be toxic to the liver.

Sources: Food and Drug Administration (*www.cfsan.fda.gov/%7Edms/ds-warn.html*) and CSPI.

"People are somewhat embarrassed when they have a problem with a supplement that they think maybe they shouldn't have been taking, like one of the weight-loss products," says Haller. "Why tell your doctor if your doctor didn't know you were taking it?"

What's more, people may not make the connection between a bad reaction and a "natural" supplement. And even if people call the consumer complaint number that's on the product label, "manufacturers sometimes don't do anything with those complaints," says Haller.

Troublesome Interactions

"There's competition in the marketplace now to give consumers the most for their dollar by offering combinations of herbs and other ingredients," says Haller. "But combining ingredients, especially herbs, isn't a good idea, because we really don't understand a lot about how they interact."

In their analysis of calls to poison control centers in the U.S., Haller and her colleagues found that multiple-ingredient supplements were more likely than single-ingredient ones to produce severe adverse effects.

No Required Warnings

"About two-thirds of the U.S. public believes that the government requires the labels of dietary supplements to include warnings about potential side effects or dangers," says Nancy Wong of the Harris Poll.

Not so. Unlike drug labels, supplement labels don't have to disclose who shouldn't take the product, what drugs it shouldn't be taken with, or other warnings.

So, for example, beta-carotene supplements labels don't have to disclose who shouldn't take the product, what drugs it shouldn't be taken with, or other warnings.

So, for example, beta-carotene supplements are unlikely to warn smokers that high doses (at least 25 mg, or 42,000 IU) may increase their risk of lung cancer. And zinc supplement labels are unlikely to disclose that too much zinc can compromise the immune system.

Unreported Problems

"The FDA maintains surveillance of prescription drugs by requiring prompt reports from manufacturers of all adverse events brought to their attention," says Arthur Grollman, chair of pharmacology at the State University of New York at Stony Brook.

"But there is no mandatory requirement for manufacturers of supplements to record, investigate, or forward to the FDA reports of adverse effects they might receive," he adds. "Under current regulations, there is no penalty for withholding these reports." Grollman wants Congress to require companies to report safety problems.

For years, Metabolife, the leading manufacturer of weight-loss pills that contain ephedra, denied that it knew of any serious complaints about its products. Then last year, lawyers who were suing the company on behalf of injured consumers learned that Metabolife had, in fact, received more than 13,000 complaints from users.

The Top Ten Supplements: How Safe?

How safe are the 10 most popular herbal supplements? Here's what you need to know. Just keep in mind that most reactions are rare; in some cases they're based on just one or two reports from physicians. Until more research is done, it's probably wise for children and pregnant or nursing women not to take any of these supplements.

Supplement	What Consumers Expect	Reported Reactions	Who Should be Especially Careful	May Interact With
Black Cohosh	To relieve symptoms of menopause.	Mild gastrointestinal distress.	Women who have had breast cancer (in an animal study, black cohosh caused cancer to spread).	No drug interactions known.
Cranberry	To prevent or treat urinary tract infections.	Regular use of cranberry concentrate tablets might increase the risk of kidney stones.	People susceptible to kidney stones.	Antidepressants and prescription painkillers.
Echinacea	To prevent or treat colds or other infections.	Minor gastrointestinal symptoms. Increased urination. Allergic reactions.	People with autoimmune diseases (like multiple sclerosis, lupus, and rheumatoid arthritis). May also trigger episodes of erythema nodosum, an inflammation that produces tender nodules under the skin.	No drug interactions known.
Garlic	To lower cholesterol levels.	Unpleasant breath odor. Heartburn and flatulence.	People who are about to have—or have just had—surgery (garlic thins the blood). Women just before or after labor or delivery.	Blood-thinning drugs like Coumadin (warfarin), heparin, or aspirin. Blood-thinning supplements like ginko or high doses of vitamin E. Chloroxazone, which is used to treat painful muscle conditions. HIV drugs.
Ginkgo Biloba	To improve memory.	Mild headache. Upset stomach. Seizures (possibly caused by contamination with ginkgo seeds, which are toxic).	People with bleeding disorders like hemophilia. People who are about to have—or have just had—surgery. Women just before or after labor or delivery. People with diabetes.	Blood-thinning drugs like Coumadin (warfarin), heparin, or aspirin. Blood-thinning supplements like high doses of vitamin E. The antidepressant trazodone. Anti-diabetes drugs. Thiazide diuretics.
Ginseng	To increase energy and relieve stress.	Insomnia. Menstrual abnormalities and breast tenderness with long-term use.	Women who had had breast cancer (ginseng stimulated the growth of breast cancer cells in test tubes). People with high blood pressure who aren't taking medication to lower it.	Any drug metabolized by the enzyme CYP 3A4 (ask your physician). MAO inhibitor drugs or digitalis. May increase the activity of insulin and oral hypoglycemics and decrease the activity of Coumadin (warfarin) and ticlopidine.
Saw Palmetto	To prevent or relieve the symptoms of an enlarged prostate.	Mild gastrointestinal distress.	People with bleeding disorders like hemophilia. People who are about to have—or have just had—surgery.	Blood-thinning drugs like Coumadin (warfarin), heparin, or aspirin. Blood-thinning supplements like ginkgo or high doses of vitamin E.
Soy Isoflavones	To relieve menopausal symptoms, prevent breast or prostate cancer, and strengthen bones.	None reported.	Women who have had—or are at high risk for—breast cancer (soy isoflavones may increase cell proliferation). Pregnant women. People with impaired thyroid function.	No drug interactions known.
St. John's Wort	To alleviate depression.	Mild gastrointestinal distress. Rash. Tiredness. Restlessness.	People with skin that's sensitive to sunlight. People taking UV treatment. People with bipolar disorder.	Ritalin, ephedrine (found in ephedra), and caffeine. May increase the activity of protease inhibitors (for HIV), digitalis (for high cholesterol), warfarin (blood-thinner), chemotherapy drugs, oral contraceptives, tricyclic antidepressants, olanzapine and clozapine (for schizophrenia), and theophylline (for asthma). May increase sensitivity to sunlight if combined with sulfa drugs, Feldene (anti-inflammatory), or Prilosec or Prevacid (for acid reflux).
Valerian	To induce sleep or relaxation.	May impair attention for a few hours.	People about to operate heavy machinery or drive.	May increase the activity of central-nervous-system depressants like barbiturates (such as Seconal) and benzodiazepines (such as Valium or Halcion).

Source: The Natural Pharmacist, Healthnotes, and CSPI.

Among them were more than 1,000 reports of significant adverse reactions, including 18 heart attacks, 26 strokes, 43 seizures, and five deaths.[3]

An angry FDA has asked the Department of Justice to pursue filing criminal charges against Metabolife officials for lying to the agency.

Unavailable Adverse Reaction Reports

For years, the Food and Drug Administration has been collecting reports of adverse reactions to dietary supplements. But last year the agency pulled the database from its Web site, saying that the information was confusing.

Last June, the FDA installed a new system (the Center for Food Safety and Applied Nutrition Adverse Events Reporting System, or CAERS) to track complaints by consumers and physicians to its MedWatch hotline (800-FDA-1088 or *fda.gov/medwatch/report/consumer/consumer.htm*).

But health professionals and the public can't view the complaints that have been submitted to CAERS.

"We're working on a way to give the public access to this information, but that's at least a year away," says FDA spokesperson Sebastian Cianci. "Until then, you need to file a Freedom of Information Act [FOIA] request to see the information."

That can take months, which is far too long to help people track down what's causing a reaction. And it certainly would have been too long for people like Jennifer Rosenthal, the California mother who paid a steep price for her lesson in supplement safety.

Notes

1. *Lancet 361*: 101, 2003.
2. Department of Health and Human Services, Office of the Inspector General: *Adverse Event Reporting for Dietary Supplements, An Inadequate Safety Valve*. OEI-01-00180, April 2001.
3. Government Accounting Office: *Dietary Supplements Containing Ephedra*. GAO-03-1042T, July 2003.

Food Colorings

Pigments make fruits and veggies extra healthful

Janet Raloff

Crop geneticist Charles R. Brown has spent a decade working to make a better potato. In the beginning, he focused on beefing up the familiar white-fleshed tuber. His strategy was to recapture healthful traits from old-style spuds from the plant's native range in South America. He examined many yellow, red, and purple potatoes, none of which grows well in a U.S. climate. While cross breeding these imports with their northern cousins, Brown and his coworkers at the U.S. Department of Agriculture laboratory in Prosser, Wash., began hearing about putative health benefits from the type of pigments, called flavonoids, that give the potatoes their color.

Flavonoids include beta-carotene and related carotenoids, which are responsible for many of the yellows, oranges, reds, and greens in produce. Other reds and most of the blues, purples, and blackish tints—especially in berries and potatoes—trace to flavonoids called anthocyanins.

These chemicals are considered antioxidants because they quash free radicals, naturally forming molecular fragments that have several damaging effects. Free radicals can kill cells, transform some of the blood's cholesterol-toting lipoproteins into agents of atherosclerosis (*SN: 4/21/01, p. 245*), and induce DNA damage that might foster cancer (*SN: 2/22/97, p. 126*).

A few years ago, Brown's group and a few others around the world began developing new lines of crops explicitly for their intense antioxidant pigments. Some early lines of red and purple potatoes are now on the market, and other colorful crops are heading that way.

Probably the most famous example is known as golden rice. It's enriched with beta-carotene, a yellow chemical from which the body fashions most of its vitamin A. Swiss and German researchers used biotechnology to design this cereal in the late 1990s to improve vitamin-poor diets in developing countries. The golden grain is still being fine-tuned for eventual commercialization.

Philipp Simon and his colleagues at a USDA lab in Madison, Wis., have been developing carotenoid-enhanced, yellow-or-ange cucumbers and red and anthocyanin-rich, dark-purple carrots. This team bred some of the carrots now on the market, which retain the traditional orange color but produce 75 percent more beta-carotene than carrots did 25 years ago. In another example of pigment boosting, researchers at Cornell University are breeding wheat with extra flavonoids.

There's currently evidence that, in addition to fighting inflammation, heart disease, and cancer, flavonoids can counter obesity and elevated blood sugar. Although scientists have presumed that flavonoids' benefits derive mainly from their antioxidant activity, some research has recently shown that the chemicals facilitate signaling between cells and silence genes that might otherwise foster disease.

Indeed, James A. Joseph of USDA's Human Nutrition Research Center on Aging at Tufts University in Boston says that this basic effect may contribute to flavonoids' broad range of activities.

With growing recognition of the health-promoting biological activity of plant pigments, many researchers are advocating that consumers expand the palette of colors on their dinner plates. For instance, Joseph wrote a book to guide people in choosing healthful foods by their colors (*The Color Code,* 2003, Hyperion Books).

Joseph acknowledges that color offers, at best, an imperfect measure of potentially beneficial antioxidant flavonoids. However, by choosing foods exhibiting a range of deep colors, he says, a person can be reasonably sure of getting a broad mix of beneficial flavonoids.

HEART-SPARING HINTS Many studies have linked anticancer benefits and protection against heart disease with diets rich in produce, especially carotenoid-rich green, leafy vegetables.

The most recent of these reports, in the Nov. 3, 2004 *Journal of the National Cancer Institute,* analyzed dietary and health data for almost 72,000 female nurses and 38,000 male health professionals. The study found significantly less risk of chronic illness, especially heart disease, in study participants eating the most fruits and vegetables. Of all foods analyzed, green leafy vegetables appeared most protective. In fact, for each daily serving of spinach or other greens consumed, an individual's risk of developing cardiovascular disease fell by 11 percent.

In 2003, Tiina H. Rissanen of the University of Kuopio in Finland and her colleagues reported that the more servings of vegetables and fruits that middle-aged men consumed, the lower their risk of dying from heart disease. The data pointed to berries, in particular, as being protective.

These findings were consistent with others published that year by an Australian team. For 6 weeks, nutrition scientists gave 32 men fruit extracts every morning and vegetable extracts every evening. Several potential heart-disease indicators, such as blood concentrations of homocysteine (*SN: 1/4/03, p.5*) and susceptibility of cholesterol to oxidation (*SN: 4/21/01, p. 245*), were far lower in men taking the supplements than in volunteers who had eaten the same diet minus the supplements.

To probe what compounds might account for such benefits, researchers have been isolating and testing the effects of various constituents of fruits and vegetables, including purified flavonoids.

DARK TINTS John D. Folts' team at the University of Wisconsin–Madison has shown that grape skins and seeds contain flavonoids that limit blood platelet clumping. That clumping is a critical step in blood clotting, but it also contributes to the formation of clots underlying heart attacks and strokes. Although the flavonoids in either skins or in seeds have proved beneficial, the best results occurred when Folts' group added extracts of both to the diets of dogs and people.

Folts suggests that extracts of grape seeds and skins could provide all the heart-health benefits that have been linked to wine and grape juice (*SN: 3/8/03, p. 155*). His group recently began studies of one commercial extract of grape seeds and skins. Such a food supplement might prove beneficial to people who'd prefer to avoid the alcohol in wine or the sugar in juice.

Pomegranates are even richer in antioxidant flavonoids, especially anthocyanins, than purple grapes are, according to research led by Michael Aviram of Rambam Medical Center in Haifa, Israel. Over the past 5 years, his team has shown that the flavonoids in pomegranate inhibit cholesterol oxidation in human blood and slow the development of atherosclerotic disease in mice.

In one recent study, Aviram's team followed volunteers who had atherosclerosis, characterized by symptoms including a narrowing of their carotid arteries. Ten of the participants drank 50 milliliters of pomegranate juice daily for 1 to 3 years. Nine others took a flavonoid-free placebo drink. Throughout the trial, all continued to receive the heart medications that their doctors prescribed.

By the end of the study, the people drinking the pomegranate juice had experienced a 20 percent drop in systolic blood pressure, while the placebo group showed no decline. Similarly, only the pomegranate group experienced a beneficial reduction in the thickness of their carotid artery walls and a dramatic drop in the oxidation-susceptibility of their low-density-lipoprotein cholesterol, the team reported in the June 2004 *Clinical Nutrition*.

Related heart benefits emerged in Chinese studies of animals treated with black-rice pigments. Black rice contains flavonoids, especially pigmented relatives of anthocyanins, also found in fruits and vegetables, explains Wenhua Ling of Sun Yet-sen University of Medical Sciences in Guangzhou. He and his colleagues fed mice and rabbits cholesterol-rich diets intended to promote heart disease. The scientists supplemented the animals' food with powdered rice bran. Half the animals got black-rice bran, the rest got equivalent amounts of pigmentfree white-rice bran. The animals ingesting black-rice supplements developed far lower concentrations of oxidation by-products in their blood and in the tissues of their arteries and experienced less artery-clogging plaque, Ling's team reported in 2002 and 2003.

Ling says he was surprised by the potency of the pigments. He and his colleagues are now conducting research in which they give black rice pigments to people with atherosclerosis.

DEEP PURPLE Plant flavonoids also show promise in other health areas. For instance, studies indicate that lycopene—the red carotenoid in tomatoes and watermelons—can prevent prostate cancer in animals and shrink prostate tumors in men (*SN: 4/24/99, p. 271*). Anthocyanins in tart red cherries seem to provide a natural inflammation-fighting alternative to aspirin (*SN: 4/17/99, p. 247*).

However, some of the most dramatic effects attributed to anthocyanins have emerged in studies of blue and purple foods. For instance, when Japanese scientists gave mice high-fat diets augmented with an anthocyanin-pigmented extract from purple corn, the animals maintained normal weights. Mice on the same diet but without the extract became obese. Moreover, only the latter group of animals developed excessive sugar and insulin concentrations in their blood, Takanori Tsuda of Doshisha University in Kyoto and his colleagues reported in 2003.

Last year, Tsuda's team showed that the purple-corn extract increased the activity of a gene that regulates the function of fat cells. It's the first food component to do so, the scientists reported in the March 26, 2004 *Biochemical and Biophysical Research Communications*. They also recommended that anthocyanins be explored as nutritional supplements for "preventing obesity and diabetes." Tsuda says, "We need to perform a human study as soon as possible."

Joseph, who is a neuroscientist, has been working with blueberries, which are rich in flavonoids. Five years ago, his team reported that adding blueberries to the diets of aging rats not only prevented further declines in memory and mental agility but also reversed those trends in the animals (*SN: 9/18/99, p. 180*).

In 2003, his team published a follow-up study in which they examined a strain of mice that normally develops Alzheimer's disease symptoms, including brain plaques and memory loss. Beginning when the mice were young, the researchers fed them 20 grams of blueberries per kilogram of food. The animals still eventually developed Alzheimer's-like brain plaques—but no memory loss. The researchers concluded that their data "indicate for the first time that it may be possible to overcome genetic predispositions to Alzheimer's disease through diet."

Some of the benefit to memory appears to trace to enhanced brain-cell signaling in animals eating the blue fruit, Joseph says. Old neurons and those in individuals with Alzheimer's disease "are like old married couples: They don't talk to each other," he says. Blueberry's flavonoids "make them [communicate] like young lovers again."

Joseph speculates that, by fostering communication between neurons, the anthocyanins or related chemicals in blueberries affect learning and memory and also spur the growth of new nerve cells, a process called neurogenesis. His group's latest studies indicate that in blueberry-fed animals, both anthocyanin concentrations and the rates of neurogenesis correlate with performance on memory tests.

AIM FOR MIXES Most flavonoid researchers argue that people should get healthy doses of these chemicals from colorful foods, not dietary supplements. Indeed, several studies have shown that megadoses of a flavonoid can trigger harmful effects, probably by boosting oxidation.

That's what biochemist Homer S. Black of Baylor College of Medicine in Houston witnessed in studies of mice. His group showed that a diet overly enriched with beta-carotene increased skin cancer resulting from ultraviolet light's oxidative damage rather than protecting against it. Black is therefore "leery of supplementing with single antioxidants," but he heartily recommends consuming a broad mix of them every day in whole foods.

Another reason for consuming antioxidants in foods rather than as supplements is that the chemistry of these agents can be influenced by what's eaten along with them. For instance, the carotenoids tinting most vegetables preferentially dissolve in lipids. Unless these pigments are eaten along with fat—such as the oil in salad dressing-the body absorbs only a small fraction of them, notes Steven J. Schwartz of Ohio State University in Columbus.

He recently showed that avocado, a high-fat fruit, facilitates carotenoid uptake by the body. In tests with 11 men and women, his team showed that adding about half an avocado to an undressed salad dramatically increased carotenoid absorption. For instance, lutein absorption more than quadrupled, and beta-carotene absorption rose 12-fold. Schwartz now recommends mashed avocado as a salad dressing.

Anthocyanins, in contrast to carotenoids, are extremely water soluble, so they don't need fat to be absorbed, reports chemist Ronald L. Prior of the USDA lab at the Arkansas Children's Nutrition Center in Little Rock.

However, adds Joseph, because these flavonoids appear to be useful to the brain and "something has to be [fat] soluble to get across the blood-brain barrier," even anthocyanins may benefit from a fat chaser. Toward that end, he suggested that the California Avocado Commission consider teaming its favorite fruit with his. The result: a recipe for avocado-blueberry smoothies (*http://www.avocado.org/recipes/view.php/Avocado/Blueberry/Smoothie?recipe_id=902*).

Now, doesn't that make a colorful image?

UNIT 6
Food Safety/Technology

Unit Selections

Key Points to Consider

- What are some of the major factors that compromise food safety?

- What action should you take to minimize your risk from exposure to environmental contaminants in the food chain?

- Survey your neighborhood supermarket about the origin of the salmon they sell.

- Check the labels of omega-3-fatty acid supplements from two different companies in reference to mercury, dioxin, and PCB content.

- What should your role be, as a consumer, in ensuring food safety from production to sale?

Student Website

www.mhcls.com/online

Internet References

Further information regarding these websites may be found in this book's preface or online.

American Council on Science and Health (ACSH)
http://www.acsh.org/food/

Centers for Disease Control and Prevention (CDC)
http://www.cdc.gov

FDA Center for Food Safety and Applied Nutrition
http://vm.cfsan.fda.gov

Food Safety Project (FSP)
http://www.extension.iastate.edu/foodsafety/

National Food Safety Programs
http://vm.cfsan.fda.gov/~dms/fs-toc.html

USDA Food Safety and Inspection Service (FSIS)
http://www.fsis.usda.gov

Food-borne disease constitutes an important public health problem in the United States. The US Centers for Disease Control has reported 76 million cases of food-borne illness each year out of which 5,000 end in death. The annual cost of losses in productivity ranges from 20 to 40 billion dollars. Food-borne disease results primarily from microbial contamination, naturally occurring toxicants, environmental contaminants, pesticide residues, and food additives.

The first Food and Drug Act was passed in 1906 and was followed by tighter control on the use of additives that might be carcinogenic. In 1958, the Delaney Clause was passed and a list of additives that were considered as safe for human consumption (GRAS list) was developed. The Food and Drug Administration (FDA) controls and regulates procedures dealing with food safety, including food service and production. The FDA has established rules (Hazard Analysis and Critical Control Points) to improve safety control and to monitor the production of seafood, meat, and poultry. Even though there have been outbreaks of food poisoning traced to errors at the commercial processing stage, the culprit is usually mishandling of food at home, in a food service establishment, or other noncommercial setting. Surveys show that over 95 percent of the time people do not follow proper sanitation methods when working with food. The US government, therefore, launched the Food Safety Initiative program to minimize foodborne disease and to educate the public about safe food handling practice. Even though animal foods are more likely to be contaminated, there has been an increase of food-born illness from fruit and vegetable consumption. Elizabeth Ward describes the sources of fruit and vegetable contamination, compares domestic and imported products, and offers strategies to minimize your risk.

Currently consumer concerns have shifted to include concerns about consuming food that may contain antibiotics, hormones, pesticides, mercury, dioxin and PCBs, and cloned animals. Crowded living conditions of animals necessitate the use of germ-fighting antibiotics that eventually become part of the food chain, increase risk of exposure to consumers, and may result in the development of antibiotic resistance. Growth hormones injected into cattle may also disrupt human hormone systems. Toxic pesticides in trace amounts found in vegetables, fruits, meats, milk and trans fat found in fast foods, bakery products, margarines and shortenings, raise our risk of chronic disease. More recently the issue of the safety of consuming farmed salmon is under question, since mercury, PCBs, and dioxin contamination is making the public and scientists uneasy about dietary recommendations. Two articles present the nutritional issues about farm-raised vs. wild fish and explain environmental contaminant bioaccumulation. They also offer suggestions as to how much fish to eat and discuss the use of fish oil supplements.

The most recent concern is the possibility that meat from cloned animals may be coming to a market near you. The FDA's Veterinary Committee has concluded that animal clones "appear to be safe" and there is no reason for product labeling. The right

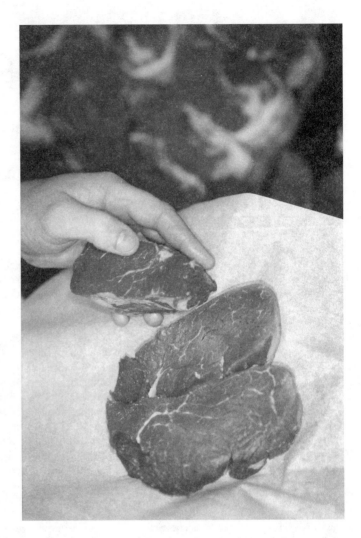

for consumers to know so that they can make their own choices, is of the utmost importance. The USDA has set the criteria for what food may be called "organic" and food makers that qualify can declare their products "certified organic." The National Organic Rule, a product of ten years of work by growers, scientists, and consumers, defines "organic" as foods that are produced without insecticides, herbicides, chemical fertilizers, radiation, genetic modification, hormones, or antibiotics. This is a breakthrough especially for consumers, since it enables them to have a good idea of what is organic and what is not.

The last article describes the history of the FDA's regulatory and monitoring function and changes the agency needs to institute to regulate the exploding dietary supplement market. The Good Manufacturing Practices regulation will set standards for handling and manufacturing supplements thus ensuring high quality.

CERTIFIED ORGANIC

STAMP OF APPROVAL: New government rules will define 'organic.' The sale of these fruits, veggies and snack foods has soared, but we still aren't sure what good they do. Here's a guide to how purer products affect the health of our families and the planet.

BY GEOFFREY COWLEY

OTTO KRAMM USED TO COME home from work at night and warn his toddlers to keep their distance until he'd bathed and changed his clothes. He wasn't just trying to keep them clean. As a vegetable farmer in California's Salinas Valley, Kramm spent his days covered in pesticides, herbicides and fungicides, and he worried about their effects on young children. "I didn't know what was on my clothes," he says, "or how it might affect the kids 15 years down the road." The more he thought about it, the less he liked the feeling. So in 1996, Kramm did something radical. He bought into a farm that was being cultivated organically. "It was scary," he says. "I couldn't fall back on the tools I'd always used to fight the pests and the weeds." But he worked out a new relationship with the soil and ended up not only cleaner but more prosperous. Today Kramm has 6,000 acres on three farms. The nation's largest organic-produce distributor, Earthbound Farm, is buying up everything he can grow. And he's never off-limits to his kids.

Organic farms are still sprouts in a forest of industrial giants. They provide less than 2 percent of the nation's food supply and take up less than 1 percent of its cropland. But they're flourishing as never before. Over the past decade the market for organic food has grown by 15 to 20 percent every year—five times faster than food sales in general. Nearly 40 percent of U.S. consumers now reach occasionally for something labeled organic, and sales are expected to top $11 billion this year. Could dusty neighborhood co-ops sell that many wormy little apples? Well, no. That was the old organic. The new organic is all about bigger farms, heartier crops, better distribution and slicker packaging and promotion. Conglomerates as big as Heinz and General Mills are now launching or buying organic lines—and selling them in mainstream supermarkets.

What exactly are consumers getting out of the deal? Until now, the definition of "organic" has varied from one state to the next, leaving shoppers to assume it means something like "way more expensive but probably better for you." Not anymore. As of Oct. 21, any food sold as organic will have to meet criteria set by the United States Department of Agriculture. The National Organic Rule—the product of 10 years' deliberation by growers, scientists and consumers—reserves the terms "100 percent organic" and "organic" (at least 95 percent) for foods produced without hormones, antibiotics, herbicides, insecticides, chemical fertilizers, genetic modification or germ-killing radiation. Food makers who document their compliance will qualify for a new USDA seal declaring their products "certified organic." "This really signifies the start of a new era," says Margaret Wittenberg of the Whole Foods supermarket chain. "From now on, consumers will get a very solid idea of what is organic and what is not."

Yet for all the clarity they provide, the standards say nothing about what's worth putting in your shopping cart. "This is not a food-safety program," says Barbara Robinson, the USDA official overseeing the effort. "We're not saying that organic food is safer or better than other kinds of food." How, then, should we read the new label?

Does "certified organic" tell us anything worth knowing about a chicken breast or a candy bar? Are organically grown grapes more nutritious than conventional ones? And is organic agriculture a viable alternative to modern factory farming? These are complicated, politically charged questions, but they're questions worth asking ourselves—both as consumers and citizens.

When the counterculture embraced organic food and farming in the early '70s, the motivation was more philosophical than practical. Maria Rodale, whose family runs the pro-organic Rodale Institute in Kutztown, Pa., sees the current boom as evidence that people are still "expressing their values about the environment and even spirituality and politics through the food choices they make." Market research suggests she's about 26 percent right. When the Hartman Group of Bellevue, Wash., surveyed consumers two years ago, only one in four cited concern about the environment as a "top motivator" for buying organic food. Flavor was a bigger concern, cited by 38 percent as reason enough to pay a premium of 15 percent or more. Sophisticated chefs have responded in droves, many now serving only fresh, seasonal food from small local growers. "The difference is huge," says Peter Hoffman, owner of New York's Restaurant Savoy and chairman of the Chefs' Collaborative. "When people taste asparagus or string beans grown in richly composted soil, they can't get over the depth and vibrancy of the flavor."

To most consumers, though, organic means healthier. Fully 66 percent of the Hartman Group's respondents cited health as a "top motivator"—as will almost any shopper on the street. "Buying an apple that has poison on it, even if you wash it you don't know how much has come off," says Wendy Abrams, a suburban Chicago mother with four kids at home. Abrams buys organic milk and stocks her pantry with Newman's Own pretzels and raisins on the theory that anything organic is less likely to harbor cancer-causing chemicals. "There have been six cases of cancer on my street," she says. "It's just weird."

All of these folks—market analysts refer to them as "true naturals," "connoisseurs" and "health seekers"—seem happy with their purchases. But are they getting what they're seeking? It's hard to argue with the connoisseurs, and not just because they know what they like. A tomato grown on a vast commercial plot is bred less for taste than for durability, notes Bob Scowcroft of the nonprofit Organic Farming Research Foundation. It has to resist disease and ship well. Organic growers, with their smaller harvests and their reliance on nearby markets, can plant delicate heirloom strains and give the fruit more time on the vine. "They pick it when it's ripe," says Marion Cunningham, author of "The Fannie Farmer Cookbook." "No one goes around picking organic fruits when they're as hard as little rocks."

Managed property, organic farms can match conventional ones for productivity, and beat them during drought conditions.

The health seekers may have common sense on their side, but no one has found a way to determine whether people eating well-balanced organic diets are healthier than those eating well-balanced conventional ones. No one denies that nonorganic produce contains pesticide residues that would be toxic at high doses. Nor is there any question that children (because of their size) consume those residues in higher concentrations than adults. But there is still no evidence that pesticides cause ill health at the doses found in food, or that people who eschew them come out ahead. Technological optimists find it ludicrous that anyone would fret over pesticide residues when the hazards of foodborne bacteria are

so much clearer. *E. coli* is "perhaps the deadliest risk in our modern food supply," says Dennis Avery of the Hudson Institute—"and its primary hiding place is the cattle manure with which organic farmers fertilize food crops." So wash your produce, but don't let it scare you. Organic or conventional, fruits and vegetables are the best fuel you can put in your body.

Dangerous bacteria are even more common in animal products, but the organic program is not a germ-control initiative. Under the new guidelines, meat and dairy labeled organic must come from creatures that are raised on organic grains or grasses, given access to the outdoors and spared treatment with growth hormones and antibiotics. Experts agree that by spiking animal feed with antibiotics, conventional farmers are speeding the emergence of drug-resistant bacteria. Buying organic is one way to vote against that practice. But in terms of your own health, you'll profit more from holding back on animal products than by eating organic ones. In one study, Danish research found that organic chickens were actually more likely than conventional ones to carry campylobacter, a pathogen that can cause severe diarrhea.

So organic food is tastier and more appealing, but not demonstrably better for you. If you're shopping with only yourself in mind, maybe you'll save your money. But if you pause to think about what you're buying into with every food purchase, organic goods start to look like a bargain. Our current agricultural system took off in the years following World War II, when farmers discovered that chemical fertilizers could force higher yields out of tired soil—and that pesticides could clear croplands of competing species. As farmers saw what the new chemicals made possible, American agriculture was transformed from a rural art into a heavy industry dominated by large corporations growing single crops on vast stretches of poisoned soil.

As any ecologist might have predicted, the new approach was hard to sustain. A small, varied farm can renew itself endlessly when managed with care. Last year's bean stocks help nourish next year's cantaloupes, and a bad year for tomatoes may be a good year for eggplant. As they lost sight of those lessons, the factory farmers grew ever more dependent on chemicals. Insects died off conveniently at

first. But each application of insecticide left a few hearty survivors, and within a few generations whole populations were resistant. Today, says Scowcroft, "we're applying three times as much chemical as we were 40 years ago to kill the same pests." It's not just insects. Conventional farmers now use herbicides to kill weeds, fungicides to kill fungi, rodenticides to kill field mice and gophers, avicides to kill fruit-eating birds and molluscicides to kill snails. Strawberry growers now favor all-purpose fumigants such as methyl bromide. "You inject it into the soil and put a tarp over it," says Monica Moore of the Pesticide Action Network of North America. "It kills everything from mammals to microbes. It's a complete biocide."

These practices may not be poisoning our food, but there is no question they're killing off wildlife, endangering farmworkers and degrading the soil and water that life itself depends on. Pesticides now kill 67 million American birds each year. The Mississippi River dumps enough synthetic fertilizer into the Gulf of Mexico to maintain a 60-mile-wide "dead zone" too choked with algae to support fish. And soil erosion threatens to turn much of the world's arable land into desert. "Conventional agriculture still delivers cheap, abundant food," says Fred Kirschenmann of the Leopold Center for Sustainable Agriculture in Ames, Iowa. "But when you factor in the government subsidies and the environmental costs, it gets very expensive. We're drawing down our ecological capital. At some point, the systems will start to break down."

Can organic agriculture save the day? Not if it's just a boutique alternative. But as demand grows, more and more farmers are taking a leap backward—and landing on their feet. They're discovering they can enrich the soil and manage some pests simply by rotating their crops. They're learning that they can often control insects with other insects—or lure them away from cash crops by planting things they prefer. Well-run organic farms often match conventional ones for productivity, even beat them when water is scarce. Creating a sustainable food supply may well require advanced technology as well as ecological awareness. But an organic ethic could be the very key to our survival.

With ANNE UNDERWOOD
and KAREN SPRINGEN

Send in the Clones

Will the FDA allow food products derived from
animal clones to be sold without any labeling requirements?

By Kate Jackson

Could food from cloned animals be coming soon to a market near you? Will you dine on roasted rack of cloned lamb, feast on ribs from a cloned pig, or down a glass of cold milk from a cloned cow? The answer is likely to be yes, but the real question is: Will you know it if you do?

A recent announcement by the FDA—based on ongoing assessments indicating that consumption of food from animal clones "appears to be safe"—suggests that it won't be long until these products are approved to enter the U.S. food supply and find their way into stores and restaurants. If that prospect makes you squeamish, this might make you downright queasy: The FDA currently sees no reason for labels that would let consumers know that they're purchasing food from animal clones.

The Ongoing Review

Somatic cell nuclear transfer is the name of the process by which animals are cloned. Through this fusion of a cell's nucleus from the body of the parent animal to an unfertilized egg cell, an identical genetic copy of the parent animal is created. The process has been used for the purpose of improving quality and increasing productivity at a cost of as much as $20,000 to clone a single

goat, pig, or cow. At this cost, it's unlikely that these animal clones will themselves enter the food supply, but their progeny are likely to reach American tables once they are approved by the government.

Before that can happen, the government must conclude its ongoing process of reviewing the scientific research concerning the safety of human consumption of cloned animal products. The FDA's risk analysis began nearly two years ago when it asked the National Academy of Sciences (NAS) to investigate the evidence. On October 31, 2003, the FDA issued a draft executive summary of its risk assessment, which it says builds upon the NAS findings. The academy determined that although animal clones "posed only a low level of food safety concern, it would be prudent to have more data in order to minimize further safety concerns." Before it could make policy decisions concerning animal clones, the FDA concluded that a risk assessment was necessary, to be followed by a review of risk management options. Information has and will continue to be communicated at public meetings and all future information will be publicly available through the FDA's Web site.

With the release of the draft executive summary, the FDA also an-

nounced that a voluntary moratorium on releasing animal clones remains in effect until further data are evaluated. The summary reveals that an advisory panel has reached the tentative opinion that food from "animal clones and their offspring is likely to be as safe to eat as food from their nonclone counterparts, based on all the evidence available." A public meeting was held November 4, 2003, at the Center for Veterinary Medicine in Rockville, Md., during which some panel members insisted on the need for further data to support the FDA's presumption of safety while others urged the agency to pay greater attention to the ethical issues surrounding animal cloning, including the suffering of cloned animals. The transcripts of this meeting explaining the review process are available online at www.fda.gov/cvm/index/vmac/VMACFall2003.htm.

The FDA is continuing to review the issues and inviting comments from the public before making a final decision. While the biotechnology industry pushes for FDA approval and suggests that cloned animals will provide a reproducible, healthful, cost-effective alternative to natural animal products, others are voicing concerns that cloning animals for food is not only potentially unsafe and perhaps unethical but also unnecessary and just plain distasteful.

Safety

The FDA's presumption of safety is based on the fact that its Veterinary Medicine Advisory Committee—like an NAS study released the previous year—could discern no difference between mature cloned animals and their counterparts in nature. Its conclusions were based on studies of cattle but extended to pigs and goats. This conclusion supports the FDA's suggestion that labels on food containing the products of animal clones would be unnecessary. If there's no difference in the products, the agency indicates, there would be no need for special labels.

> **The FDA currently sees no reason for labels that would let consumers know that they're purchasing food from animal clones.**

In a swift response to the FDA's announcement of its tentative support of cloning, George Siemon, CEO of Organic Valley, told the press, "American families should not be guinea pigs for corporate greed. Contrary to what the FDA says, there is no level of 'acceptable risk' when it comes to putting unproven science on the table for dinner."

When the FDA comments that consumption of cloned products appears to be safe, adds Michael Levine, president, Organic Meat Company, a wholly owned subsidiary of Organic Valley, it's taking a leap of faith that hurdles a chasm of uncertainty. The agency indicates that it has no reason to believe cloned products are unsafe. That, suggests Levine, isn't evidence that they are safe. "What makes me particularly uncomfortable," he says, "is that there's a lack of knowledge, so consequently we can't find the risks

because we don't understand it well enough."

The notion that since science can't distinguish a difference between natural and cloned animals there must not be a difference "borders on ignorance and egotism," says Levine. "We know what we know, and beyond that, we'll find out." Rather than cater to business interest, he insists, we should err on the side of caution.

Ethics and the Unknown

According to Levine, "There is an enormous amount of uncertainty as to where this will lead." Once cloned products are released, there's no returning, he suggests. "You can't call it back," he says. "Once it's out and the genetic material is allowed to blend with regular genetic material, then it essentially infects."

"Whether it's genetically engineered crops, cross-pollinating with wild weeds, genetically modified salmon breeding with wild fish, or future concerns with clone mammals, the risks to the balance in ecosystems worldwide are great," said Siemon. Ethical concerns have been raised as well about the welfare of the animals themselves, many of which are born with deformities or disease as a result of the cloning technology.

The Yuck Factor

Levine believes the prospect of eating the products of cloned animals makes people uncomfortable enough that there will be a strong consumer outcry regarding the need for labeling. "It's one thing when it's a tomato, but when it's a living, breathing animal—a created, processed creature—that's something else," he says. Once a need for labeling is established and people see the labels, he speculates, people won't want the products. Much like irradiated foods, says Levine, "there's enough uncertainty and discomfort at the consumer level that it will prevent it from widespread distribution."

Wahida Karmally, DrPH, RD, CDE, director of nutrition, Irving Center for Clinical Research at Columbia University, took an informal survey of colleagues, asking whether or not they'd eat cloned animals or products from cloned animals. Most, she says, were not so inclined. However, among her sampling were three doctors, each of whom had no qualms about it. The scientists among the group claimed they could see no difference, while those opposed to eating cloned animal products cited concerns about safety and the unknowns. Some, in addition, merely question the need for cloning, asking, "Why not leave animal reproduction to nature?"

Karmally, herself not a big meat eater, says she finds the idea distasteful. Although she has no reason to believe these products are hazardous to human health, she's concerned that the government's assessment discusses the appearance rather than the certainty of safety. Why, she wonders, do they just appear to be safe, and what's preventing the government from using more conclusive language? "I'm not totally convinced that it's without hazards, but I really don't know," says Karmally.

"Ultimately what will happen if the business interests push through ... somehow they'll be able to disguise it and then it's out there and there's nothing we'll be able to do because the market, in face of ignorance, will accept it," she continues. "Knowledge, though, is a remarkably powerful tool, and if consumers have the knowledge that it's out there, I believe they will opt not to participate."

Necessity

Like her colleagues, Karmally questions the necessity for cloning in the first place, asking, "Don't we have enough production?" Katherine Tallmadge, American Dietetic Association spokesperson, agrees. "We have plenty of food. Why do we need to clone?"

"Obviously from my perspective, the organic protocol and the organic system is the right way to raise animals," says Levine. "But even conventionally speaking, the quality level of animals is high enough. There's no need."

Labeling

Even many who believe there's no harm to human health and/or for concern about eating the products of animal clones believe the public has a right to know where their food comes from. "I think we should let people decide whether they want to eat [food from cloned] animals," says Karmally, "People need to make informed decisions." Echoes Tallmadge, "The more educated the consumer is, the better, so the more labeling, the better." One reason labels may be important, says Karmally, is to assure consumers that the cloned animal has the equivalent nutrient content. They may want to know that the cloned product offers the same amount of protein, for example.

Even though Levine clearly believes that if animal clone products are released into the food supply they should be labeled, he's uncomfortable with the statement. "I'd rather say it should never get to that."

Making Choices

If products from animal clones are permitted to enter the food supply and the FDA determines that labeling is necessary, consumers will be able to recognize cloned products and make their own choices. If these products are permitted without labeling, only consumers who purchase organic meat products will be certain that their food is not from animal clones. "Buying organic is a safety valve across so many different levels," says Levine. "The organic protocol is about raising animals and crops in harmony with nature, as nature intended. So you don't have any of these issues because they're not within the organic system."

Staying Tuned

The FDA risk assessment will continue and its findings will be published on the agency's Web site, possibly by early this year, after the public has had an opportunity to comment. The FDA will then look at risk management and regulatory options. To stay current, follow the risk assessment process or offer comment on the FDA's Web site at www.fda.gov/cvm.

— Kate Jackson is a staff writer for *Today's Dietitian*.

Seafood Safety

Is Something Fishy Going On?

Matthew Robb

When New York writer Nancy Peske shops for groceries, her 5-year-old son Dante is foremost in her mind.

Hoping to prepare the most nutritious meals possible, Peske sidesteps the processed foods, bypasses the fatty snacks, ignores the siren song of refined sugars, and instead fills her cart with the freshest ingredients from her favorite Manhattan health food store.

Peske considers herself an informed consumer—that is, until she reaches the seafood counter. A lifelong fish lover, she is baffled by recent advisories warning of mercury and other seafood contaminants. Not knowing whom to trust amid a flurry of diverging opinions, Peske has chosen to essentially abstain.

The decision, she says, wasn't easy.

"My father was a fisherman. We grew up in Milwaukee and enjoyed fresh fish pulled right from Lake Michigan and other nearby lakes—lots of northern pike and trout." Pausing to reflect, the 41-year-old continues: "I was always aware of the pollutants that ended up in fish. My father would tell me not to eat the dark meat near the skin. I've also edited nutrition books, so I know the key issues. I'm especially concerned because Dante is a growing kid."

Peske's dilemma mirrors uneasiness among consumers nationwide. Wanting to eat a delicious product once depicted as a miracle food, today growing numbers of Americans are wondering which species are safe—and which should be avoided even with a 10-foot fishing pole. Seeking commonsense guidance, we polled a range of experts to get their thoughts on this long-simmering controversy.

Assessing Benefits, Balancing Risks

For Peske and others with elevated cholesterol, saying no to fish may carry its own risks. "I feel like I'm between a rock and a hard place," she acknowledges. "I know the omega-3 fatty acids are important, but how do I get fish oil into me and my family without getting all those toxins?"

Of particular concern to public interest groups and government regulators is the contaminant mercury, along with polychlorinated biphenyls (PCBs), polybrominated diphenyl ethers (PBDEs), and dioxins. In its organic form—and at high enough exposures—methylmercury is a neurotoxin linked with birth defects, brain damage in children, and serious impairment in adults. According to the British journal *The Lancet,* human exposure to mercury can be "almost exclusively" linked to fish. Experts trace the pollution "point source" to emissions from power plants and incinerators dotting the globe.

In February, the U.S. Environmental Protection Agency (EPA) estimated that approximately 630,000 children are born each year "at risk for lowered intelligence and learning problems caused by exposure to high levels of mercury in the womb." The EPA also estimates that roughly 7 million women and children are eating mercury-contaminated fish at or above levels it considers safe. Researchers note that mothers who eat contaminated fish or shellfish pass up to one-half of the "toxic load" to their nursing babies.

In February, the FDA reported that newborns often have higher mercury levels than their mothers.

Mercury contamination is found in both recreational (fresh water) and commercial fish. In late August, the EPA reported that a record one-third of U.S. lake waters (14 million acres) and one-quarter of its riverways (850,000 miles) are so tainted with mercury (or other contaminants) that children and pregnant women should reduce eating fish from these sources. Notably, these recreational fish comprise a small percentage of overall U.S. consumption.

Against a backdrop of dueling epidemiologists and squabbling biostatisticians, all parties agree on this: Larger, older predatory fish tend to "bioaccumulate" more mercury than smaller, younger stock. In March, the FDA joined the EPA to caution children and women—specifically women who might become pregnant, are pregnant, or are nursing—to completely avoid the "Big Four": shark, swordfish, king mackerel, and tilefish. The advisory also cautioned this group to eat only modest amounts of albacore tuna and tuna steak. In February 2003, the British Food Safety Agency explicitly warned this same group that tuna "could present a health hazard."

Describing fish and shellfish as "an important part of a healthy diet," the FDA/EPA advisory nevertheless set dietary limits to "reduce exposure to the harmful effects of mercury." The current government recommendation is that women of childbearing age and young children should eat no more than 12 ounces per week of any type of fish. In Restaurant Land—where 8-ounce adult portions are commonplace—this translates into one to two servings per week for women. On the FDA's elite "dean's list" are shrimp, cod, catfish, pollock, trout, and salmon.

Tuna Troubles?

Advocacy groups are particularly concerned about tuna—fresh or canned—because Americans eat lots of it and it continues to fly under most consumers' radar. Surprisingly, premium albacore (or "white") tuna contains more mercury than "light" tuna, explaining why the FDA/EPA advisory recommended to women and children no more than 6 ounces per week, or one can. In July, food-safety officials at Consumers Union of U.S., Inc.—publisher of *Consumer Reports*—recommended that women of childbearing age eat no more than 3 ounces of albacore weekly and young children none. Advocacy groups thus talk of the "Big Five," saying tuna should be added to the FDA/EPA list because consumers tend to eat oversized portions and because advocates believe keeping one's mercury exposure below the FDA's maximum limit is prudent.

Regulators and other researchers, meanwhile, counter that hard scientific data should guide public health advisories and that the FDA/EPA advisory "action levels" factor in a wide safety margin. The U.S. Tuna Foundation goes a step further, asserting that mercury levels in albacore are "well below government standards." The Consumers Union notes that the U.S. government has set no official safety standards for mercury in albacore or any other fish.

The FDA/EPA landmark March mercury advisory comes on the heels of other key findings. Two of note:

• The journal *Science* recently reported that cultivated (or "farm-raised") salmon—especially Atlantic stock—is sufficiently tainted as to possibly nullify any health benefits. Critics respond that the amount of mercury found even in farm-raised salmon is miniscule.

• An August report from the College of William & Mary advises consumers not to be concerned over trace amounts of flame retardants (PBDEs) found in wild and farmed salmon.

Making Sense of It All

Confronted with a riptide of contradictory facts, opinions, and thready suppositions, the layperson is understandably confused, says Melinda Johnson, RD.

As spokesperson for the American Dietetic Association, she counsels, "We should focus on reliable, valid recommendations based on good science, not on one-time uncontrolled studies that make headlines. We shouldn't scare people away from certain foods." What worries Johnson is the possibility that consumer overload—a media blitz that whipsaws fish lovers with a confusing "good fish-bad fish" debate—will turn them away from a healthful food source. She adds, "It's important to wait for the science to catch up with the early claims."

But according to Jackie Savitz, pollution campaign director and senior scientist for Washington, D.C.-based Oceana, the hard data are available and conclusive. "There are over 2,000 fish advisories for mercury in this country right now," she says. "The FDA demands a lot of evidence but doesn't have a systematic, active testing program. When the FDA is willing to issue an advisory—in the face of intense political pressure—you know you really have a problem because it's survived that regulatory morass.

Larger, older predatory fish tend to "bioaccumulate" more mercury than smaller, younger stock.

"Tuna is also a big problem," Savitz continues. "Few people eat much swordfish, but many people eat tuna every day—people on fixed budgets, people with kids, people who are dieting. The best thing to do is to eat fish lower on the food chain. Avoid the 'big fish with teeth'—swordfish, shark, king mackerel, tilefish—and tuna. Consumers hear that there are contaminants in seafood and think, 'Oh, there is nothing that I can eat.' But there are a lot of different kinds of fish and shellfish out there that are low in contaminants and high in omega-3 fatty acids." The bottom line, she says, is the need for better regulation, more communication, and less pollution.

"The Great Mimicker"

Dietitian Chuck Balzer, MS, RD, acquired his schooling in mercury the hard way. In late 2001, the lifelong swordfish and tuna fanatic developed a frightening condition. "My legs had this tingling,

burning, sometimes shooting-pain sensation—even at rest," he recalls. As his mystery condition progressed, Balzer began feeling weaker, shakier. When physicians started conducting diagnostic workups for multiple sclerosis, a panicky Balzer started downloading information on disability.

His answer finally arrived in early 2002, when an emergency department physician, acting on a hunch, tested a "twitching" Balzer for mercury poisoning. The lab test detected mercury at roughly five times the upper normal range. After unsuccessful treatment by his general physician, the frantic dietitian opted for controversial intravenous chelation therapy. By summer 2003, he was again mercury-free and biking, walking, and playing beach volleyball.

"Mercury is called 'the great mimicker,'" Balzer notes. "I suspect lots of people with mercury poisonings are being treated for other disorders. Today, I'm seafood-free and supplement with omega-3 capsules." Balzer's personal struggle graphically illustrates why the FDA/EPA placed swordfish on its "hands-off" list.

Eat More Fish?

Nutrition consultant Joyce A. Nettleton, DSc, RD, sees the ocean half-full—maintaining that the risks from contaminants in most seafood types for most people are minimal to nonexistent. Quoting Renaissance physician-surgeon Paracelsus, she says, "It's the dose that makes the thing a poison." Consumer advocates agree on this point but debate safety levels.

"If you're going to encourage people to avoid certain fish or not to eat something that's as healthful as seafood—which we eat so little of in this country—you better have good grounds for doing so, and those grounds just aren't there," she says. "The bottom line is that people are not getting sick from eating too much fish, [but] they are compromising their health from eating too little fish."

Nettleton, a spokesperson for the tuna industry and author of the 1995 book *Omega-3 Fatty Acids and Health*, says she supports the FDA/EPA advisory.

"Most data," she says, "indicate that most people aren't consuming anything near the amounts [of mercury] that would compromise their health." She deems it "perfectly safe" for pregnant women to consume up to 12 ounces of canned tuna per week—although the FDA/EPA

Seafood Mercury Content

Fish/Shellfish	Mean Level Parts Per Million	Mercury Content
Tilefish	1.45	High
Swordfish	1.0	High
King Mackerel	0.73	High
Shark	0.96	Low
Red Snapper*	0.6	Low
Orange Roughy*	0.58	Low
Bass (saltwater)*	0.49	Low
Marlin*	0.47	Low
Tuna	0.32	Low
Lobster (North American)	0.31	Low
Grouper	0.27	Low
Brook Trout	0.26	Low
Halibut	0.23	Low
Mahi Mahi*	0.19	Low
Canned Tuna	0.17	Low
Crab	0.09 to 0.18, depending on type	Very Low/Nondetectable
Catfish	0.07	Very Low/Nondetectable
Scallops	0.05	Very Low/Nondetectable
Salmon	ND	Very Low/Nondetectable
Oysters	ND	Very Low/Nondetectable
Shrimp	ND	Very Low/Nondetectable
Clams*	ND	Very Low/Nondetectable

*Data based on limited samples
—Source: FDA

chose, in its advisory, the more conservative terminology, "reduce exposure to the harmful effects of mercury." On the topic of wild and farm-raised salmon, she says, "I recommend both without qualification." She continues, "The levels [of contaminants] found in commonly consumed fish are a fraction of what the World Health Organization and the FDA consider to be safe limits." Nettleton also points to a recent university study showing ultra-premium "troll-caught albacore," harvested young from the Pacific Northwest, has much lower mercury levels. A 7.5-ounce can of this "gourmet" product sells online for $3.75.

Simmons College nutrition professor Teresa Fung, ScD, RD, LDN, takes a pragmatic approach. "For nonpregnant, nonlactating adults who only occasionally consume fish," she says, "I am not concerned about the kind of fish they eat, unless they have other sources of mercury exposure. Frequent fish consumers should look into the FDA mercury advi-

sory. For pregnant, lactating women and young children, they should especially be careful of mercury. Occasional consumption of low-mercury tuna should not be of concern. However, I would err on the side of caution and only consume the other types of tuna on rare occasions." Expanding her view, she comments, "Fish are an excellent source of omega-3 fatty acids. And salmon is an excellent source of vitamin D."

Agreed, says Katherine L. Tucker, PhD, professor of nutritional epidemiology at Tufts University in Boston. "My position is that people should eat fatty fish; the benefits outweigh the risks," she says. "The other side, however, is the risk of PCBs and dioxins that accumulate in these fatty fish." Tucker points to a colleague's study that "showed pretty clearly" that farmed salmon have higher contaminant levels than wild salmon. Wild salmon caught in Chile appear safest, followed by Alaska salmon. Trailing behind are Atlantic farm-raised salmon.

The problem: contaminated feed. "The very fat that protects our heart and probably our brains is contaminated with PCBs and dioxins," she says. "The problem is we don't know who is susceptible to these contaminants, and they are very expensive and difficult to analyze." In the final analysis, Tucker offers this advice: Eat fish, enjoy fish, but choose wisely.

Fish Oil Supplements

The March 2003 Harvard Health Letter notes that the health value of seafood is mainly derived from the well-studied omega-3 fats: eicosapentaenoic acid and docosahexaenoic acid. Some observers, however, wonder about industry oversight. "[Fish oil capsules are] an option," Nettleton says. "But they don't do anything to improve one's dietary habits and there's no assurance ... that what you're buying contains what the label says."

Savitz disagrees. "Fish oil in capsules is most likely taken from fish lower on the food chain than tuna. Those fish have not bioaccumulated as much as the fish for which the FDA has issued advisories." She echoes other experts by saying that consumers should not be scared away from the vast smorgasbord of healthful fish and shellfish.

Pulling back from the ensuing debate, what is the take-home message for today's dietitian?

Avoid the Big Four fish, monitor (and possibly minimize) your intake of tuna, watch for local fish advisories, and enjoy the rest. Our experts underscore the fact that no food—indeed, nothing in life—is risk-free and that fish and shellfish confer vital health benefits to a nation reeling from obesity, heart disease, diabetes, and more.

— *Matthew Robb is a freelance writer residing in suburban Washington, D.C.*

Suspect Produce

How To Be Safe From Contaminated Fruits, Vegetables

Elizabeth M. Ward, M.S., R.D.

No doubt you're aware there are risks from eating contaminated meat, poultry, seafood or eggs. But it may come as a shock to learn that fruits and vegetables can harbor some of the same bacteria, viruses and parasites. Moreover, when produce is eaten raw, you can't rely on cooking to kill the bugs.

According to the Centers for Disease Control and Prevention, tainted food causes an estimated 76 million cases of illness in the U.S. each year, though the majority of cases go unreported. While most foodborne illness is mild, older adults and people with reduced immunity are usually hit the hardest.

Even though animal foods are more likely to be contaminated, there's been a definite upswing in foodborne illnesses traced to fruits and vegetables. Does that mean you should avoid eating raw produce? Not at all. But there are precautions you should take. *EN* investigates how best to protect yourself against the growing threat of tainted produce.

Contamination Happens. In recent years, numerous microbes have made their way onto fresh fruits and vegetables. In the late 1990's, raspberries from Guatemala contaminated with the *Cyclospora* parasite gave nearly 1,400 people diarrhea. A few years later, *Salmonella*-tainted cantaloupes wreaked havoc, while just last summer, *Salmonella* on Roma tomatoes was to blame for making more than 600 people sick in the U.S. and Canada. And in perhaps one of the worst cases of produce contamination, Mexican-grown scallions were guilty of transmitting the hepatitis A virus to diners a few years back.

Just Say No to Sprouts

Sprouts may seem like a healthful addition to stir-fries, salads and sandwiches, but they are some of the riskiest foods around. The last 10 years has seen more than 1,600 people in the U.S. become ill from eating raw or lightly cooked sprouts, including alfalfa, clover and mung bean sprouts.

During that time, sprouts accounted for an astounding 40% of all major foodborne outbreaks traced to fresh produce, according to the Food and Drug Administration. *Salmonella* and *E.coli* 0157:H7 were often the culprits.

Despite efforts by government and industry to improve sprout safety, contamination has not decreased, often because the seeds themselves are contaminated. Plus the typical moist growing conditions only encourage bacterial growth. The FDA warns: Don't eat sprouts of any kind.

—E.M.W.

How do fruits and vegetables become carriers of disease? Many types of produce, such as melons, some berries and lettuce, are prone to contamination because they grow close to the ground where bacteria and other germs reside. Fruits and vegetables are also vulnerable to contamination from unsanitary water on farms; lettuce that's "triple washed" isn't clean if the water is not clean. This is more of a problem outside the U.S.

Often, produce becomes contaminated through contact with human hands—farm workers or foodservice personnel for example. At the supermarket, dozens of shoppers may handle unwrapped apples, pears and potatoes before you take them home.

Imports vs. Domestic. In a way, healthier eating habits have contributed to a riskier fruit and vegetable supply. A steadily increasing demand for fresh fruits and vegetables, especially out of season, means suppliers turn to imports. What's wrong with foreign produce? Many of the countries we get our fruits and vegetables from fall short of stringent U.S. standards. In fact, the Food and Drug Administration has found imported produce from 21 countries to have four times the contamination rate of domestic produce.

"The benefits from eating fruits and vegetables far outweigh any risk."

However, don't let that statistic lull you into a false sense of security about domestic produce, which is

Reduce Your Produce Risk

- **Purchase produce that's not bruised or damaged.** Germs thrive in moist areas caused by damage.
- **Eat in season.** Buy local produce.
- **Consider eating more of your vegetables cooked rather than raw,** especially if you are older or have compromised immunity. Frozen vegetables and canned fruits (in its own juice) are nutritious too.
- **Choose juice and cider that's been pasteurized** to kill *E. coli* bacteria.
- **Avoid buying cut-up produce,** like chunks of melon. It's another opportunity for contamination. Plus enzymes released when produce is cut trigger the deterioration process, inviting microbial growth.
- **Refrigerate produce,** like berries, that deteriorates quickly.
- **Clean equipment** (knives, cutting boards) before cutting up produce.
- **Wash your hands for at least 20 seconds** with warm, soapy water before handling food; dry with a clean towel. Wash again during food preparation if you touch raw meat, poultry, seafood or eggs, use the bathroom or touch a pet.
- **Avoid cross-contamination** by designating one cutting board for produce and another for meat.
- **Don't wash produce until you're ready to eat it.** Fruits and vegetables have a coating that imparts protection until you wash it off.
- **Rinse "prewashed" veggies,** just to be sure.
- **Wash especially well produce with layers or crevices** where dirt and germs can hide, such as lettuce, cabbage, scallions and raspberries.
- **Discard outer leaves** of leafy greens like lettuce and spinach.
- **Scrub fruits and vegetables with skins and rinds,** such as cantaloupe, oranges and avocados, under cool running water before cutting into them, so the knife won't transfer germs from the outer rind or skin to the inside.
- **Refrigerate cut produce promptly.**

certainly not immune from germs. In 1996, *E. coli* O157:H7, the virulent strain of this fecal bacterium, found its way onto California-grown lettuce, probably at the farm.

Organic Solution? If all this makes you want to buy organic, it's not quite as simple as that. While *EN* is a fan of organic farming to promote soil fertility and avoid unnecessary pesticide use, organic produce is not necessarily safer from microbial contamination. Once organic fruits and vegetables leave the farm, they are subject to the same contamination pitfalls as other produce. That's why it's so important to wash produce well.

Some critics charge organic produce is actually *more* likely to be contaminated, because organic farmers use manure as fertilizer, and manure is a documented source of *E. coli*. But both organic farmers and conventional farmers often use manure. Farms producing certified organic crops, however, must follow strict guidelines that prohibit the use of raw manure within 90 days of harvest. And proper composting of manure actually reduces bacterial contamination.

The Bottom Line. It's ironic that the very foods experts say promote good health might also threaten it. Still, the benefits gained from eating fruits and vegetables far outweigh any risk. Research links diets rich in fruits and vegetables to less risk of heart disease, cancer and obesity.

The 2005 Dietary Guidelines for Americans call for five or more cups of fruits and vegetables each day. You just need to be sure those choices are safe ones and that you handle them with care (see "Reduce Your Produce Risk,").

Ensuring the Safety of Dietary Supplements

Michelle Meadows

When taken appropriately, some dietary supplements have clear benefits. Folic acid lowers the risk of some birth defects. Calcium supplements can strengthen bones and help prevent osteoporosis. But some dietary supplements pose health risks. They may be improperly manufactured or handled, or their ingredients may cause harmful effects on the body.

Under the Dietary Supplement Health and Education Act of 1994 (DSHEA), dietary supplements are regulated like foods. Unlike new drugs, dietary supplements don't generally have to go through review by the Food and Drug Administration for safety and effectiveness or be "approved" before they can be marketed. But manufacturers must provide premarket notice and evidence of safety for any supplements they plan to sell that contain dietary ingredients that were not on the market before DSHEA was passed.

The FDA evaluates the safety of dietary supplements after they are on the market primarily through research and adverse event monitoring. Those who market and make dietary supplements are responsible for ensuring that any claims are substantiated with adequate evidence, and they cannot claim that the dietary supplements will treat or cure any disease.

Monitoring Industry

The dietary supplement industry has changed a lot in the last decade. When DSHEA was passed, there were about 4,000 dietary supplements on the market. Now there are about 29,000 on the market, with another 1,000 new products introduced each year, according to a recent Institute of Medicine report that was sponsored by the FDA. "We have seen a huge growth in the industry over the last 10 years, including the introduction of products that seem far removed from the vitamins and minerals of the pre-DSHEA days," says Dr. Lester M. Crawford, Acting FDA Commissioner. "Unlike most foods, some dietary supplements are pharmacologically active." When a substance is pharmacologically active, it can cause changes in the body. Such a substance could be toxic on its own or cause dangerous interactions with over-the-counter or prescription drugs.

The FDA is developing regulations on the standards for manufacturing and handling dietary supplements.

Ephedra, which was often marketed for weight control and improved energy, was linked to cardiovascular problems, such as increased blood pressure and irregular heart rhythm. In the first formal action to stop the sale of a dietary supplement since DSHEA was passed, the FDA banned ephedra last year. "This is an example of how we can get a dietary supplement off the market if we have solid scientific proof that it does more harm than good," Crawford says.

The dietary supplement industry has changed a lot in the last decade.

Manufacturers and retailers can make claims about the impact of dietary supplements on the structure or function of the body, but these claims must be truthful. An example of such a claim is "calcium builds strong bones." The FDA plans to issue guidance for what data substantiates these types of claims. The agency has worked closely with the Federal Trade Commission to aggressively enforce the law against dietary supplements that are labeled with fraudulent health claims. In April 2004, the FDA sent warning letters to 16 firms, asking them to stop making false claims for weight loss.

From November 2003 to April 2004, the FDA inspected 180 domestic dietary supplement manufacturers, sent 119 warning letters to dietary supplement distributors, refused entry to 1,171 foreign shipments of dietary supplements, and seized or supervised the voluntary destruction of almost $18 million worth of mislabeled or adulterated dietary supplement products.

In March 2004, the FDA requested that 23 companies stop distributing dietary supplements containing androstenedione, also known as "andro." Widely marketed to athletes and body builders, androstenedione has been touted as a way to increase muscle growth and reduce fat. However, it acts like a steroid in the body and increases the risk of serious diseases. For example, women who use these products may be at increased risk for breast cancer and endometrial cancer. Children who use these products are at risk of early onset of puberty and of premature cessation of bone growth.

Additionally, the FDA is developing regulations for industry on good manufacturing practices (GMPs) for dietary supplements. When finalized, the rule will set standards for the manufacturing and handling of dietary supplements to ensure that consumers are provided with high-quality dietary supplements.

"The GMP regulation is the linchpin for properly regulating dietary supplements," Crawford says. "It gives FDA benchmarks for regulating dietary supplements and it gives clear instructions to the industry on how to manufacture products that meet rigorous quality standards."

Continuing Research

Crawford says that these initiatives are an important part of the agency's science-based approach to regulating dietary supplements. He also notes that the FDA was pleased to welcome Barbara O. Schneeman, Ph.D., as the new director of the Office of Nutritional Products, Labeling, and Dietary Supplements, part of the FDA's Center for Food Safety and Applied Nutrition. Schneeman has an extensive background in nutrition science and has served on the faculty of the University of California, Davis, since 1976.

The FDA continues to collaborate with federal research partners at the National Institutes of Health and other organizations to gather evidence about the safety and effectiveness of dietary supplements. "In evaluating dietary supplements, we look at scientific information from a range of sources," Crawford says, "including published research, evidence-based reports, and data about the pharmacology or toxicology of a compound." Crawford notes that the agency has particular interest in gathering safety data about certain dietary supplements suspected to pose human health risks, including:

- an ephedra substitute called *Citrus aurantium*, also known as bitter orange, which may present health risks similar to ephedra
- usnic acid, marketed for weight loss and linked to liver damage
- kava, a botanical ingredient that has caused liver failure
- pyrrolizidine alkaloids, which are found in some plants and have been shown to have toxic effects that can cause liver damage.

The FDA recommends that consumers talk with a health care provider before using a dietary supplement. People who think they have been harmed by a dietary supplement should contact their health providers, and also report it to the FDA's MedWatch program by calling (800) FDA-1088 (332-1088), or visiting *www.fda.gov/medwatch/*.

From *FDA Consumer*, July/August 2004. Published by U.S. Food and Drug Administration.

UNIT 7

World Hunger and Malnutrition

Unit Selections

Key Points to Consider

- How extensive is global hunger and malnutrition?

- What is the role of global food companies in world hunger and malnutrition?

- Offer several solutions to decreasing or eliminating food insecurity and malnutrition.

- What are some steps you can take to reduce water consumption?

- What sort of role will genetically modified food have in feeding people in developing countries?

Student Website
www.mhcls.com/online

Internet References
Further information regarding these websites may be found in this book's preface or online.

Population Reference Bureau
http://www.prb.org
World Health Organization (WHO)
http://www.who.int/en/
WWW Virtual Library: Demography & Population Studies
http://demography.anu.edu.au/VirtualLibrary/

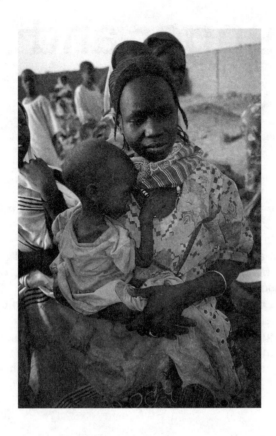

The cause of malnutrition worldwide is poverty. The United Nations Food and Agriculture Organization (FAO) determined that a body mass index (BMI) (body weight divided by the square root of height) of 18.5 is indicative of chronic energy deficit in adults. Approximately 840 million people are malnourished in the developing world; Asia has the largest number and children under 5 years of age are the most susceptible. Infectious disease kills approximately 10 million children each year. Thus, the director general of FAO launched, in 1994, a special Programme for Food Security (SPFS) for low-income, food-deficit countries (LIFDCs), which was endorsed by the World Food Summit held in Rome in 1996. They pledged to increase food production and access to food in LIFDCs so that the number of malnourished people would be reduced by half. They set goals to increase sustainable agricultural production within the cultural, political, and economic millieu of the country to improve access to food, increase the role of trade, and to deal effectively with food emergencies.

Malnutrition is also the main culprit for lowered resistance to disease, infection, and death—especially in children. The malnutrition-infection combination results in stunted growth, lowered mental development in children, lowered productivity, and higher incidence of degenerative disease in adulthood. This directly affects the economies of developing countries. Over one billion people globally suffer from micronutrient malnutrition frequently called "hidden hunger." Additionally, partnerships between the public and private sectors may prove valuable in combating malnutrition. Solutions to the above problems such as building sustainability through indigenous knowledge and practices that are

community based and environmentally friendly such as biofortification and dietary diversification, may combat hunger and nutrient deficiencies.

Nutrient deficiencies magnify the effect of disease and result in more severe symptoms and greater complications of the disease. For example, vitamin A deficiency leads to blindness in about 250,000–300,000 children annually, and exacerbates the symptoms of measles. Iron deficiency, which is widespread among pregnant women and those in the child-bearing years in developing countries, increases the risk of death from hemorrhage in their offspring and reduces physical productivity and learning capacity. Finally, iodine deficiency causes brain damage and mental retardation. It is estimated that 1.5 billion people are at risk for iodine deficiency disorders.

Malnutrition does not only affect children and adults in developing countries but is also prevalent in this country. Thirty million Americans, of whom 11 million are children, experience food insecurity and hunger. In a country where one-fifth of the food is wasted and 130 pounds of food per person is disposed of, it is unacceptable that Americans go hungry. The primary nutrient deficiencies in this country and in developing countries are iron deficiency anemia—common in infants, young children, and teens—and lead poisoning. Undernourished pregnant women give birth to low-weight babies who suffer developmental delays and increases in mortality rate. Another group in the United States that experiences health problems due to hunger is the elderly. Inadequate supermarket access to low- income, urban areas creates a crisis. Strategies to bringing supermarkets back are critical for the poor. Many charities and relief funds are working together to alleviate hunger in America.

A recent paradox some of the poorest countries are facing along with food insecurity and malnutrition is obesity and malnutrition. The World Health Organization in their recent report on "Diet, Nutrition and the Prevention of Chronic Disease" question the role and contribution of global food companies on the increasing incidence of obesity in developing countries. The creation of the Mega Country Health Promotion Network by the WHO to identify public health strategies that involve public and private partnerships to find solutions to the obesity problem is expected in the future. Not only is this paradox observed in developing countries, but has also been documented in the US. Health professionals need to understand the relationship among food insecurity, hunger poverty, and obesity as they strive to help the poor.

Biotechnologists believe that genetically modified (GM) foods such as rice that is fortified with beta-carotene and iron may not only help feed the world, but also eradicate nutritional deficiencies. Additionally, GM foods may decrease damage to crops from pests, viruses, bacteria, and drought. Yet it seems too good to be true. If farmers cannot afford to grow GM crops or afford to buy the food, if the infrastructure for transport and distribution is not available, then the products may never reach the consumers. Since the safety of humans and the efficacy for the environment of GM crops has not been adequately studied, many scientists and consumers believe that genetic engineering is by no means the panacea for hunger. The potential of GM foods to cause allergies is real. It is so real, that the US Environmental Protection Agency, gathered scientists from universities and government laboratories to discuss strategies in assessing the allergenic potential of GM foods. The debate of the health risks of GM foods and the need for labeling will rage for years to come.

Undernourishment around the world

Hunger and mortality

Millions of people, including 6 million children under the age of five, die each year as a result of hunger. Of these millions, relatively few are the victims of famines that attract headlines, video crews and emergency aid. Far more die unnoticed, killed by the effects of chronic hunger and malnutrition, a "covert famine" that stunts their development, saps their strength and cripples their immune systems.

Where prevalence of hunger is high, mortality rates for infants and children under five are also high, and life expectancy is low (see map and graphs). In the worst affected countries, a newborn child can look forward to an average of barely 38 years of healthy life (compared to over 70 years of life in "full health" in 24 wealthy nations). One in seven children born in the countries where hunger is most common will die before reaching the age of five.

Not all of these shortened lives can be attributed to the effects of hunger, of course. Many other factors combine with hunger and malnutrition to sentence tens of millions of people to an early death. The HIV/AIDS pandemic, which is ravaging many of the same countries where hunger is most widespread, has reduced average life expectancy across all of sub-Saharan Africa by nearly five years for women and 2.5 years for men.

Even after compensating for the impact of HIV/AIDS and other factors, however, the correlation between chronic hunger and higher mortality rates remains striking. Numerous studies suggest that it is far from coincidental. Since the early 1990s, a series of analyses have confirmed that between 50 and 60 percent of all childhood deaths in the developing world are caused either directly or indirectly by hunger and malnutrition.

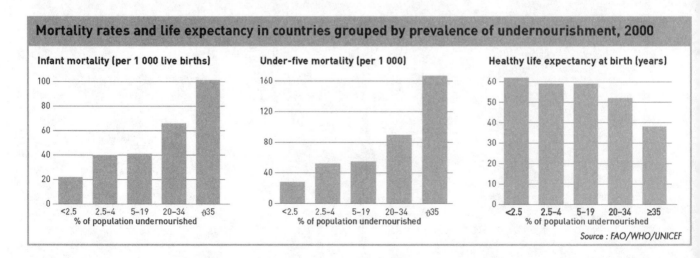

Mortality rates and life expectancy in countries grouped by prevalence of undernourishment, 2000

Infant mortality (per 1 000 live births) — % of population undernourished

Under-five mortality (per 1 000) — % of population undernourished

Healthy life expectancy at birth (years) — % of population undernourished

Source : FAO/WHO/UNICEF

Correspondence between high rates of chronic hunger and childhood mortality, 2000

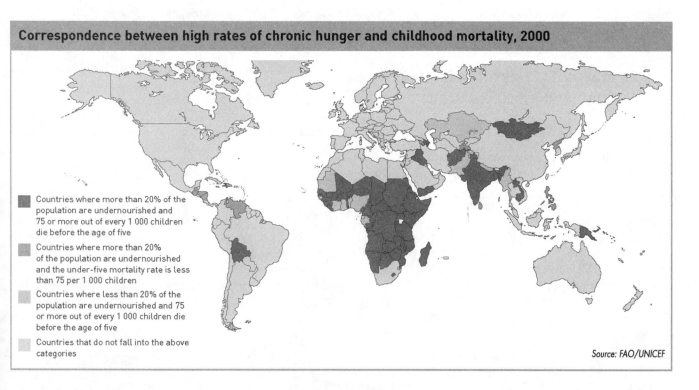

Countries where more than 20% of the population are undernourished and 75 or more out of every 1 000 children die before the age of five

Countries where more than 20% of the population are undernourished and the under-five mortality rate is less than 75 per 1 000 children

Countries where less than 20% of the population are undernourished and 75 or more out of every 1 000 children die before the age of five

Countries that do not fall into the above categories

Source: FAO/UNICEF

Hunger and child mortality

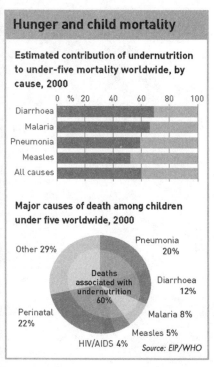

Estimated contribution of undernutrition to under-five mortality worldwide, by cause, 2000

Diarrhoea
Malaria
Pneumonia
Measles
All causes

Major causes of death among children under five worldwide, 2000

Other 29%
Pneumonia 20%

Deaths associated with undernutrition 60%

Diarrhoea 12%

Perinatal 22%
Malaria 8%
Measles 5%
HIV/AIDS 4%

Source: EIP/WHO

Proportion and number of underweight children, 1997–99

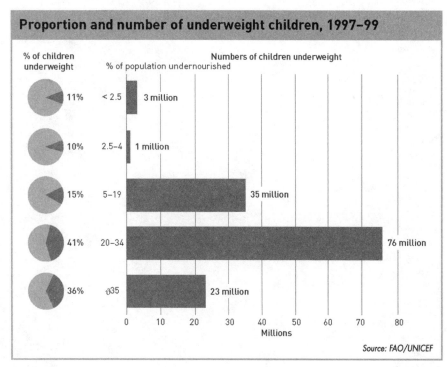

% of children underweight

Numbers of children underweight
% of population undernourished

% of children underweight	% of population undernourished	Number
11%	< 2.5	3 million
10%	2.5–4	1 million
15%	5–19	35 million
41%	20–34	76 million
36%	≥35	23 million

Millions

Source: FAO/UNICEF

Relatively few of those deaths are the result of starvation. Most are caused by a persistent lack of adequate food intake and essential nutrients that leaves children weak, underweight and vulnerable.

As might be expected, the vast majority of the 153 million underweight children under five in the developing world are concentrated in countries where the prevalence of undernourishment is high (see graph above).

Even mild-to-moderate malnutrition greatly increases the risk of children dying from common childhood diseases. Overall, analysis shows that the risk of death is 2.5 times higher for children with only mild malnutrition than it is for children who are adequately nourished. And the risk increases sharply along with the severity of malnutrition (as measured by their weight-to-age ratio). The risk of death is 4.6 times higher for children suffering from moderate malnutrition and 8.4 times higher for the severely malnourished.

Common diseases often fatal for malnourished children

Infectious diseases are the immediate cause of death for most of the 11 million children under the age of five who die each year in the developing world. But the risk of dying from those diseases is far greater for children who are hungry and malnourished.

The four biggest killers of children are diarrhoea, acute respiratory illness, malaria and measles. Taken together, these four diseases account for almost half of all deaths among children under the age of five. Analysis of data from hospitals and villages shows that all four of these diseases are far more deadly to children who are stunted or underweight.

In the case of diarrhoea, numerous studies show that the risk of death is as much as nine times higher for children who are significantly underweight, the most common indicator of chronic undernutrition. Similarly, underweight children are two to three times more likely to die of malaria and acute respiratory infections, including pneumonia, than well-nourished children.

Lack of dietary diversity and essential minerals and vitamins also contributes to increased child and adult mortality. Iron deficiency anaemia greatly increases the risk of death from malaria, and vitamin A deficiency impairs the immune system, increasing the annual death toll from measles and other diseases by an estimated 1.3–2.5 million children.

Improving nutrition to save lives

The weight of evidence clearly argues that eliminating hunger and malnutrition could save millions of lives each year. That conclusion has been confirmed by a study that examined factors that had helped reduce child mortality during the 1990s. Topping the list were the decline in the proportion of children who were malnourished and lacking access to adequate water, sanitation and housing.

The Scourge of "Hidden Hunger": Global Dimensions of Micronutrient Deficiencies

G. KENNEDY, G. NANTEL AND P. SHETTY

The most recent estimates from FAO indicate that 840 million people do not receive enough energy from their diets to meet their needs. The overwhelming majority of these people—799 million—live in developing countries. The global toll of people affected by micronutrient deficiency is estimated to be even higher and probably exceeds two billion. Micronutrient deficiencies can exist in populations even where the food supply is adequate in terms of meeting energy requirements. In these situations, people are not considered "hungry" in the classical sense, but their diets may be grossly deficient in one or more micronutrients. Blindness and goitre are two of the most visible external manifestations of micronutrient deficiency, and have helped to bring it into the limelight. However, they represent only a fraction of the problem, and subclinical deficiencies afflict a much larger proportion of the population. Today, the consequences of subclinical deficiency are becoming better understood and monitored, but they often go unnoticed within the community in spite of their insidious effects on immune system functioning, growth and cognitive development. It is for these reasons that micronutrient deficiencies have been referred to as "hidden hunger".

Micronutrient deficiencies are most prevalent in areas where the diet lacks variety, as is the case for many individuals in developing countries. When people cannot afford to diversify their diets with adequate amounts of fruits, vegetables or animal-source foods that contain large amounts of micronutrients, deficiencies are inevitable. In addition, a minimum amount of fat or vegetable oil is required in the diet for adequate absorption of the fat-soluble vitamins A, D, E and K.

Grave consequences, including continued and sustained loss of productivity, permanent mental disability, blindness, depressed immune system function and increased infant and maternal mortality can result from micronutrient deficiencies. The heaviest toll from these dietary deficiencies is borne disproportionately by women and children. Death and the disabilities caused by micronutrient deficiencies need not occur, because there are several short- and long-term strategies that can be employed to prevent the development of these deficiencies. Many actions can be undertaken by the communities them selves, once they recognize and understand the problem. This article provides an overview of the global prevalence of micronutrient malnutrition and discusses approaches that may be used to address the situation while emphasizing the role of food-based strategies favoured by FAO.

Global prevalence of hidden hunger

Micronutrients are the essential vitamins and minerals required by human beings to stimulate cellular growth and metabolism. Nineteen vitamins and minerals are considered essential for physical and mental development, immune system functioning and various metabolic processes.[1] Deficiencies of iron, iodine and vitamin A are the most widespread forms of micronutrient malnutrition with public health consequences. Other micronutrients have been shown to play a role in preventing specific disease conditions (e.g. folic acid and calcium) or in promoting growth (e.g. zinc). The global prevalence of zinc and folate deficiency has not yet been established, but it is predicted to be significant, as micronutrient deficiencies rarely occur in isolation. One reason is that deficiencies usually occur when the habitual diet lacks diversity or is overly dependent on a single staple food, as is the case with monotonous cereal- or tuber-based diets (FAO/WHO, 2002). Situations of food insecurity, where populations do not have enough to eat, will also inevitably result in micronutrient deficiency.

Iron, vitamin A and iodine deficiencies are the three micronutrient deficiencies of greatest public health significance in the developing world.

IRON

Iron deficiency anaemia

Anaemia is defined as a reduction in the oxygen-carrying capacity of red blood cells, which occurs as a result either of decreased haemoglobin or of a reduction in the total number of red blood cells (i.e. a decline in red blood cell mass). Iron deficiency is the most common cause of anaemia, although anaemia can also occur as a result of vitamin B$_{12}$ or folate deficiencies, con genital hereditary defects in red cells, reproductive blood losses, or from infection by malarial parasites or infestations of the gut by parasites such as hookworm. The level of haemoglobin in the blood is the most commonly used indicator to screen for iron deficiency anaemia (IDA), and is thus the indicator for which there is the most data worldwide. The true prevalence of iron deficiency in a population, however, will be larger than the level of clinically detectable iron deficiency anaemia (WHO, 2001a), because most individuals are likely to be iron deficient long before there is a detectable drop in blood haemoglobin levels.

When people cannot afford to diversify their diets with adequate amounts of fruits, vegetables or animal-source foods that contain large amounts of micronutrients, deficiencies are inevitable

Nutritional iron deficiency, or habitual iron intake that is insufficient to cover requirements, is the most common cause of iron deficiency (FAO/WHO 2002). Dietary sources of iron are present in two forms, haem and non-haem iron. Haem iron, found in animal-source foods such as meat, poultry and fish, has greater bioavailability than does non-haem iron, found in cereals, pulses, fruits and vegetables. There are many dietary factors that can either inhibit or enhance absorption of non-haem iron. Iron absorption is inhibited by phytate, found in whole grains, seeds, nuts and legumes, and by the phenolic compounds (tannins) present in tea, coffee and red wine. By contrast, iron absorption is enhanced when consumed with ascorbic acid, present in many fruits and vegetables. Iron deficiency becomes more common when an individual's iron requirements are increased owing to physiological demands such as pregnancy, menstrual loss or periods of growth, or when iron is lost because of parasitic infections (hookworm or malaria). As a consequence of these compounding factors, people living in environments prone to infection from malaria and hookworm, and whose habitual diet is high in phytate with few animal-source foods are more likely to become iron deficient.

IDA is considered as a micronutrient deficiency of public health significance not only because it is widespread, with an estimated two billion persons affected worldwide, but also because of its serious consequences in both adults and children. IDA is more prevalent in women than in men, and is also prevalent among children and the elderly. IDA during pregnancy can result in serious consequences for both mother and baby. Iron-deficient women have a higher mortality risk during childbirth and an increased incidence of low-birth-weight babies (WHO, 2002). Figure 1 illustrates the prevalence of IDA in pregnant women. Southeast Asia shows the highest prevalence of anaemia in women, with over 50 percent of pregnant women affected (Mason *et al.*, 2001). In addition to the effects of anaemia during pregnancy, much more is now known of the deleterious effects of anaemia on the cognitive performance, behaviour and physical growth of infants and children of preschool and school age (WHO, 2001a). IDA in adults diminishes their stamina and work capacity by as much as 10-15 percent, and it has been estimated that this deficiency provokes losses in gross domestic product of up to 1.5 percent (FAO, 2002).

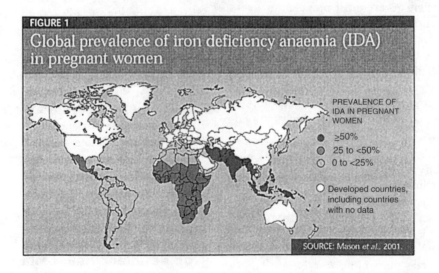

FIGURE 1

Global prevalence of iron deficiency anaemia (IDA) in pregnant women

PREVALENCE OF IDA IN PREGNANT WOMEN

- ≥50%
- 25 to <50%
- 0 to <25%
- Developed countries, including countries with no data

SOURCE: Mason *et al.*, 2001.

IODINE

Iodine deficiency

Iodine is an essential mineral required by the body to synthesize thyroid hormones, the most important of which is thyroxine, a metabolism-regulating substance. The iodine content of plant foods is heavily influenced by the presence of iodine in the soil or environment. Seaweed concentrates iodine from seawater and therefore constitutes a rich source of this nutrient. Seaweed and seafood, in general, are good dietary sources of iodine. Eggs, meat, milk and cereals also contain small amounts of iodine. Populations with little access to ocean fish or other marine products, for example persons living in mountainous areas, are the most likely to show iodine deficiencies resulting from a lack of natural dietary sources of iodine.

Clinical iodine deficiency is detected by the presence of goitre (swelling of the thyroid gland). Subclinical iodine deficiency can be detected by measuring urinary iodine or assessing thyroid function. Figure 2 shows the global prevalence of goitre. The latest estimates indicate that 741 million people, or 13 percent of the world's population, are affected by goitre (WHO, 2001b). As with IDA, the true prevalence of iodine deficiency is even more widespread than the numbers of those affected with goitre would seem to indicate; however, there are no global estimates for prevalence of low urinary iodine, which is the best subclinical indicator.

The most devastating consequence of iodine deficiency is reduced mental capacity. Fifty million people worldwide are mentally handicapped as a result of iodine deficiency (WHO, 2002). According to one source, it has been estimated that 100 000 children are born each year with irreversible brain damage because their mothers lacked iodine prior to and during pregnancy (ICCIDD, 2002). Maternal iodine deficiency can also lead to spontaneous abortions, stillbirth and impaired foetal development. In infancy and childhood, this deficiency is manifested by poor mental development and growth defects. Persons living in communities with endemic iodine deficiency may show an intelligence quotient 13.5 points lower than persons from similar communities with adequate iodine supplies (WHO, 2001b). Iodine deficiency is the most preventable cause of brain damage and one of the easiest disorders to prevent: it suffices to add small amounts of iodine to frequently consumed foods such as common table salt.

VITAMIN A

Vitamin A deficiency

Vitamin A is required by all body tissues for normal growth and tissue repair. The visual and immune systems are particularly dependent upon this vitamin for normal functioning. Vitamin A in the form of retinol is present in a variety of foods including eggs, milk and fish, or in its precursor form as carotene in yellow fruits and vegetables, green leafy vegetables and red palm oil. Retinol forms of vitamin A are more readily absorbed by the body than carotene, although the bioavailability of carotene can be enhanced by consuming dietary sources of fat at the same time. The efficiency in converting carotene (and other carotenoids) into the active form of the vitamin is now thought to be considerably poorer than previously assumed; this topic is currently an active area of investigation.

Blindness resulting from vitamin A deficiency (VAD) has been largely responsible for sensitizing communities and raising international awareness of the devastating consequences of this deficiency. VAD is still the leading cause of preventable blindness in children. However, clinical forms of the deficiency are now becoming less frequent, and detection of subclinical deficiency is gaining

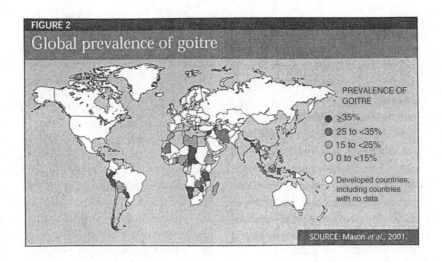

FIGURE 2
Global prevalence of goitre

PREVALENCE OF GOITRE
- ≥35%
- 25 to <35%
- 15 to <25%
- 0 to <15%
- Developed countries, including countries with no data

SOURCE: Mason *et al.*, 2001.

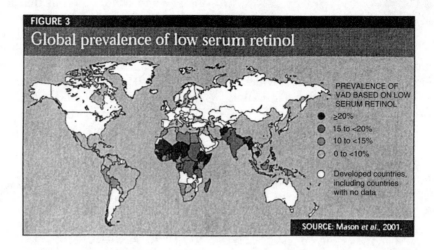

FIGURE 3
Global prevalence of low serum retinol

PREVALENCE OF VAD BASED ON LOW SERUM RETINOL

≥20%
15 to <20%
10 to <15%
0 to <10%
Developed countries, including countries with no data

SOURCE: Mason et al., 2001.

more importance (Mason *et al.*, 2001). Optimal vitamin A status is necessary for the immune system to function normally. Subclinical deficiency has been linked to increased childhood illness and death. It is estimated that improving the vitamin A status of children would decrease overall child mortality rates by 25 percent, measles death rates by 50 percent and death caused by diarrhoea by 40 percent (UNICEF, 2002).

Previously, the most common indicators used to assess VAD were clinical signs affecting the eye. Collectively known as xerophthalmia, these range from relatively mild, rever sible conditions to permanent blindness as a result of keratomalacia (irreversible corneal damage). Subclinical deficiency can be detected through measurement of serum retinol. This indicator can be used to identify populations at risk from increased morbidity and mortality and can also be used to classify the severity of the problem. The World Health Organization (WHO) recommends that VAD be regarded as a severe public health problem in populations where more than 20 percent of the children have serum retinol levels equal to or lower than 0.7 mmol/l (WHO, 1996). Figure 3 shows the global prevalence of low serum retinol.

Other micronutrients

Deficiencies of the micronutrients vitamin A, iron and iodine are those considered to be of the greatest public health significance. However, much more is now being discovered about the vital role of other important nutrients for growth, development, immune system functioning and prevention of birth defects; zinc and folate are two of these.

Zinc. Global attention to zinc deficiency has accelerated rapidly over the past 15 years. However, there is still no information about the prevalence of this deficiency, although it is assumed to be widespread in areas lacking dietary diversity. Zinc is an essential component in over 300 enzymes needed by the body for metabolism (FAO/WHO, 2002). The best dietary sources of zinc are meat, particularly organ meats, and shellfish, while eggs and dairy products are also relatively good sources of zinc. The bioavailability of zinc is inhibited by phytate, which is present in large amounts in cereals and legumes. Thus people whose diet contains only minor amounts of animal-source foods (including dairy products), with large amounts of staple grains and pulses, will be at greater risk of zinc deficiency. Research is emerging on the role of zinc deficiency and the impact of zinc supplementation on pregnancy outcomes for both mother and foetus, and on the morbidity, growth and neuro-behavioural development of children. The clearest indicator of zinc deficiency is stunted child growth; there is evidence that zinc supplementation can improve the growth of stunted children (Brown and Wuehler, 2000). Some benefits in relation to incidence and prevalence of diarrhoea have also been noted with zinc supplementation. Evidence linking zinc to improvement in pregnancy outcomes and cognitive development of children is not strong, and more research is needed in these areas (Brown and Wuehler, 2000). Most importantly, there is a need to develop simple low-cost methods for assessing the zinc status of individuals so that a better assessment of the global prevalence of zinc deficiency can be conducted.

Folate. Folate is required for the synthesis of nucleic acids. Deficiency can arise from insufficient dietary intake as well as malabsorption resulting from gastrointestinal disorders and secondary deficiencies of B_6 and B_{12}, or iron (Stover and Garza, 2002). Liver is considered to be the richest source of this nutrient; folate is also present in a variety of vegetables. Folate has received considerable attention for its role in the prevention of foetal neural tube defect, a condition associated with inadequate folate stores in early pregnancy. Thus folate status before conception and during early pregnancy has become the focus of much of the discussion on this nutrient. There is increased risk of foetal neural tube defects if the folate status of pregnant women shifts from adequate to poor (FAO/WHO, 2002). It is for this reason that folate supplementation for women planning a pregnancy and during the first trimester has become a recommendation in many countries. An important distinction to note with folate is that recommendations during early conception are designed to prevent deficiency and are recommended even for people whose folate status is considered adequate. The supplementation strategy in this case focuses on prevention rather than correction of problems. Even though there has not been a large effort to determine the global prevalence of folate deficiency, the FAO/WHO Expert Consultation on Human Vitamin and Mineral Requirements has recommended that further investigation be conducted into the relationship between folate deficiency and incidence of neural tube defects in developing countries (FAO/WHO, 2002).

Progress in controlling micronutrient deficiencies

Micronutrient deficiencies remain a significant global public health concern. Although scientific knowledge is sufficient to solve the problems of micronutrient deficiencies, operational impediments prevent the implementation of solutions. Impediments include lack of political commitment and poor use of resources (Underwood, 1999). A recent report by the Micronutrient Initiative undertook a thorough analysis of trends in the prevalence of the three major deficiencies. This analysis revealed reductions in the prevalence of clinical VAD and significant improvements in goitre rate in countries with substantial iodization programmes, such as Bolivia, Cameroon, Peru and Thailand but virtually no progress in the control of IDA (Mason *et al.*, 2001). However, it is equally important to note the difficulties encountered in estimating the global reduction of micronutrient deficiencies, owing to underestimation in past evaluations, lack of comparable information from one survey to another and improved detection skills in recent surveys (WHO, 2001b; Hunt and Quibria, 1999; Mason *et al.*, 2001).

The importance of collecting data on subclinical and process indicators is becoming increasingly evident. Table 1 provides a list of clinical, subclinical and process (or programmatic) indicators for vitamin A, iron and iodine deficiencies. Process indicators are being increasingly utilized to detect programmatic improvements in control strategies, and are frequently included in nationally representative surveys such as multiple cluster indicator surveys or demographic and health surveys. When systematically collected, these indicators can also be used to demonstrate progress and are often easier to collect than clinical and subclinical indicators.

Innovative and multisectoral approaches to controlling micronutrient deficiencies have contributed to observed improvement in the global situation. One of the more successful recent strategies in the control of VAD has been to link the distribution of vitamin A capsules to national immunization days. The United Nations Children's Fund (UNICEF) estimates that 11 countries had vitamin A supplementation coverage rates of 70 percent or more for the targeted population of children under five years of age in 1996, and by 1999, 43 countries had reached this level of coverage (UNICEF, 2001). In the case of iodine deficiency, an estimated 72 percent of households in developing countries now use iodized salt, compared to 20 percent a decade ago (UNICEF, 2001).

Strategies to address micronutrient malnutrition

Three of the main strategies for addressing micronutrient malnutrition are dietary diversification, fortification (including biofortification) and supplementation. Most micronutrient deficiencies can be effectively addressed through dietary diversification. Fortification strategies are needed in areas where the traditional diet lacks a specific nutrient, such as iodine. Food-based approaches to

TABLE 1

Examples of indicators commonly used to detect vitamin A, iron and iodine deficiencies			
TYPE OF INDICATOR	**DEFICIENT MICRONUTRIENT**		
	Vitamin A	Iron	Iodine
Clinical	Xerophthalmia and Bitot's spots	Haemoglobin, haematocrit	Goitre, visible or palpable
Subclinical	Serum retinol	Serum ferritin	Urinary iodine
Process/ Programmatic	Percentage of preschool children receiving vitamin A capsules	Percentage of households consuming adequately iodized salt	Percentage of pregnant women receiving iron supplementation

fulfilling micronutrient requirements have received strong support as a sustainable means of meeting the nutritional needs of population groups (WHO/FAO, 1996; FAO/WHO, 2002). These strategies are discussed in more detail below.

Supplementation

Supplementation is a technical approach in which nutrients are delivered directly by means of syrup or pills. Supplementation is most appropriate for targeted populations with a high risk of deficiency or under special circumstances, such as during pregnancy or in an acute food shortage. Under normal circumstances, supplementation programmes are used only as a short-term measure and are then replaced with long-term, sustainable food-based measures such as fortification and dietary modification, usually by increasing food diversity.

Fortification

Fortification strategies utilize widely accessible, commonly consumed foods to deliver one or more micronutrients. The most widespread effort to date has been fortification of salt with iodine. However, many other foods may be used as vehicles for a variety of micronutrients. Some of the more common combinations are wheat products (cereal, bread or pasta) with one or more nutrients including calcium, iron, niacin, riboflavin, thiamine and zinc. Milk can be fortified with vitamin D; fruit and fruit juices have been fortified with calcium and vitamin C. Fish sauce and soy sauce are also recognized as good fortification vehicles, and trials are under way to determine the efficacy of these foods as fortification tools (Mannar and Gallego, 2002; Chen, 2003).

Successful employment of fortification strategies requires centralized processing facilities, mechanisms for quality control, and social marketing and public education strategies (Nantel and Tontisirin, 2002; Uauy et al., 2002). The required infrastructure is often weak or lacking in developing countries, which reduces the potential for the success of fortification measures. Adequate income and marketing channels are essential if these strategies are to succeed, but the poor and nutritionally vulnerable are frequently less able to purchase fortified food products. Moreover, infrastructure, including roads and transportation systems, is weak in many developing countries. In order for fortification programmes to be successful, these issues need to be addressed, particularly in rural and remote areas, where the majority of the populations at high risk live.

Biofortification

Consumption of a wide variety of foods, including those that contain an array of micronutrients, is still seen as the best long-term sustainable solution to eradicate hidden hunger. Along the path to achieving this goal, biofortification may help to improve the health and welfare of many populations. Biofortification, or plant breeding for the specific purpose of enhancing the nutritional properties of crop varieties, reflects the new application of an ancient technique. For centuries, farmers have bred crops to enhance specific traits such as improved yield, drought tolerance or insect resistance. Recently, breeding trials have been undertaken for the specific purpose of enhancing the nutritional value of crops with the specific objective of improving human nutrition. Gene-marking techniques make it possible for scientists to identify the specific plant genetic material that controls nutrient content so as to select the most beneficial ones for breeding purposes. Using genes that contain nutritionally superior traits has enabled scientists to produce crop varieties with higher nutrient content. There have been some reported successes, including high-protein maize, high-carotene sweet potato and cassava, and iron-enhanced rice (IFPRI, 2002).

Dietary diversification

Dietary diversity can be augmented by expanding the production, processing, marketing and consumption of a wide variety of foods. In treating the problem of micronutrient deficiencies, food-based approaches that focus on improving overall dietary quality, rather than merely delivering a single nutrient, are particularly useful. Several factors lend support to this approach. First, there are complex nutrient-nutrient interactions that increase bioavailability when nutrients are consumed simultaneously. For example, iron absorption is increased when it is combined with vitamin C (FAO, 1997). New evidence about the protective role of phytochemicals and antioxidants continues to emerge. These protective chemicals are easily obtained by consuming a wide variety of fruits and vegetables. Scientific knowledge linking nutrition and disease continues to evolve and expand, implicating an even wider range of nutrients with a variety of roles in health maintenance. Rickets, a disease associated with vitamin D deficiency, has now been connected to diets low in calcium. Demonstrating the existence of dependent relationships heightens the importance of promoting food-based approaches that focus on achieving sustained improvements in the overall diet.

There are several low-cost, food-based measures that can be promoted at the community level to improve micro nutrient status, some of which are presented in Box 1. Culturally appropriate dietary modifications should be developed to help people identify con crete actions that can improve both dietary supply and the absorption of micronutrients. This information needs to be disseminated to the public through traditional information channels.

BOX 1

Community-based strategies to improve micronutrient status

- Encouraging exclusive breastfeeding up to six months of age and continued breastfeeding for older infants
- Identifying and promoting use of culturally appropriate weaning foods rich in micronutrients
- Identifying and promoting use of traditional green leafy vegetables and fruits to add diversity to the diet
- Preserving micronutrients in fruits and vegetables by using solar drying or canning technologies
- Promoting small-scale community gardens
- Rearing small livestock
- Improving year-round supply of micronutrient rich foods

SOURCE: Adapted from FAO/ILSI (1997).

Factors for success: increased collaboration and political commitment

Developing communities face multiple problems. Therefore focusing on a single micronutrient deficiency or on a single strategy is not the most effective means to eliminate micronutrient deficiencies. The problems often result from a wider set of factors including health care, education, sanitation, water supply and housing (Nantel and Tontisirin, 2002). Complementary public health interventions that can help reduce micro nutrient mal nutrition include deworming, malaria prophylaxis, improved water and sanitation facilities and childhood immunization. Successful strategies are those that address all these issues in an integrated and coordinated fashion. Holistic strategies, using a mixture of direct and indirect interventions and public health measures, as well as education and awareness campaigns, have proved to be the most successful in reducing micronutrient malnutrition (Under wood, 1999). Communities themselves are best suited to determine which corrective actions to employ to address their problems. Collecting process indicators at this level can help direct community actions. The role of government and government counter parts is to support these actions through political commitment, training and the provision of basic services, including attention to micronutrients.

References

Brown, K. & Wuehler, S., eds. 2000. *Zinc and human health.* Ottawa, Micronutrient Initiative.

Chen, Chunming. 2003. Iron fortification of soy sauce in China. *Food, Nutrition and Agriculture,* 32, pp. 76–82.
FAO. 1997. *Human nutrition in the developing world,* by M. Latham. Rome.
FAO. 2002. *State of Food Insecurity in the World 2002.* Rome.
FAO/ILSI (International Life Sciences Institute). 1997. *Preventing micronutrient malnutrition: a guide to food-based approaches. A manual for policy makers and programme planners.* Rome/Washington, DC, FAO/ILSI.
FAO/WHO. 2002. *Human vitamin and mineral requirements.* Report of a joint FAO/WHO expert consultation. Rome.
Hunt, J. & Quibria, M., eds. 1999. *Investing in child nutrition in Asia.* Manila, Asian Development Bank.
ICCIDD (International Council for the Control of Iodine Deficiency Disorder). 2002. IDD fact card. New Orleans, ICCIDD Communications Focal Point, Tulane University School of Public Health and Tropical Medicine (available at www.tulane.edu/~icec/aboutidd.htm; accessed end May 2003).
International Food Policy Research Institute (IFPRI). 2002. *Biofortification: harnessing agricultural technology to improve the health of the poor* (available at www.ifpri.org/themes/grp06/papers/biofort.pdf; accessed end May 2003).
Mannar, V. & Gallego, E. 2002. Iron fortification: Country level experiences and lessons learned. *J. Nutr.,* 132: 856S–858S.
Mason, J.B., Lotfi, M., Dalmiya, N., Sethuraman, K., & Deitchler, M.; with Geibel, S., Gillenwater, K., Gilman, A., Mason, K. & Mock, N. 2001. *The micronutrient report: current progress in the control of vitamin A, iodine, and iron deficiencies.* Ottowa, Micronutrient Initiative/International Development Research Center (available at http://www.micronutrient.org/frame_HTML/resource_text/publications/mn_report.pdf; accessed end May 2003).
Nantel, G. & Tontisirin, K. 2002. Policy and sustainability issues. *J. Nutr.,* 132: 839S–844S.
Stover, P. & Garza, C. 2002. Bringing individuality to public health recommendations. *J. Nutr.,* 132: 2476S–2480S.
Uauy, R., Hertrampf, E. & Reddy, M. 2002. Iron fortification of foods: Overcoming technical and practical barriers. *J. Nutr.,* 132: 849S–852S.
Underwood, B. 1999. Perspectives from micronutrient malnutrition elimination/eradication programmes. *MMWR—Morbidity and Mortality Weekly Report,* 48: 37–42.
United Nations Children's Fund (UNICEF). 2001. *Review of the achievements in the implementation and results of the World Declaration on the Survival, Protection and Development of Children and Plan of Action for Implementing the World Declaration on the Survival, Protection and Development of Children in the 1990s.* Report of the Secretary General to the United Nations General Assembly, 27th Special Session. New York.
UNICEF. 2002. *Vitamin A global initiative* (available at www.unicef.org/vitamina; accessed end May 2003).
USAID (The United States Agency for International Development). 1992. *Economic rationale for investing in micronutrient programs: A policy brief based on new analyses.* Washington, DC, United States Agency for International Development, Bureau for Research and Development, Office of Nutrition, Vitamin A Field Support Project.
WHO (World Health Organization). 1996. *Indicators for assessing vitamin A deficiency and their application in monitoring and evaluating intervention programmes.* WHO/NUT/96.10. Geneva.
WHO. 2001a. *Iron deficiency anaemia: Assessment, prevention and control—a guide for programme managers.* Geneva.
WHO. 2001b. *Assessment of iodine deficiency disorders and monitoring their elimination—a guide for programme managers.* Second edition. Geneva.
WHO. 2002. Turning the tide of malnutrition, responding to the challenge of the 21st century (available at www.who.int/nut/documents/nhd_brochure.pdf; accessed end May 2003).
WHO/FAO. 1996. *Preparation and use of food-based dietary guidelines.* Geneva.

Note

[1]Vitamins A, B4, B12, C, D, E and K; thiamine, riboflavin, niacin, pantothenic acid and biotin, folate and folic acid, calcium, iodine, iron, magnesium and zinc.

Gina Kennedy is a Consultant in the Nutrition Planning, Assessment and Evaluation Service (ESNA) at FAO, **Guy Nantel** is a Senior Officer, ESNA and **Prakash Shetty** is Chief of ESNA.

Pushing Beyond the Earth's Limits

The future will see not just more mouths to feed, but a growing demand for higher-quality, more resource-intensive food. The world's farmers may not be up to the many challenges of meeting those demands.

By Lester R. Brown

During the last half of the twentieth century, the world economy expanded sevenfold. In 2000 alone, its growth exceeded that of the entire nineteenth century. Economic growth, now the goal of governments everywhere, has become the status quo. Stability is considered a departure from the norm.

As the economy grows, its demands are outgrowing the earth, exceeding many of the planet's natural capacities. While the world economy multiplied sevenfold in just 50 years, the earth's natural life-support systems remained essentially the same. Water use tripled, but the capacity of the hydrological system to produce fresh water through evaporation changed little. The demand for seafood increased fivefold, but the sustainable yield of oceanic fisheries was unchanged. Fossil-fuel burning raised carbon dioxide (CO_2) emissions fourfold, but the capacity of nature to absorb it changed little, leading to a buildup of CO_2 in the atmosphere and a rise in the earth's temperature. As human demands surpass the earth's natural capacities, expanding food production becomes more difficult.

Losing Agricultural Momentum

Environmentalists have been saying for years that, if the environmental trends of recent decades continued, the world would one day be in trouble. What was not clear was what form the trouble would take and when it would occur. Now it has become increasingly clear that tightening food supplies will be our greatest trouble and that it will emerge within the next few years. In early 2004, China's forays into the world market to buy 8 million tons of wheat marked what could be the beginning of the global shift from an era of grain surpluses to one of grain scarcity.

World grain production is a basic indicator of dietary adequacy at the individual level and of overall food security at the global level. After nearly tripling from 1950 to 1996, the grain harvest stayed flat for seven years in a row, through 2003, showing no increase at all. And production fell short of consumption in each of the last four of those years. The shortfalls of nearly 100 million tons in 2002 and again in 2003 were the largest on record.

Consumption exceeded production for four years, leading world grain stocks to drop to the lowest level in 30 years. The last time stocks were this low, in 1972–1974, wheat and rice prices doubled. Importing countries competed vigorously for inadequate supplies. A politics of scarcity emerged, and some countries, such as the United States, restricted exports.

In 2004, a combination of stronger grain prices at planting time and the best weather in a decade yielded a substantially larger harvest for the first time in eight years. Yet even with a harvest that was up 124 million tons from that in 2003, the world still consumed all the grain it produced, leaving none to rebuild stocks. If stocks cannot be rebuilt in a year of exceptional weather, when can they?

From 1950 to 1984, world grain production expanded faster than population, raising the grain produced per person per year from 250 kilograms to the historic peak of 339 kilograms—an increase of 34%. This positive development initially reflected recovery from the disruption of World War II, and then later solid technological advances. The rising tide of food production lifted all ships, largely eradicating hunger in some countries and substantially reducing it in many others.

But since 1984, growth in grain harvests has fallen behind growth in population. The amount of grain produced per person fell to 308 kilograms in 2004.

Africa is suffering the most, with a decline in grain produced per person that is unusually steep and taking a heavy human toll. Soils are depleted of nutrients, and the amount of grainland per person has been shrinking steadily due to population growth in recent decades. But in addition, Africa must now contend with the loss of adults to AIDS, which is depleting the rural workforce and undermining agriculture. In two of the last three years, grain production per person in sub-Saharan Africa has been below 120 kilograms—dropping to a level that leaves millions of Africans on the edge of starvation.

Several long-standing environmental trends are contributing to the global loss of agricultural momentum. Among these are the cumulative effects of soil erosion on land productivity, the loss of cropland to desertification, and the accelerating conversion of cropland to nonfarm uses. All are taking a toll, although their relative roles vary among countries.

In addition, farmers are seeing fewer new technologies to dramatically boost production. The high-yielding varieties of wheat, rice, and corn that were developed a generation or so ago doubled and tripled yields, but there have not been any dramatic advances in the genetic yield potential of grains since then.

Similarly, the use of fertilizer has now plateaued or even declined slightly in key food-producing countries. The rapid growth in irrigation that characterized much of the last half century has also slowed. Indeed, in some countries the irrigated area is shrinking.

And now, two newer environmental trends are slowing the growth in world food production: falling water tables and rising temperatures. The bottom line is that it is now more difficult for farmers to keep up with the growing demand for grain. The rise in world grainland productivity, which averaged over 2% a year from 1950 to 1990, fell to scarcely 1% a year in the last decade of the twentieth century. This will likely drop further in the years immediately ahead.

If the rise in land productivity continues to slow and if population continues to grow by 70 million or more per year, governments may begin to define national security in terms of food shortages, rising food prices, and the emerging politics of scarcity. Food insecurity may soon eclipse terrorism as the overriding concern of national governments.

Food Challenges Go from Local to Global

The world economy is making excessive demands on the earth. Evidence of this can be seen in collapsing fisheries, shrinking forests, expanding deserts, rising CO_2 levels, eroding soils, rising temperatures, falling water tables, melting glaciers, deteriorating grasslands, rising seas, rivers that are running dry, and disappearing species.

Nearly all of these environmentally destructive trends contribute to global food insecurity. For example, even a modest rise of 1°F in temperature in mountainous regions can substantially increase rainfall and decrease snowfall. The result is more flooding during the rainy season and less snowmelt to feed rivers during the dry season, when farmers need irrigation water.

Or consider the collapse of fisheries and the associated leveling off of the oceanic fish catch. During the last half century, the fivefold growth in the world fish catch that satisfied much of the growing demand for animal protein pushed oceanic fisheries to their limits and beyond. Now, in this new century, we cannot expect any growth at all in the catch. The Food and Agriculture Organization warns that all future growth in animal protein supplies can only come from that produced on land, not the sea, putting even more pressure on the earth's land and water resources.

Until recently, the economic effects of environmental trends, such as overfishing, overpumping, and overplowing, were largely local. Among the many examples are the collapse of the cod fishery off Newfoundland from overfishing that cost Canada 40,000 jobs, the halving of Saudi Arabia's wheat harvest as a result of aquifer depletion, and the shrinking grain harvest of Kazakhstan as wind erosion claimed half of its cropland.

Now, if world food supplies tighten, we may see the first global economic effect of environmentally destructive trends. Rising food prices could be the first economic indicator to signal serious trouble in the deteriorating relationship between the global economy and the earth's ecosystem. The short-lived 20% rise in world grain prices in early 2004 may turn out to be a warning tremor before the quake.

Two New Challenges

As world demand for food has tripled, so too has the use of water for irrigation. As a result, the world is incurring a vast water deficit. But the trend is largely invisible because the deficit takes the form of aquifer overpumping and falling water tables. Falling water levels are often not discovered until wells go dry.

The world water deficit is a relatively recent phenomenon. Only within the last half century have powerful diesel and electrically driven pumps given us the pumping capacity to deplete aquifers. The worldwide spread of these pumps since the late 1960s and the drilling of millions of wells have in many cases pushed water withdrawal beyond the aquifers' recharge from rainfall. As a result, water tables are now falling in countries that are home to more than half of the world's people, including China, India, and the United States—the three largest grain producers.

Groundwater levels are falling throughout the northern half of China. Under the North China Plain, they are dropping 1–3 meters (3–10 feet) a year. In India, they are falling in most states, including the Punjab, the country's breadbasket. And in the United States, water levels are falling throughout the southern Great Plains and the Southwest. Overpumping creates a false sense of food security: It enables us to satisfy growing food needs today, but it almost guarantees a decline in food production tomorrow when the aquifer is depleted.

It takes a thousand tons of water to produce a single ton of grain, so food security is closely tied to water security. Seventy percent of world water use is for irrigation, 20% is used by industry, and 10% is for residential purposes. As urban water use rises while aquifers are being depleted, farmers are faced with a shrinking share of a shrinking water supply.

Meanwhile, temperatures are rising and concern about climate change is intensifying. Scientists have begun to focus on the precise relationship between temperature and crop yields. Crop ecologists at the International Rice Research Institute in the Philippines and at the U.S. Department of Agriculture (USDA) have jointly concluded that each 1°C rise in temperature during the growing season cuts 10% off the yields of wheat, rice, and corn.

Over the last three decades, the earth's average temperature has climbed by nearly 0.7°C; the four warmest years on record came during the last six years. In 2002, record-high temperatures and drought shrank grain harvests in both India and the United States. In 2003, Europe bore the brunt of the intense heat. The record-breaking August heat wave claimed 35,000 lives in eight nations and withered grain harvests in virtually every country from France to Ukraine.

In a business-as-usual scenario, the earth's average temperature will rise by 1.4°–5.8°C (2°–10°F) during this century, according to the Intergovernmental Panel on Climate Change. These projections are for the earth's average temperature, but the rise is expected to be much greater over land than over the oceans, in the higher latitudes than in the equatorial regions, and in the interior of continents than in the coastal regions. This suggests that increases far in excess of the projected average are likely for regions such as the North American breadbasket—the region defined by the Great Plains of the United States and Canada and the U.S. corn belt. Today's farmers face the prospect of temperatures higher than any generation of farmers since agriculture began.

The Japan Syndrome

When studying the USDA world grain database more than a decade ago, I noted that, if countries are already densely populated when they begin to industrialize rapidly, three things happen in quick succession to make them heavily dependent on grain imports: Grain consumption climbs as incomes rise, grainland area shrinks, and grain production falls. The rapid industrialization that drives up demand simultaneously shrinks the cropland area. The inevitable result is that grain imports soar. Within a few decades, countries can go from being essentially self-sufficient to importing 70% or more of their grain. I call this the "Japan syndrome" because I first recognized this sequence of events in Japan, a country that today imports 70% of its grain.

In a fast-industrializing country, grain consumption rises rapidly. Initially, rising incomes permit more direct consumption of grain, but before long the growth shifts to the greater indirect consumption of grain in the form of grain-intensive livestock products, such as pork, poultry, and eggs.

Once rapid industrialization is under way, the grainland area begins to shrink within a few years. As a country industrializes and modernizes, cropland gets taken over by industrial and residential developments and by roads, highways, and parking lots to accommodate more cars and drivers. When farmers are left with fragments of land that are too small to be cultivated economically, they often simply abandon their plots, seeking employment elsewhere.

As rapid industrialization pulls labor out of the countryside, it often leads to less double cropping, a practice that depends on quickly harvesting one grain crop once it is ripe and immediately preparing the seedbed for the next crop. With the loss of workers as young people migrate to cities, the capacity to do this diminishes. As incomes rise, diets diversify, generating demand for more fruits and vegetables. This in turn leads farmers to shift land from grain to these more profitable, high-value crops.

Japan was essentially self-sufficient in grain when its grain harvested area peaked in 1955. Since then the grainland area has shrunk by more than half. The multiple-cropping index has dropped from nearly 1.4 crops per hectare per year in 1960 to scarcely one crop today. Some six years after Japan's grain area began to shrink, the shrinkage overrode the rise in land productivity and overall production began to decline. With grain consumption climbing and production falling, grain imports soared. By 1983, imports accounted for 70% of Japan's grain consumption, a level they remain at today.

South Korea and Taiwan are tracing Japan's pattern. In both cases, the decline in grain area was followed roughly a decade later by a decline in production. Perhaps this should not be surprising, since the forces at work in the two countries are exactly the same as in Japan. And, like Japan, both South Korea and Taiwan now import some 70% of their total grain supply.

Based on the sequence of events in these three countries that affected grain production, consumption, and imports—the Japan syndrome—it was easy to anticipate the precipitous decline in China's grain production that began in 1998. The obvious question now is which other countries will enter a period of declining grain production because of the same combination of forces. Among those that come to mind are India, Indonesia, Bangladesh, Pakistan, Egypt, and Mexico.

Of particular concern is India, with a population of nearly 1.1 billion now and growing by 18 million a year. In recent years, India's economic growth has accelerated, averaging 6%–7% a year. This growth, only slightly slower than that of China, is also beginning to consume cropland. In addition to the grainland shrinkage associated with the Japan syndrome, the extensive overpumping of aquifers in India—which will one day deprive farmers of irrigation water—will also reduce grain production.

Exactly when rapid industrialization in a country that is densely populated will translate into a decline in grain production is difficult to anticipate. Once crop production begins to decline, countries often try to reverse the trend. But the difficulty of achieving this can be seen in Japan, where a rice support price that is four times the world market price has failed to expand production.

The China Factor

China—the most-populous country in the world—is now beginning to experience the Japan syndrome. The precipitous fall in China's grain production since 1998 is perhaps the most alarming recent world agricultural event. After an impressive climb from 90 million tons in 1950 to a peak of 392 million tons in 1998, China's grain harvest fell in four of the next five years, dropping to 322 million tons in 2003. For perspective, this decline of 70 million tons exceeds the entire grain harvest of Canada.

The decline resulted when China's farmers began converting cropland to nonfarm uses and shifting grainland to higher-value fruits and vegetables. And, as happened in Japan, better jobs in some of the more prosperous regions lured away the rural labor needed for multiple cropping, thus reducing productivity.

China is also losing grainland to the expansion of deserts and the loss of irrigation water, due to both aquifer depletion and di-

The Japan Syndrome

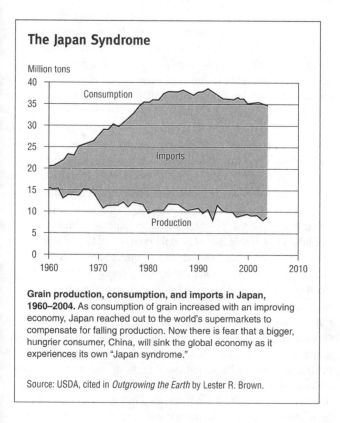

Million tons

Grain production, consumption, and imports in Japan, 1960–2004. As consumption of grain increased with an improving economy, Japan reached out to the world's supermarkets to compensate for falling production. Now there is fear that a bigger, hungrier consumer, China, will sink the global economy as it experiences its own "Japan syndrome."

Source: USDA, cited in *Outgrowing the Earth* by Lester R. Brown.

version of water to cities. Unfortunately for China, none of the forces that are shrinking the grainland area are easily countered.

Between 1998 and 2003, five consecutive harvest shortfalls dropped China's once massive stocks of grain to their lowest level in 30 years. With stocks now largely depleted, China's leaders—all of them survivors of the great famine of 1959–1961, when 30 million people starved to death—are worried. For them, food security is not a trivial issue.

China desperately wants to reverse the recent fall in grain production and has tried to encourage farmers to grow more grain. In March 2004, Beijing expanded the agricultural budget by one-fifth ($3.6 billion) and raised the support price for the early rice crop by 21%. These two emergency measures did reverse the grain harvest decline temporarily, but whether they can reverse the trend over the longer term is doubtful.

When China turns to the outside world for commodities, it can overwhelm world markets. When wheat prices within China started climbing in the fall of 2003, the government dispatched wheat-buying delegations to Australia, Canada, and the United States. They purchased 8 million tons, and overnight China became the world's largest wheat importer. China has been the world's fastest-growing economy since 1980, and the economic effects of this massive expansion can be seen in the rest of the world.

But China is also putting enormous pressure on its own natural resource base. The northern half of the country is literally drying out. Water tables are falling, rivers are going dry, and lakes are disappearing. The World Bank warns of "catastrophic consequences for future generations" if China's water use and supply cannot quickly be brought back into balance. More immediately, if China

cannot quickly restore a balance between the consumption of water and the sustainable yield of its aquifers and rivers, its grain imports will likely soar in the years ahead.

For people not living in China, it is difficult to visualize how quickly deserts are expanding. Like invading armies, expanding deserts are claiming ever more territory. Old deserts are advancing and new ones are forming, like guerrilla forces striking unexpectedly, forcing Beijing to fight on several fronts. Throughout northern and western China, some 24,000 villages have either been abandoned or partly depopulated as drifting sand has made farming untenable.

China's food problems now are not hunger and starvation, as the nation now has a substantial cushion between consumption levels and minimal nutrition needs. Rather, the concern is rising food prices and the effect that this could have on political stability. China's leaders are striving for a delicate balance between food prices that will encourage production in the countryside but maintain stability in the cities.

If smaller countries like Japan, South Korea, and Taiwan import 70% or more of their grain, the impacts on the global economy are not so dramatic. But if China turns to the outside world to meet even 20% of its grain needs—which would be close to 80 million tons—it will create a huge challenge for grain exporters. The resulting rise in world grain prices could destabilize governments in low-income, grain-importing countries. The entire world thus has a stake in China's efforts to stabilize its agricultural resource base.

The Challenge Ahead

We must not underestimate the challenges that the world faces over the next half century. There will be a projected 3 billion more people to feed, and 5 billion who will want to improve their diets by eating more meat, which requires more grain (as livestock feed) to produce. Meanwhile, the world's farmers will still be fighting soil erosion and the loss of cropland to nonfarm uses, as well as newer challenges, such as falling water tables, the diversion of irrigation water to cities, and rising temperatures.

The World Food Summit of 1996 in Rome set a goal of halving the number of hungry people by 2015. That would require reducing the ranks of the hungry by 20 million a year. While some progress was made in the 1990s, it has not been enough. And things have gotten even worse: By the end of the century, the number of hungry people in the world began to increase, rising to 798 million in 2001. This increase in hunger is not too surprising, given the lack of growth in the world grain harvest during this period.

Looming over this darkening horizon is the prospect that other countries will soon fall victim to the Japan syndrome of accelerating economic growth and shrinking grain harvests. Will India's grain production peak and start declining in the next few years, much as China's did after 1998? Or will India be able to hold off the loss of cropland to nonfarm uses and the depletion of aquifers long enough to eradicate most of its hunger? There are signs that the shrinkage in India's grain area—a precursor to the shrinkage of overall production—may have begun.

Because aquifer depletion is recent, it is taking agricultural analysts into uncharted territory. Water tables are falling simultaneously in many countries and at an accelerating rate, but we cannot be certain exactly when aquifers will be depleted and precisely how much this will reduce food production. And in a world of rising temperatures, there is added reason to be concerned about world food security.

On another front, in Africa the spread of HIV/AIDS is threatening the food security of the entire continent as the loss of able-bodied field workers shrinks harvests. In sub-Saharan Africa, disease begets hunger and hunger begets disease. In some villages, high HIV-infection rates have claimed an entire generation of young adults, leaving only the elderly and children. Without a major intervention from the outside world, the continuing spread of the virus—combined with the hunger that is cutting life expectancy in half in some countries—could take Africa back to the Dark Ages.

In a world where the food economy has been shaped by an abundance of cheap oil, tightening world oil supplies will further complicate efforts to eradicate hunger. Modern mechanized agriculture requires large amounts of fuel for tractors, irrigation pumps, and grain drying. Rising oil prices may soon translate into rising food prices.

Feeding the World

If grain imports continue to grow in Asia, where half the world's people live, and if harvests continue to shrink in Africa, the second-most populous continent, we have to ask where tomorrow's grain will come from. The countries that dominated world grain exports for the last half century—the United States, Canada, Australia, and Argentina—may not be able to export much beyond current levels.

The United States has produced as much as 350 million tons of grain a year several times over the last two decades, though never much more than this. The country exported about 100 million tons of grain a year two decades ago, but only an average of 80 million tons in recent years, as demand has increased domestically. The potential for expanding grain production and export in both Canada and Australia is constrained by relatively low rainfall in their grain-growing regions. Argentina's grain production has actually declined over the last several years as land has shifted to soybeans, principally used for feeding livestock rather than people.

> "In a world of rising temperatures, there is added reason to be concerned about world food security."

By contrast, Russia and Ukraine should be able to expand their grain exports, at least modestly, as population has stabi-

lized or is declining. There is also some unrealized agricultural production potential in these countries. But northern countries heavily dependent on spring wheat typically have lower yields, so Russia is unlikely to become a major grain exporter. Ukraine has a somewhat more promising potential if it can provide farmers with the economic incentives they need to expand production. So, too, do Poland and Romania.

Yet, the likely increases in exports from these countries are small compared with the prospective import needs of China and, potentially, India. It is worth noting that the drop in China's grain harvest of 70 million tons over five years is equal to the grain exports of Canada, Australia, and Argentina combined.

Argentina can expand its already large volume of soybean exports, but its growth potential for grain exports is limited by the availability of arable land. The only country that has the potential to substantially expand the world's grainland area is Brazil, with its vast cerrado—a savannah-like region on the southern edge of the Amazon basin. Because its soils require the heavy use of fertilizer and because transporting grain from Brazil's remote interior to distant world markets is costly, it would likely take substantially higher world grain prices for Brazil to emerge as a major exporter. Beyond this, would a vast expansion of cropland in Brazil's interior be sustainable? Or is its vulnerability to soil erosion likely to prevent it from making a long-term contribution? And what will be the price paid in the irretrievable loss of ecosystems and plant and animal species?

In sum, ensuring future food security is a formidable, multifaceted problem. To solve it, the world will need to:

- Check the HIV epidemic before it so depletes Africa's adult population that starvation stalks the land.
- Arrest the steady shrinkage in grainland area per person.
- Eliminate the overgrazing that is converting grasslands to desert.
- Reduce soil erosion losses to below the natural rate of new soil formation.
- Halt the advancing deserts that are engulfing cropland.
- Check the rising temperature that threatens to shrink harvests.
- Arrest the fall in water tables.
- Protect cropland from careless conversion to nonfarm uses.

About the Author

Lester R. Brown is president of the Earth Policy Institute, 1350 Connecticut Avenue, N.W., Suite 403, Washington, D.C. 20036.

This article draws from his most recent book, *Outgrowing the Earth: The Food Security Challenge in an Age of Falling Water Tables and Rising Temperatures* (W.W. Norton, 2005), which is available from the Futurist Bookshelf, www.wfs.org/bkshelf.htm. For additional information, visit www.earth-policy.org/Books/Out/index.htm.

Food Security, Overweight, and Agricultural Research—A View from 2003

ABSTRACT: Some of the poorest countries of the world are facing an apparent paradox. Food insecurity, undernutrition, and overweight exist side by side within the same country. Indeed, food-insecure households often contain an overweight member. Data from 11 mega-countries (countries with a population of more than 100 million) will be presented to illustrate the magnitude of the problem. These 11 countries represent more than 60% of the world's population. Agriculture is still a dominant industry. The links between food insecurity, nutritional status, and agriculture will be presented.

E. KENNEDY, D.SC.

Introduction

Enormous progress has been made since the 1974 World Food Summit. Dramatic increases in food supplies have occurred, in part due to effective investment in agricultural research. In addition over the past 30 years progress has been made in improving nutrition globally. For example, in developing countries, stunting in preschool-aged children decreased from 47.1% in 1980 to 32.5% in 2000

However, we now have a different dilemma. Increasingly, countries are finding that food insecurity and undernutrition exist side by side with problems of overnutrition and chronic disease.

The purpose of this paper is to examine the links between food security, overweight, and agriculture.

The double burden of disease

The phenomenon of hunger and malnutrition existing in the same countries and the same households with overweight and chronic disease has been labeled "the double burden of disease." World Health Organization (WHO) and the Food and Agriculture Organization of the United Nations (FAO) in 2003 released their report "Diet, Nutrition and the Prevention of Chronic Disease."

The old view of overweight and obesity was that these were problems for middle- and upper-income countries. The new view is that developing countries are increasingly suffering from high levels of overweight and obesity and other chronic diseases. This issue of dramatic rise in overweight and obesity is a message that has not gotten out to many policy makers and implementers in developing countries.

The WHO/FAO report highlights the fact that, in 2001, 60% of all deaths are due to chronic diseases; this represents 46% of the global burden of disease. By 2020, 75% of deaths worldwide are estimated to be due to noncommunicable diseases.

The challenge for international institutions, researchers, and national policy officials is, "How can food and agricultural policy meet the needs of the poor and undernourished while also tackling the problem of overweight and obesity?"

Mega Country Health Promotion Network

Indonesia is but one country that reflects the "double burden of disease"; in Indonesia, 1 out of 10 households has both underweight and overweight in the same family. Rates of overweight have been increasing worldwide. In Brazil, 49% and 45% of men and women, respectively, are overweight in urban areas. The rates in Brazil for overweight in rural areas are somewhat lower. In urban India, 19.9% of women are overweight and in Russia, 30.3% and 50.3% of men and women are overweight.

Thus, in December 2001, WHO created the Mega Country Health Promotion Network. The network includes 11 countries with populations of more than 100 million. These 11 countries represent more than 60% of the world's population. The 11 countries include: China, Japan, Bangladesh, India, Pakistan, Indonesia, Brazil, Mexico, Nigeria, Russia, and the USA. The purpose of this network is to identify public health strategies to decrease the burden of chronic disease including overweight and obesity.

Data from each of the 11 countries indicate that:

(1) There is a continuum in each country going from under-nutrition to over-nutrition. It is no longer an "either/or situation" for under- and over-nutrition. The point on this continuum where each country falls varies.

(2) The poor in each country, increasingly, have a greater risk of overweight and obesity.

(3) Urbanization of the population has brought about changes in diets and physical activity.

In this nutrition transition that is occurring worldwide, urban diets have shifted from basic staples to refined grains and more fats and sugars. There are now increased levels of total fat and saturated fat in the diet. The old view was that increases in fat in the diet were associated with middle and upper income countries and households. The new view is that fat consumption is not linked to national GNP. This pattern globally is similar to what occurred in the USA between the 1950s and 1970s. During this period in the US the dietary patterns of lower- and upper-income households became more similar.

The challenge for the Mega Country Health Promotion Network is to identify newer paradigms and approaches for promoting healthy lifestyles. The essential components of these approaches are:

- Comprehensive—many sectors need to be involved in the solution; no one approach by itself is likely to be successful.
- Each country must select the optimal mix of actions and policies to put in place.
- Public–private partnerships will be an important part of the strategies used.

The first core guiding principle in prevention of overweight and obesity is that Food Security is the foundation to good health and good nutrition. Even where overweight and obesity exists the poor are most at risk of food insecurity.

There has been a marked change globally in how we define and measure food insecurity. It's what some are calling the "newer faces of food security." Food security requires enough food—both quantity and quality—for an active and healthy life—but also that food be obtained in a socially acceptable manner. Therefore, households that need to rely on emergency food supplies—such as soup kitchens—are not food-secure, even where their energy intakes may be adequate.

In addition, international organizations such as the FAO are exploring newer methods for measuring food insecurity. The classic measure of food insecurity, kcals per individual, in the modern environment no longer sufficiently captures food insecurity. At the World Food Summit Plus Five meeting in Rome in June 2002, there was in-depth discussion of the use of qualitative or semi-quantitative measures of food insecurity that allow us to measure on a continuum from food-secure to food-insecure to food-insecure with hunger.

Role of agricultural research

In dealing both with problems of food insecurity/hunger and over-weight/obesity, agricultural research will continue to be essential. There are 4 key areas where the need for agricultural research is essential:

(1) Agricultural research will continue to be essential in increasing food supplies worldwide. All of the projections from FAO for meeting increasing demands for food supplies worldwide are premised on continued investment in agricultural research. Just a word of caution, we cannot be complacent about the support for agricultural research. Even when I was in USDA, we would regularly be asked if the support for agricultural research was still needed, given the overall sufficiency of world food supplies. My answer was an unequivocal, absolutely "yes".

(2) For small-farm households dependent on own farm production, agricultural research will continue to be needed to increase returns to land and returns to labor from agriculture.

(3) A general benefit to society is the low food prices that accrue from successful agricultural production.

(4) Finally, agricultural research through more effective agricultural technologies can help smooth out variations in food production, which can lead to seasonal variations in food prices.

There are other areas where agricultural research can make significant contributions. The potential for agricultural research to provide more nutritious foods at a low cost is enormous. This can be a particularly important role of agricultural research for the poor consumers. For example, lowering the price of fruits and vegetables to consumers would be an important way to improve the micronutrient content of the diet.

There are indirect effects of agricultural research that often are less apparent. Clearly, some farms in developing countries are so small as to be uneconomical. Agricultural research by promoting growth in the agricultural sector would also spur growth in the rural and urban nonfarm economy. The nonfarm economy increasingly will have to provide employment for the very small farmers who will need both farm and nonfarm income to have sufficient income. Of course, the rural poor rely on the nonfarm sector for employment as well as employment as hired labor on farms.

What else?

There are other factors influencing people's lifestyle choices that affect what we call "Healthy Lifestyles". Some of these factors include:

Access—this includes both physical access (are the foods available in the marketplace?) and economic access (can the consumer afford them?).

Culture—what people are used to eating, realizing that culture can change over time and people's preferences are obviously also subject to change over time.

Sedentary Lifestyles—which is a modern phenomenon.

Taste—which does not have to be explained. Changes in physical activity patterns have been changing rapidly throughout the world; this is true in both urban and rural areas, although the changes in relative energy expenditure are greater in the urban areas. Changes in level of energy output are:

Work-related levels of energy expenditure are declining—even in traditional occupations, such as agriculture. I chaired the FAO/WHO/IUNS expert consultation on Energy in Human Nutrition—

the report is soon to be released. Using more precise measures of energy expenditure, we find that for many activities, energy expenditures have been overestimated in the past.

Transportation-related energy expenditures have also changed. Again, this is a phenomenon worldwide. I like to use the personal example of Beijing. When I started going there in the last 1980s, walking was the common mode of transportation, then replaced by bicycles, now being replaced by cars.

Leisure-related activities are also changing to become less energy-intensive.

The combination of less intensive work, transportation, and leisure have meant that many people are consuming more kcals than is needed for energy expenditure. Hence overweight and obesity are increasing.

Policy and research challenges

The challenge for policy makers and research is to identify policies, programs, and approaches that deal with the new lifestyle realities. Consumers worldwide have gotten what they have asked for, cheaper food supplies, and a less energy-intensive lifestyle. How do we take this reality and think about ways to promote healthy lifestyles for healthy people?

A key part of this challenge is that there are fewer successful nutrition interventions for the urban poor. Even interventions that have been used in rural areas have focused on undernutrition, not overnutrition and chronic disease. Therefore, an essential first step is to identify models for healthy lifestyle promotion. Clearly, there is general agreement that this will involve a combination of a healthful diet and physical activity. But what is it we are asking policy makers and implementers to actually do?

It is likely that we will find common elements in interventions that "work". These include being comprehensive. It is unlikely that a single intervention or approach, by itself, will work. Agriculture is a key sector in the solution; but increasingly we see a need to link agriculture to other sectors.

Finally, policy makers, given resource constraints, including lack of money, are interested in exploring the potential of public–private partnerships for promoting healthy lifestyles—healthy people. The potential of public–private partnerships is enormous; we now need some success stories.

Edited by Manfred Kroger, Ph.D., Editor of the Proceedings of the 12th World Congress of Food Science and Technology

Author Kennedy is with the International Life Sciences Institute, One Thomas Circle, Washington, D.C. (E-mail: ekennedy@ilsi.org).

Towards the Summit commitments

Confronting the causes of malnutrition: the hidden challenge of micronutrient deficiencies

Over 2 billion people worldwide suffer from micronutrient malnutrition, often called "hidden hunger". Their diets supply inadequate amounts of vitamins and minerals such as vitamin A, iron, iodine, zinc, folate, selenium and vitamin C. Deficiencies usually occur when the habitual diet lacks diversity and does not include sufficient quantities of the fruits, vegetables, dairy products, meat and fish that are the best sources of many micronutrients.

Vitamin A and mortality, 1992

A World Health Organization study concluded that an improved vitamin A nutriture could prevent 1.3 to 2.5 million deaths each year among children aged six months to five years in the developing world.

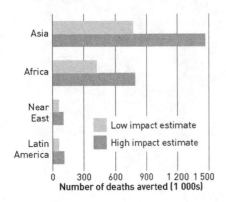

Asia
Africa
Near East
Latin America

Low impact estimate
High impact estimate

0 300 600 900 1 200 1 500
Number of deaths averted (1 000s)

Source: WHO

Micronutrients are essential for human growth and development as well as normal functioning. The three most common forms of micronutrient malnutrition are deficiencies of vitamin A, iodine and iron. In developing countries, deficiencies of micronutrients often are not present in isolation but exist in combination (see map).

Children and women are the most vulnerable to micronutrient deficiencies—children because of the critical importance of micronutrients for normal growth and development, women because of their higher need for iron, especially during childbearing years and pregnancy.

"We will implement policies aimed at . . . improving . . . access by all, at all times to sufficient, nutritionally adequate and safe food . . ."

Between 100 and 140 million children suffer from vitamin A deficiency. That figure includes more than 2 million children each year afflicted with severe visual problems, of whom an estimated 250 000 to 500 000 are permanently blinded.

Lack of vitamin A also impairs the immune system, greatly increasing the risk of illness and death from common childhood infections such as diarrhoea and measles (see graph).

Prevalence of micronutrient deficiencies in developing countries

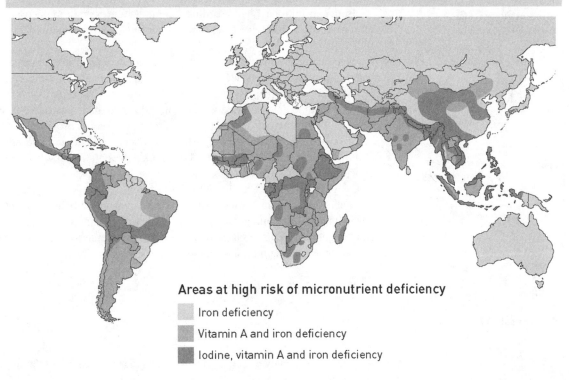

Areas at high risk of micronutrient deficiency

Iron deficiency

Vitamin A and iron deficiency

Iodine, vitamin A and iron deficiency

Source: USAID

Dietary diversification reduces vitamin A deficiency

Home gardens boost consumption of micronutrient-rich food

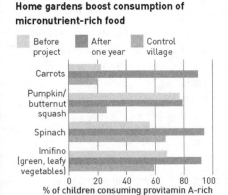

Source: Faber et al.

A home gardening programme focusing on production and consumption of vegetables rich in vitamin A and its precursor, beta carotene, has been successfully demonstrated by the Medical Research Council of South Africa in a mountainous, rural village in KwaZulu-Natal.

Prior to the programme, the diet of children in the village consisted mainly of maize porridge, bread and rice. The lack of variety and vitamin-rich foods resulted in high incidence of vitamin A deficiency. The programme changed that by promoting cultivation of vegetables, such as carrots, pumpkins and spinach, that are rich in beta carotene and by teaching villagers, especially women, the importance of including them regularly in their diet.

After only one year, the percentage of children consuming vitamin-A rich vegetables had increased significantly. And the increased diversity in their diets led to measurable improvements in vitamin A status.

The most devastating consequence of iodine deficiency is reduced mental capacity. Some 20 million people worldwide are mentally handicapped as a result of iodine deficiency, including 100 000 born each year with irreversible brain damage because their mothers lacked iodine prior to and during pregnancy.

Iron deficiency and the anaemia it causes are the most widespread of all forms of micronutrient malnutrition. Anaemia results in fatigue, dizziness and breathlessness following exertion.

Children with anaemia are less able to concentrate and have less energy for play and exploratory behaviours. In adults, anaemia diminishes work capacity and productivity by as much as 10–15 percent. And for pregnant women, anaemia substantially increases the risk of death in childbirth, accounting for up to 20 percent of maternal deaths in Asia and Africa.

The three main strategies for reducing micronutrient deficiencies are dietary diversity and food fortification along with supplements.

Most micronutrient deficiencies could be eliminated by modifying diets to include a greater diversity of nutrient-rich foods. Promoting home gardens, community fish ponds, and

Biofortification increases nutrient content of staple foods

Varietal differences suggest high biofortification potential for rice

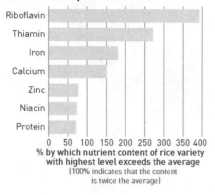

% by which nutrient content of rice variety with highest level exceeds the average
(100% indicates that the content is twice the average)

Source: FAO

Both conventional plant breeding techniques and genetic engineering can be used to develop varieties of staple food crops that are enriched with essential minerals.

"Golden rice" offered proof that biotechnology can produce both nutrients and controversy. Golden rice owes its colour and its name to beta carotene, introduced by transplanting genes from daffodils and bacteria. Critics have charged that the enriched rice will not provide enough beta carotene to satisfy vitamin A requirements. But supporters argue that it could provide 15 to 20 percent of daily requirements and significantly reduce the incidence and severity of vitamin A deficiency, particularly if consumed in conjunction with other nutrient-rich foods.

Conventional plant breeding also holds promise for enhancing the nutrient content of staple foods. Varieties of crops differ considerably in the quantities of nutrients that they contain (see graph). Advances in plant breeding techniques and biotechnology may make it possible to cross varieties that are relatively rich in micronutrients with high-yielding varieties preferred by farmers.

Iodine deficiency disorders

Access to iodized salt, 1995–98

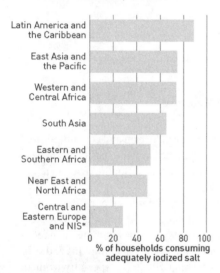

% of households consuming adequately iodized salt

NIS = newly independent states   *Source: FAO*

Iodine deficiency disorder (IDD) is particularly prevalent in the mountainous regions of the world.

The areas with the most severe deficiencies include the Himalayas, the Andes, the European Alps and the vast mountains of China. IDD is also common in frequently flooded lowlands. In both mountains and flooded areas, iodine that is naturally present in the soil is leached away, reducing the iodine content in locally grown crops.

Iodization of salt has virtually eliminated IDD in the mountainous regions of industrialized countries in Europe and North America. Three-quarters of the countries in the developing world have enacted legislation for iodizing salt, mostly over the past 15 years. More than two-thirds of households now get adequately iodized salt. But access varies considerably (see graph). Increasing access to iodized salt and improving quality control of its iodine content hold the key to eliminating iodine deficiency worldwide.

livestock and poultry production can contribute to increasing dietary diversity, while improving food supplies and incomes at the same time (see box on dietary diversification).

Another important food-based strategy is food fortification. The most successful of these initiatives is fortification of salt with iodine (see box). Other micronutrients can also be supplied to populations by enriching widely consumed foods such as milk and flour. In addition, recent advances in crop breeding and biotechnology have heightened the prospects for "biofortification"—developing crops with higher concentrations of micronutrients (see box).

Supplementation involves treating and preventing micronutrient deficiencies by administering capsules, tablets, syrups or other preparations. This medical approach is the method of choice when the deficiency is severe and life-threatening or when access to regular intake of the deficient micronutrient is limited. Use of high-dose vitamin A supplements can reduce mortality from acute measles by up to 50 percent.

Successful campaigns to eliminate micronutrient deficiencies often combine all of these strategies. Vitamin A intake, for example, can best be increased over the long term by adding nutrient-rich foods to the diet and fortifying staple foods, while providing supplements to high-risk groups in vulnerable areas.

Contribution of Indigenous Knowledge and Practices in Food Technology to the Attainment of Food Security in Africa

RUTH ONIANG'O, JOSEPH ALLOTEY, SERAH J. MALABA

ABSTRACT: Indigenous knowledge and practices are important aspects of a society's culture and its technology. They include accumulated knowledge, as well as skills and technology of the local people, usually derived from their direct interaction with their local environment. These aspects need due recognition and full understanding and utilization because of the valuable contributions to food security, especially in African communities. Africa's people have traditionally utilized indigenous knowledge, skills and structures, most often locally developed and handed down in the course of centuries. Insufficient attention has been given to this local knowledge within the mainstream food security development and management interventions. However, there is now increasing awareness of the fact that technology includes not only energy sources and tools, but also knowledge and skills, as well as social organizations. It is, therefore, imperative to approach indigenous communities as partners and collaborators in all food security endeavors in order to realize the objective of sustainability. African communities offer a vast array of indigenous knowledge and practices in food technology that are favorable to the food supply, as well as to food quality and food safety and thus directly contribute to food security. As such, indigenous knowledge and practices in food technology that have proved capable of ensuring food security need to be implemented before considering the introduction of external ones if food security is to be realized in Africa. Emphasis of the same should be especially made for foods that are adapted to local conditions thus improving food access, safe food availability, and utilization to meet local and regional needs. This paper seeks to outline the numerous contributions and enormous potentials that indigenous knowledge and practices in food technology have in ensuring food security in Africa.

Introduction

Africa experiences the stark reality of hunger in the midst of plenty. Since the early 1970s, Africa has periodically experienced episodes of drought with famine, civil unrest with food deficits, and structural adjustment programs with food distribution dislocations. Indeed, during these last 3 decades, Africa has prominently featured as a basket case; and food aid has almost become a fixture of the social condition of several African countries [1].

Specifically, between 1990–1992 and 1997–1999, food deprivation has increased in practically all African countries with the exception of a few, such as, Sudan, Chad, Nigeria, and Ghana [2]. Almost one-half of the sub-Saharan African population is food-insecure, and about one-third of the pre-school children are malnourished. More than 4 million preschool children die every year, mostly from nutrition-related illnesses [3].

This state of human condition was never the case in Africa. In 1938 Africa exported cereals; in 1950 Africa was self-sufficient; in 1976 Africa was importing 10 million tons of cereals a year; in 1978, 13 million tons of cereals imported; in 1983, 31 million tons of cereals imported; from 1983–1985 disastrous drought and food shortages were experienced in Africa [4]

The food quantity, food quality, and nutritional insecurity that Africa faces today can be mitigated and sustainably reversed. As food is uniquely part of a people's integral culture, as well as a key socio-cultural survival mechanism, a manifest change can be realized through the appreciation of Africa's indigenous knowledge.

Indigenous knowledge (IK)

Indigenous knowledge is knowledge that is unique to a given culture or society [5]. Communities use IK at the local level as the basis of decision making pertaining to vital activities in which food security is included. As such, IK is the most important and often only asset for many poor, rural societies and its significance increases as other resources disappear or dwindle.

Building on this IK to ensure food security in Africa can be particularly effective as this is an asset that the people of Africa control and certainly one with which they are very familiar. Utilizing IK will help increase the sustainability of food security efforts because the IK integration process provides for mutual learning and adaptation, which in turn contributes to the empowerment of local communities. Building on IK systems will empower local communities in Africa, enabling them to shape their own food security agenda by actively participating in it.

IK in agriculture

Traditional agricultural practices provide valuable lessons to be learned from local farmers who, through their own innovations and experimentation on farms, have perfected tools such as the hoe and the plough, developed seeds and plants through preservation and selection, and designed crop mixtures and rotations leading to improved productivity.

Practices like fallow, mixed farming, and intercropping were contained in the IK systems long before the introduction of the Green Revolution. These practices provide advantages that are now recognized for ensured fertility of soils, control of pests as well as variety of food sources, among others [6].

Classically, in subsistence agriculture, farmers grew and used traditional food crops because the practice was familiar. They understood traditional food plants, selected varieties to meet the needs and constraints of their environment, and trusted seed from their own land races to produce a reliable crop [6].

Many of these traditional plants make an important contribution to crop productivity. Grown as rotation crops between successive main crops, they may have the advantage of reducing the build-up of pests and diseases. When interplanted they may act as an ecological barrier to diseases. By acting as ground cover, traditional food plants help to prevent soil erosion, reduce evaporation and suppress weed growth. Grown as green manure and ploughed in, traditional plants can increase soil organic matter and improve soil structure. In addition, legumes fix atmospheric nitrogen, enriching the soil for the following crop or for nearby plants [7].

It is necessary to understand the knowledge of traditional agriculture. This knowledge should be harnessed to ensure food security. Besides, the farmers who have been involved in the selection and conservation of food plants need to be recognized for their role in the conservation of germplasm used in breeding programmes while being encouraged to continue conservation of such germplasm.

Africa's indigenous knowledge has thrived over the years. So far over 90% of the food production in sub-Saharan Africa

is attributed to traditional peasant or low-resource farmers. These farmers rely on age-tried methods that depend on expansion of area under cultivation to achieve about 80% of the annual increases in food and agricultural production. Knowledge of things around us can be put to effective use in satisfying our everyday needs [8]

Africa's indigenous food crops

Africa's traditional food crops are underexploited, yet they have been accepted by communities through habit and tradition and are appropriate as well as desirable food sources. In terms of technology input, subsistence agriculture in African tropics has totally depended on traditional farming methods and low inputs of labor-saving technologies [9].

People are accustomed to traditional food crops, know how to cultivate them and prepare them, and enjoy eating dishes made from them. For example, to see them through the hungry season, rural people grow traditional food plants near their homes. Many of these crops are drought-resistant, can be grown without expensive inputs, and have good storage qualities [7].

Traditional food crops fall into 2 broad categories: those consumed as traditional dietary staples, such as cassava, yam, plantain, sweet potato, millets, and sorghum, and those that serve as ingredients in accompanying relishes and sauces, which include a wide variety of legumes, oilseeds, seeds, and vegetables [7].

Traditional staples

Roots, tubers, bananas, and plantains account for some 40% of total food supplies (in terms of food energy) for about one-half of the population of sub-Saharan Africa, where overall food supplies are at very low levels [7]. The major root and tuber crops grown in Africa include cassava, yam, sweet potatoes, and cocoyams. Cassava and yams are among the principal staple crops in many countries on the west coast of Africa, including Nigeria, Cameroon, Ghana, Benin, Togo, and Cote d' Ivoire [10]. Cassava is grown and consumed extensively in Zaire also. On the other hand, in East Africa and Madagascar, cassava and sweet potatoes are important crops and constitute major staples [11].

Traditional staples are known to be more resilient to domestic climate. Roots and tubers are the major contributors to food security, particularly in years of cereal crop failures. Most countries have grown more roots and tubers to combat famine, hunger, and mitigate drought impact [12]. These crops have low input requirements, which is desirable among poor farmers.

Oil crops

Oil crops are essential components of food security, because of their high energy value and the high protein value of the meals, especially the leguminous crops such as soybeans, groundnuts, beans, and peas. Countries on the coastal fringes of West Africa grow palm oil, coconut palms, cotton crops, and sunflower, which can also provide both oil and meals [12]. The processing of nuts and oil seeds that include groundnuts, sunflower seed, sesame seed, olive oil, and palm oil enables Africa to meet part of its vegetable oil requirements. These should be effectively exploited, as there is great potential.

Fruits and vegetables

Africa is endowed with a large variety of fruits and vegetables. Indigenous vegetables are plants whose fruit, leaves, pods, or roots are consumed as relish and they have originated in Africa or have been cultivated in Africa over a long period of time [13]. They include crops that are wild, semi-wild, or domesticated.

Indigenous fruits and vegetables are noted for meeting the energy and protein requirements of populations. These plants also have the vitamins that provide the necessary nutrients the populace need, especially in the region's harsh environment [14]. Traditional green leafy vegetables are rich sources of vitamin A, C, folic acid, thiamine, vitamin B2, niacin, calcium, phosphorus, iron, and zinc. They contribute significantly as sources of protein. The protein is high in lysine, an amino acid insufficient in diets based on most cereals and root crops [15].

Traditional vegetables are familiar in terms of taste, methods of cultivation, and preparation. They are cheaper to grow, as they require minimal labor and management and very little cultivation. Most, especially *Solanum nigrum* and *Amaranthus*, may be harvested severally as need arises. In addition to the afore-mentioned, traditional vegetables are much more resistant to diseases, nutrient deficiency, and water stress than the exotic vegetables [12].

The post-harvest technology and processing methods employed with these fruits and vegetables are diverse, varying from simple mechanical equipment and sun-drying techniques to highlevel technology. Fruits and vegetables are processed into products such as jams, jelly, fruit preserves sauces, juices, nectars, squashes, wines, vinegar, dried and pickled vegetables, sauces, and flour.

Milk

Traditionally, milk is churned to make butter and sour milk, which are especially popular in southern Sudan and among pastoralists all over Africa [7]. The Somali community adds the aromatic hoary basil (*Ocium americanum*) to milk as a flavoring agent. To most pastoralists, fresh blood obtained by darting the jugular vein of an animal (usually a cow) is an important food, especially in times of food shortage. Blood is normally mixed with milk and stirred vigorously into a uniform brown mixture [7].

The nomadic tribes of Sudan make a type of cheese called *kush*, which is eaten with sorghum porridge. The camel herders put milk into a bag that is fastened to the saddle of a camel, and the milk (*gariss*) is allowed to ferment.

In undocumented instances, a cheese-like product, *wagashi*, is prepared from cow milk. Preheated fresh cow milk is coagulated with juice from the leaves of *Calotropis pro-*

cera and put in a basket to drain before it is formed into round balls. *Wagashi* is then fried and is consumed in the place of meat with gravy. In addition, among some communities in Kenya, fresh or sour milk is added to African leafy vegetables to enhance taste and vitamin C bioavailability, boost protein intake, and allow long shelf-life as is the case when sour milk is added.

Meat

Traditionally, in Africa meat from cattle, sheep, goats, and pigs is used unprocessed. However, generally, meat is preserved by drying, smoking, or salting [7].

In Ethiopia and northern Kenya, among the pastoralists, meat that is cut into long pieces (*quanta*) is smeared with powdered pepper, salted, and dried by hanging it above the fireplace for 5-7 days [14]. Among the Somali, dried meat (*otkac* or *nyirnyir*) is prepared from camel meat (*hilib* gel). Strips of sun-dried meat are cut into small pieces that are fried (usually in oil with garlic and *iliki*) and immersed in camel ghee (*subag*). *Nyirnyir* can last for several months and is usually eaten with tea, honey, chapatti, and *enjera* [7]. Quails, which are wild birds that resemble small chickens, are also considered a delicacy in East Africa [7].

Insects

Despite their vast numbers, insects represent an underexploited resource in many parts of Africa. About 500 insect species are known to be consumed worldwide [16]. Insects eaten include green bugs (*Hemiptera*), termites (*Isoptera*), various caterpillars, crickets, and grasshoppers. These insects are widely used in the rural areas of the north-eastern part of southern Africa and may make an important contribution to the protein and fat of the local diet [18].

During the rainy season, the flying reproductive forms of termites emerge from termite mounds. These are trapped, dried or roasted, and eaten or preserved in honey, or used as a snack and occasionally in sauces. A variety of caterpillars are also harvested and eaten [7].

Fish

Fresh water and sea fish constitute an important source of protein in the diets of many African populations, although consumption of fish by low-income groups has not progressed significantly [10]. However, the poor in Kenya's Nyanza Province mostly eat minnows/whitebait (*omena*) because they are cheap and plentiful.

Processing methods used to prevent fish spoilage include salting, drying, smoking, pickling, fermentation, canning, and freezing. Fish is salted by rubbing dry salt into the flesh, or by immersing the fish in brine while natural air-drying of fish uses the combined action of the sun and wind, whereby fish to be dried are put on a raised platform or racks. Fish-smoking in traditional smoking kilns is a widely employed practice in Africa. In most tropical developing fisheries, however, smoking is used not only to impart desirable flavors, but also, and more more importantly, to accelerate the drying process. Smoked products in tropical countries have storage properties, which enable them to be marketed without the use of sophisticated refrigeration systems. Smoking is often combined with a period of sun-drying and/or preliminary brining. The temperature of smoking varies from place to place depending on consumer preference and the type of smoking kiln or oven available for use. Most products, however, are hot- smoked, with the smoking temperature cooking the product.

Documented practices of IK

The traditional technologies for processing perishable foods or for the pre-treatment of originally unpalatable foods such as cassava have created stable foodstuffs that are not only edible but also nutritious and enjoyable. A few of these have been documented as successes of IK:

Sun-drying of fruits, vegetables, and edible insects

In Zimbabwe, older women sun-dry food in 2 main ways. One method is to immerse fresh vegetables in salted boiling water for a few minutes and then to dry them in the sun for about 3 days. These are then stored in a safe, dry place. This method is also used to dry edible insects such as white ants, termites, and caterpillars [18].

Another method is to directly spread the food in the sun. The food is first salted if there is danger of decaying during the drying process, as is the case with mushrooms and tomatoes. Food drying is an important activity for women as they bear responsibility for food preparation, even during the dry seasons [11].

Palm wine making technique

Kongo-lori farmers from the South of Congo-Brazzaville in the Democratic Republic of Congo have maintained palm wine making techniques from the 16th century [18]. These techniques have enabled them to produce much appreciated wines. The palm wine is produced locally and sold in cities and rural areas in cans containing 10 liters. The wines are appreciated and in demand by local populations, and constitute an important market in the capital city of Brazzaville [18].

Palm produce

Extraction of kernels from the palm fruit involves crude processing, which in the case of oil extraction implies boiling or fermenting the fruit, depulping by pounding or mashing with the feet in a container, and squeezing the depulped fiber by hand to obtain the oil. The palm nuts obtained during the process are dried, usually for a month and later cracked between stones or with the aid of stones to extract the palm kernel. The fruit of the oil palm is useful not only for its oil which is used in the production of edible oil, fats, and soups, but also for its press cake which is used to supplement animal feeds [19]. Palm kernel press cake is cheaper than other feeds and contains a favorable calcium-to-phosphorus ratio and for this reason it makes a valuable contribution to protein build-up of a compound animal feed.

Salt production

The Moundang and Toupouri people, who live in the Mayo-Kebbi district in the nothern province of Cameroon, have developed a technology to make salt from dry stalks of sorghum plants [18]. The stalks are gathered and burned, and the remaining ash is sieved and boiled in water until it becomes whitish. After cooling, the liquid is left to coagulate. At that stage, it is ready for consumption as a substitute for salt. This salt, called *garlaka*, is produced by women who are said to earn up to 250.000 cfa francs per year in selling it [18].

Small-scale community vegetable and fruit gardens

Community and family vegetable and fruit gardens play a significant role in increasing small-scale production of micronutrient-rich foods. The home garden is the most direct means of supplying families with most of the nonstaple foods they need year-round [11]. Growing of vegetables as intercrops, that is, mixing vegetables among trees or staple crops, eases land constraints [11].

Solar drying techniques

In many African countries, women use solar drying techniques for fruits, vegetables, mushrooms, and tubers. Drying is also often used to preserve meat, fish, and roots. Cassava and bananas are also preserved by fermentation followed by drying, as is the case with *gari* and the preservation of *ensete*, a banana-type plant [11]. Reducing the moisture in food prevents growth of the microorganisms that cause foods to decay. At the same time, enzymatic and biochemical activities are practically stopped or reduced at very low levels. Foods preserved by drying can be kept at ambient temperatures for long periods and provide nutrients when fresh produce is not available [7].

Storage of roots, tubers, bananas, and plantains

Fresh roots and tubers are highly perishable and cannot be stored for long periods. Cassava, for example, has to be processed within 48 hours of harvesting to avoid deterioration of quality [10]. Fresh cassava, therefore, is best left unharvested until needed. As they exhibit a period of dormancy, curing extends the storage life of sweet potatoes and yams. As an alternative, yams, cocoyams, and cassava may be stored in underground pits after harvesting [7]. In some instances, root crops such as cassava can be grown as a food reserve, left in the ground for up to 2 y and used as the main source of energy during lean times [7].

In West Africa, yams are stored for 6 to 9 mo but if they begin to run low, fruits, seeds, and nuts that grow in abundance at different times of the year usually supplement them [7].

Processing of these crops is generally conducted on a small scale in the rural areas. The unit operations in regard to the processing of roots and tubers include peeling, cleaning, grating, fermentation, de-watering, heating or roasting, milling, and sieving.

Cereal and legume grains

For these crops, the drying stage is all-important to reduce attack and damage by insects and fungi. Threshing or shelling follows after which the grains are then stored in traditional grain cribs [11]. These operations reduce the fiber content and may extend the storage life of the foodstuff. In humid areas, the cribs are ventilated to facilitate both the drying and storing of grain. Some cribs are raised on a platform and a fire is lit under the structure for insect control by natural fumigation. Smoke enters through holes into the platform and escapes through the roof. Thus, the wall must have few openings, so the structure will function as a chimney. Before consumption, many grains are ground, pounded or milled, and sieved to provide various grades of flour.

Cowpeas and other grain legumes may be treated as follows: soaked in water and boiled; roasted; milled into flour; fried in oil; steamed. These processing techniques are employed to eliminate anti-nutritive factors and improve the overall value of the food. Cowpeas are eaten in the form of oily seeds, green pods, green seeds, and tender green leaves. Dry cowpeas are processed into a wide variety of dishes, ranging from soups to snacks. The utilization of cowpeas is limited to perishable traditional food products that are processed as and when needed by traditional methods. The utilization of cereals such as maize follows a variety of processing procedures including soaking, dehulling, grinding, roasting, boiling, fermentation, and germination. Cereals and legumes can be utilized in making various combinations of food mixtures and such mixtures can be used as a basis for infant and children foods, which are equally good as imported foods.

Hunting and foraging

Hunting and gathering are food procuring methods which do not involve production in the sense of investing in the environment and waiting to harvest whatever has withstood the constraints of drought and pests. Hunting communities had hunting guilds and closely monitored traditional practices of group hunting ensured that the environmental resources were well maintained. Great care was taken not to kill unnecessarily. Very young or pregnant animals were not killed and this ensured constant renewal of edible wild animals. Hunting was not performed carelessly or too frequently [11].

Fermentation

Fermentation is widely employed in Africa to preserve vegetables, meat, fish, roots, and tubers, and also to manufacture alcoholic beverages [10].

Fermentation is a traditional way of preserving vegetable surpluses which, when used, enhances the overall flavor of the meal. The technique provides a suitable environment for lactic acid bacteria to grow, thus imparting an acid flavor to the vegetable.

On the other hand, roots and tubers are mainly fermented to add variety to the diet. Cassava and sweet potatoes are the most commonly fermented ones. Two well known types of fermented cassava are *gari* and *fufu*, products of natural fermentation.

Fermentation also provides a low-cost way of preserving meat and fish, as well as adding variety to the diet. There is a wide range of fermented meat products from Sudan that include fermented strips of fatty meat, and similar products made from intestines and offal [10]. Fermented meat products, by comparison with fermented products of other food commodities, are less widely reported.

Alcoholic beverages constitute the largest category of fermented products in Africa [10]. Most of these beverages are processed from fruits. Banana beer, a popular drink in Uganda, Rwanda, Burundi, Gabon, and Cameroon, is made by allowing banana juice to ferment. Palm wine and coconut wine are made through the same process. The examples cited are few of many hundreds of foods produced by fermentation processes that are consumed all over Africa.

Qorasum

Qorasum is a woman's indigenous food preservation technology that is used for storage and preservation of food, particularly milk. It can extend the life of fresh milk in the desert for up to 24 h. Yogurt and sour milk can be preserved for up to 2 mo. *Qorasum* is also used to impart flavor and aroma to foods and it also ensures the proper maintenance of vessels of food storage. It plays a critical role in the preservation of milk, fat, and meat products, all of which are vital in pastoralist nutrition.

A dried taproot of the maderra tree (*Cordia sinensis*) is split into several pieces, 6 inches long and 1 inch thick. The ends of these faggots are placed in the fire until they ignite. They are then pulled out of the flame, and the flame blown out and are popped one by one into the open container. The lid is closed and the vessel shaken for several minutes, taking the lid off intermittently to release pressure before repeating the process again. After several rounds of shaking and releasing pressure, the pieces are poured out and placed carefully back into the fire to begin the process from fire to shaking to fire again, 3 to 5 times. When the last piece has come out of the container, a sort of rag pounded from bark and soaked in fat is used to clean the inside of the container after which it is ready to store milk. Variations of this process are repeated all day long by pastoral women all over Kenya. The Gabra call this technology *qorasum* [20].

In most parts of Africa, the bulk of the agricultural produce is processed using simple indigenous knowledge and practices. Women use these techniques predominantly and they provide income and employment. For example, cereals and legumes play an important role in the diet of the majority of the population and in issues related to their production, storage, marketing, and processing are very important. The outcome expected is to provide Africans with adequate and nutritionally balanced diets at affordable prices, both now and in the future. The cereals grown in Ghana can be used in many various foods using indigenous knowledge and technology. Some of the foods from maize include fried cakes (*akpiti*), steamed or baked dumplings (*abolo*), boiled maize porridge, cornwine (*nmeda*), or just corn on the cob. Legumes are used in various forms in Ghana, such as boiled beans, cakes (*akara*), bean stews, bambara porridge (*aboboe*), roasted or boiled groundnuts, groundnut paste, groundnut soup, and groundnut cakes. Certainly in Africa indigenous knowledge and practices cannot be overlooked.

Conclusion

The indigenous knowledge and practices outlined by this paper present an opportune basis on which food security interventions in Africa may be built as they have the potential, if exploited, to ensure food security in Africa. The challenge, however, is that systematic documentation of IK has not been done. This is largely attributed to its oral and rural nature that makes it largely invisible. Moreover, the introduction of "western food" constitutes a threat to indigenous food crops that have survived the test of time. This, therefore, calls for research and adequate citation of IK before its appreciation and incorporation in the existing interventions. As IK is dynamic and based on innovation, adaptation, and experimentation, it presents an existent possibility for improving food and livelihood security in Africa. In addition, greater recognition must be accorded IK if its potential is to be exploited.

Notes

1. http://www.ift.org/iftsa/featurearchive/africa.html
2. COASAD/UN-HABITAT. 2002. Food Security in English-Speaking African Countries. Report of the Proceedings of a Joint COASAD/UN-HABITAT Workshop on Food Security for Parliamentarians from English-Speaking African Countries, Gigiri, Nairobi, Kenya, 30 April–2 May, 2002.
3. Toward Eradicating Hunger and Poverty. Life and Work of Per Pinstrup-Andersen and Anwar Dil. 2003.
4. African Farmer Nr1 p. 5–12. 1988.
5. Grenier L. 1998. Working with indigenous knowledge: A Guide for Researchers. IDRC, Ottawa.
6. Kabuye CHS. 2002. Indigenous knowledge for biodiversity and development. Proceedings of the national workshop on indigenous knowledge, National Museums of Kenya.
7. Katz HS, Weaver WW. 2003. Encyclopedia of food culture Volume 1.
8. Okigbo BN. 1987. Overview of technical crisis in subsistence Agriculture. In: Amoako-Atta B, editor. Subsistence Agriculture in Africa: Problems and Prospects. UNESCO/ABN. p 57–92.
9. Nyiira ZM. 1987. The status of subsistence Agriculture in Africa. In: Amoako- Atta B, editor. Subsistence Agriculture in Africa: Problems and Prospects. UNESCO/ABN. p 28–56.
10. RANDFORUM/UNDP. 1995. Sourcebook on African Food Technology. Production and Processing Technologies for Commercialization.
11. FAO. 1997. Agriculture, food and nutrition for Africa. A Resource Book for Teachers of Agriculture.
12. Scott GJ, Rosegrant MW, Ringler C. Roots and Tubers for 21st Century: Trends, Projections and Policy Options. 2020 Vision for Food, Agriculture and the Environment. Discussion Paper 31.
13. Schippers RR. 2000. African Indigenous Vegetables. An Overview of the Cultivated Species Natural Resources Institute, Univ. of Greenwich.
14. UNDRO. 1988. Peasant Survival Strategies in Ethiopia. *UNDRO News* No.8 (July/August).
15. JICA-Dept. of Social Services (K). Traditional vegetables in Kenya. User's Manual.
16. Groombridge B. 1992. Global biodiversity. Status of the Earth's living resources.
17. Crafford JE. 1991. Insects as a source of food, folklore and folk taxonomy in Venda. Proceedings of the Eighth Entomological Congress.
18. http://www.worldbank.org/afr/ikdb/ik_results.cfm
19. Kuku FO, Umeh EO. 1979. The effect of five lipolytic mold species on the protein content of palm kernels. Tech Rep Nr 7. Rep Nig Stored Prod Res Inst 1976–77. p. 75–7.
20. Ramos Elorduy de Conconi J. 1996. Insect consumption as a means of national identity. In: Jain SK. Ethnobiology in Human Welfare. p 9–12.

Edited by Manfred Kroger, Ph.D., Editor of the Proceedings of the 12th World Congress of Food Science and Technology

Author **Oniang'o** is Professor of Food Science and Nutrition, Editor-in-Chief, African Journal of Food, Agriculture, Nutrition and Development (AJFAND) and Chair, Kenya Union of Food Science and Technology (KUFoST). Author **Allotey** is Associate Professor, Post Harvest Food Systems, Univ. of Botswana, Private Bag 0022, Gaborone, Botswana. Author **Malaba** is Student Intern, African Institute of Knowledge Management. Authors **Oniang'o and Malaba** are with the Rural Outreach Program: Josem Trust Place, Ground Floor, Bunyala Road, Upper Hill, P.O. Box 29 Nairobi, KENYA. Direct inquiries to author Oniang'o (E-mail: oniango@iconnect.co.ke).

Taking Steps Toward Adequate Supermarket Access

Philadelphia is tackling a problem that plagues low-income areas of many cities throughout the United States: inadequate access to affordable and nutritious food.

Mary Anne Clairmont, RD

Food insecurity threatens the health of millions of American families every year. Americans with low incomes are most vulnerable to unreliable food sources.

Inadequate access to supermarkets elevates the rate of diet-linked disease, which threatens both adults and children, among people who live in poor communities and creates a food crisis. This crisis must be confronted and dealt with by providing a secure and stable food source in neglected neighborhoods.

Supermarkets are the answer to this crisis. However, they have all but disappeared from many urban areas and it is no simple matter to bring them back to inner cities. No group knows this better than the Philadelphia Food Trust.

SUPERMARKET CAMPAIGN OF PHILADELPHIA'S FOOD TRUST

"Food retailers have redlined low-income neighborhoods," says Hannah Burton, the program coordinator for the Supermarket Campaign of Philadelphia's Food Trust. Founded in 1992, the trust's mission is to ensure that everyone in the city has access to affordable, nutritious food. The trust directs programs on several fronts, including the Supermarket Campaign, to accomplish its mission.

Burton joined The Food Trust as program coordinator for the Supermarket Initiative in 2002 during the birth of the Supermarket Campaign. " 'Food for Every Child' was intentionally created and chosen as a tagline to motivate public officials to action," she says. "But the risks to the health and nutrition of children and the needs of the children in Philadelphia are very real." A report that was researched and written by staff of The Food Trust shows that the shortage of supermarkets is definitely a big issue impacting the health of Philadelphians, especially poor children.[1]

According to Burton, Philadelphia's poverty status is not much different from most other major cities across the country, but it has the second-lowest number of supermarkets per capita of all the major cities in the nation. (See "Supermarket Scarcity in Major Cities" for facts about other cities.) "There are large areas of Philadelphia with only a few supermarkets and many neighborhoods where there are no supermarkets at all," Burton says. "People who live in large areas all over the city have to shop in small corner stores where the prices are high and the selection of food is limited. These are the people who can least afford to pay high prices—residents with the lowest incomes who can't afford to travel to supermarkets where prices are better. This uneven distribution of food in Philadelphia has a tremendous negative effect on large numbers of low-income people."

Burton believes the public sector has a responsibility to provide a safe and stable food supply in underserved communities, and that's why The Food Trust is calling "upon the city and state governments to take the lead in developing a public-private response to this problem."

FOOD MARKETING TASK FORCE

In April 2002, the Philadelphia City Council Committee on Public Health and Human Services held a hearing on the issue of access to proper nutrition for low-income children and families. The hearing was held in response to the public health epidemic of poor access to nutritious foods resulting in malnutrition and diet-related disease in Philadelphia. The hearing was the first step in an effort to increase public awareness, initiate dialogue about solutions, and create change. As a response to the call to action begun by this hearing, the Food Marketing Task Force was created in April 2003 to further the goals of the Supermarket Campaign. The Food Marketing Task Force is chaired by Christine James-Brown, president and CEO of the United Way of Southeastern Pennsylvania, and

Walter Rubel, director, government and community affairs of Acme Markets.

Philadelphia's poverty status
is not much different from most
other major cities across the country,
but it has the second-lowest number of
supermarkets per capita of all
the major cities in the nation.

The Food Marketing Task Force examines the barriers and opportunities to increasing the availability of food in Philadelphia's neighborhoods and reports back to City Council and the mayor's office. The task force was formed to produce a report recommending both short- and long-term policies to improve the availability of affordable and nutritious food in those areas of the city that are underserved.

The task force staff has held meetings with supermarket industry representatives to discuss barriers and opportunities for inner-city supermarkets. They have also met with the Wharton Real Estate department to discuss supermarket requirements and considerations for inner-city sites and to learn about the acquisition and development process.[2]

WHY DID SUPERMARKETS LEAVE CITIES?

Philadelphians are not alone in their struggle to find a decent, affordable place to shop. Millions of Americans experience hunger. When the degree of nutrition required for good health is not met, hunger prevails. Access to an affordable, nutritious food supply is a basic right of every human being. This right is threatened by the national trend of supermarket redlining.

This trend began during the 1960s, as major supermarket chains pulled up stakes in inner cities and set up full amenity, 24-hour mega stores in the suburbs. As inner-city stores closed, urban residents found themselves either traveling farther to purchase wholesome, reasonably priced groceries or paying extravagant prices for inferior processed foods at corner stores. Supermarket closures usually occur in low-income, inner-city neighborhoods. This means that those who can least afford it are forced to pay more for their groceries and travel farther to get them.[3]

Redlining usually calls to mind visions of insurance companies, realtors, and banks refusing to grant reasonable insurance policies, mortgages, and loans to inhabitants of specific communities. Now these visions include the crumbling shells of urban supermarkets. The supermarket business has drawn borders signifying where wholesome, nutritious, economical food is and has not provided for communities throughout the country.[3]

The result of supermarket redlining is that low-income shoppers are cut off from easy access to nutritious, affordable food. As food becomes more inaccessible, the number of those suffering from hunger increases throughout the country.[3]

BRINGING THEM BACK

The Food Marketing Task Force and the Supermarket Campaign have been crucial to paving the way for negotiations with a medium-sized chain that's interested in establishing stores in Philadelphia. "There are dollars to be made by the supermarket, but they need the right conditions to operate their business," says Burton. "We understand they have to make a profit. We are not asking them to give us anything. We are offering the supermarkets an opportunity to partner with us and serve underserved communities, making a profit in the process."

The task force recognizes that there are unique marketing challenges in a city compared to a suburb, where populations tend to be more homogenous. "The urban population is more diverse with more ethnic groups and different preferences," Burton says. "You may have Hispanic, Asian, and African American customers with strong preferences all shopping at your store."

The costs involved in building and operating a store in a city can also be a challenge. "The public sector can help by offering tax incentives, expediting zoning permits, and putting together attractive incentive packages that make owners want to do business here," Burton suggests. "Changing public transportation routes is another strategy to assure supermarket owners that customers will have easy access to their store."

Another option is to meet them halfway—literally. Instead of bringing supermarkets all the way into communities, people can be transported to the closest supermarkets. This can be accomplished with shuttles, adjusted public transportation schedules, or ride share programs. The public sector, private sector, or a creative mix that is the most beneficial to all parties concerned can fund these strategies. This will meet the goal of "ensuring that everyone has access to affordable, nutritious food," albeit through a different route.

SETTING AN EXAMPLE

The successful efforts of the Food Marketing Task Force and the Supermarket Campaign have been discovered by other communities throughout Pennsylvania and have served as a model solution for their own food security problems.

Norristown is a community of 31,282 citizens and the county seat for Montgomery County, which borders the city of Philadelphia. At one time, Norristown housed a thriving downtown business district, three movie theaters, three general hospitals, and one of the largest government psychiatric hospitals in the country. A large shopping mall

Supermarket Scarcity in Major Cities[4]

- Boston has the least number of supermarkets per person; since 1970, 34 of the 50 supermarkets in Boston have closed.
- In Los Angeles, where 1,068 stores once existed, by 1990, only 694 stood.
- In Chicago, more than 1,000 supermarkets could be found in 1970 and now less than 500 remain.
- In the Tenderloin section of San Francisco, no supermarkets exist.
- In San Francisco's Bay View Hunter's Point, there is only one discount supermarket.

in a neighboring town and ever-increasing suburban sprawl eventually led to the decline of the town.

"It's been seven years since we had a supermarket in Norristown," says Rochelle Griffin-Culbreath, Norristown borough councilwoman. "So many of our residents have to walk to the store to buy food, [but] they can only get to convenience stores and 'dollar stores' that sell high-sodium convenience foods. A large percentage of our population is elderly with high rates of heart disease, high blood pressure, and diabetes, so these stores are selling food that is plaguing our community."

Griffin-Culbreath hopes to attract Supremo, a chain of grocery stores serving the Hispanic population that recently opened a store in North Philadelphia. She looks at the Supermarket Campaign of Philadelphia's Food Trust process as a model for Norristown to follow. "You have to consider the business issues, the costs of doing business for the supermarkets, and make it worth their while," she says. "They are not going to build a store unless they will make money, so you have to learn about their parking needs, tax incentives, and suitable sites," she says.

Griffin-Culbreath explains that she began looking into the town's supermarket crisis because "residents were asking, 'Why don't we have any supermarkets?'" She has sent out requests for proposal that contain attractive packages to potential supermarket chains to entice them to build in Norristown.

Burton confirms that in addition to Norristown, there are supermarket initiatives in Allentown, Pa., and Erie, Pa. Rep Frank Oliver of the Pennsylvania House prepared a report that cited a link between diet-related diseases and a lack of grocery stores in low-income neighborhoods. The report called on state government and municipalities to find ways to attract full-service grocery stores into low-income urban neighborhoods. It recommended the State Department of Community and Economic Development and local governments create economic incentives to bring supermarkets back into urban neighborhoods and eliminate the existing tax and regulatory barriers.

The Pennsylvania Supermarket Access Campaign has been created by The Food Trust, Pittsburgh's Just Harvest, and Harrisburg's Pennsylvania Hunger Action Center to bring together government leaders, health professionals, food retailers, business experts, and community activists to address the problem. The campaign's objectives include involving "leaders from local and state government in meeting communities' needs for fresh, affordable food at a reasonable price"; and analyzing and understanding "the relationship between supermarket access, income, and diet-related disease in rural and urban areas of Pennsylvania."

"I know of no other state that has identified a role for state government," Burton says. "It's groundbreaking and exciting."

—*Mary Anne Clairmont, RD, is the nutritionist at Fairmount Behavioral Health System and owner of Take Two Nutrition, a nutrition consulting company in Plymouth Meeting, Pa.*–

Helping Solve Hunger in America

ROBERT FORNEY

June 5, 2003, is National Hunger Awareness Day, designed to help raise awareness that hunger exists in America.

Americans know that there is hunger in underdeveloped and war-torn countries around the globe, but they may not realize that there is hunger in the United States as well. In a focus group conducted in 2001 by the Advertising Council, the nation's leading producer of public-service advertisements, one participant said, "If there were hungry children in America, we'd know about it. The press would report on it, and we would feed those children and solve the problem."

Besides arranging for food donations, food industry professionals can help solve hunger in a number of ways.

The fact is that there is hunger in America. Last year, the U.S. Dept. of Agriculture reported that 33 million Americans were food insecure—they didn't know if they would be able to buy the food they needed to feed their families. The Census Bureau announced last fall that, for the first time in a decade, the number of people living in poverty had grown and real earnings had dropped for the average American worker. America's Second Harvest, the nation's largest hunger-relief charity, reported in its landmark study, *Hunger in America: 2001,* that it feeds 23 million hungry Americans, 9 million of whom are children.

Amid the stress of the war and terrorism, American families are facing a more personal sort of stress. More than two million jobs have been lost in the past two years. Discouraged workers have exhausted their savings and emptied their retirement accounts. They have been forced to ask family and friends for aid. And when all other resources are gone, they turn to hunger-relief charities to feed their families. These new demands at food pantries, soup kitchens, and shelters have strained the hunger-relief system.

America's Second Harvest, a national umbrella organization dedicated to creating a hunger-free America, supports a network of more than 200 regional food banks and food-rescue organizations that collect, sort, warehouse, and then distribute the food and personal-care products that are donated by companies across the country. More than 50,000 hunger relief charities in the U.S. depend on organizations affiliated with America's Second Harvest for the food they give directly to hungry Americans. These include national organizations such as Catholic Charities, the Red Cross, Meals on Wheels, and the Salvation Army, as well as community and faith based organizations created to help people on a local level.

America's Second Harvest makes it easy for food manufacturers, producers, retailers, and restaurants to donate food they cannot sell. Sometimes, food ends up in packages that are mislabeled, dented, or underfilled; or products are the wrong shape, size, or color; or there may just be more on hand than can be sold before its shelf life expires; or excess product may be left over from events. Companies willing to donate such products can call 800-771-2303, and America's Second Harvest will make arrangements to accept delivery of the donation, make arrangements for shipping to a regional affiliate that can distribute the food, and provide receipts acknowledging the donation.

Last year, America's Second Harvest network distributed 1.8 billion lb of food—including 17,820 lb of product donated by the exhibitors at the close of the Institute of Food Technologists' 2002 Annual Meeting & Food Expo® last June. Every day, America's Second Harvest works with industry professionals to capture potential waste and distribute it through its network of hunger-relief agencies that serve every county in America.

Besides arranging for food donations, food industry professionals can help solve hunger in a number of ways. They can make sure that meetings are held at facilities that participate in "food rescue" programs so that leftovers are distributed to hunger-relief organizations; volunteer at a soup kitchen; teach parents how to prepare healthy meals; add a panel about how food industry people can help end hunger at professional conferences; or invite a local, regional, or national hunger-relief professional to be a guest speaker at meetings.

Food industry professionals can also share their expertise with America's Second Harvest by volunteering to serve on Corporate Inspection Teams that visit regional food banks and share their knowledge of logistics, marketing, storage, and other food-specific business matters. They can also volunteer to participate in two national programs that particularly depend on the support of foodservice professionals. The first program, Community Kitchen, is a technical training course that provides unemployed people with foodservice skills. These programs rely to a great extent on professionals who are willing to volunteer to share their knowledge with students. The second program is called Kids Cafe. There are more than 600 of these after-school feeding programs at America's Second Harvest affiliates across the country. They, too, seek professional volunteers to help plan new kitchens at local Kids Cafes, provide menu or foodservice assistance, and teach participating children about nutrition and food preparation.

More information about these and other ways to help solve hunger in America can be obtained by contacting America's Second Harvest at 312-263-2303 or visiting www.secondharvest.org.

Robert Forney is President and CEO, America's Second Harvest, 35 E. Wacker Dr., Suite 2000, Chicago, IL 60601.

Assessment of Allergenic Potential of Genetically Modified Foods: An Agenda for Future Research

Speakers and participants in the workshop "Assessment of the Allergenic Potential of Genetically Modified Foods" met in breakout groups to discuss a number of issues including needs for future research. These groups agreed that research should progress quickly in the area of hazard identification and that a need exists for more basic research to understand the mechanisms underlying food allergy. A list of research needs was developed. *Key words:* biotechnology, food allergy, genetically modified food, hazard identification, research needs. *Environ Health Perspect* 111: 1140–1141 (2003). doi:10.1289/ehp.5815 available via *http:/dx.doi.org/*[Online 19 December 2002].

MaryJane K. Selgrade,[1] Ian Kimber,[2] Lynn Goldman,[3] and Dori R. Germolec[4]

Potential benefits that may be derived from biotechnologies involving genetically modified organisms could be enormous. Potential risks of allergenicity possibly associated with their use will likely be manageable, provided appropriate information is available to decision makers. At the end of the workshop "Assessment of the Allergenic Potential of Genetically Modified Foods," speakers and participants met in small groups to discuss information needs. Five groups considered the following key issues: *a*) use of human clinical data, *b*) animal models to assess food allergy, *c*) biomarkers of exposure and effect, *d*) sensitive populations, *e*) dose-response assessment, and *f*) postmarket surveillance. The groups were asked to consider two general questions: On the basis of current information, what can we do to assess the potential allergenicity of genetically modified food, and what do we need to know to improve this process, i.e., what are the most critical research needs? The first question is the topic discussed in another article in this mini-monograph (Germolec et al. 2003). The research needs are the topic of this article. Just as research provided the tools to generate genetically modified food, it can also provide the tools needed for effective safety evaluation and risk assessment/management.

Regulatory problems are rarely stated in scientific terms. The problem in this case is we wish to avoid inadvertently introducing an allergenic protein into the food supply. One task for this workshop was to translate this problem into research needs. Because there is a sense of urgency to develop tools for hazard identification, much of the conversation revolved around the short-term research required to develop test methods for this purpose. This discussion focused largely on the potential allergens and how to distinguish these from other proteins. However, it was recognized also that more long-term (basic) research is needed on the characteristics of food allergens, allergic disease, and the mechanisms underlying susceptibility to food allergy. This discussion considered more broadly the factors leading to allergic sensitization, including the nature of the allergen, and how genetics, life stage, and other environmental influences might affect susceptibility.

Hazard Identification: Immediate Needs

Research needed to improve hazard identification fell into three categories:

development of animal models, identification and characterization of food allergens, and establishment of well-defined clinical serum banks. All were deemed important to improve the Food and Agriculture Organization of the United Nations/World Health Organization (FAO/WHO) decision tree (FAO/WHO 2001) or to replace it with a better approach. Also discussed was the need to improve human skin test technology for incorporation in a decision tree. Animal models are needed that could be used not only for hazard identification purposes but also to determine relative potency, to derive sensitization and elicitation thresholds, and to define the conditions under which tolerance (failure to develop an allergic response to potential food allergens) is induced. Identification, characterization, purification, and banking of food allergens (and nonallergens) are needed for two reasons: to provide positive (and negative) controls for animal and serum bank tests and for use in defining the characteristics that confer on food proteins the ability to induce allergic sensitization, that is, to establish structure-activity relationships. Serum from clinically well-defined allergic individuals needs to be banked for use in

Table 1. Summary of research needs.

Hazard identification
    Development, evaluation, and validation of animal models
    Establishment of clinically well-defined banks of human serum containing antibodies to allergens
    Improved human skin test technology
    Identification, purification, and banking of both known protein allergens and proteins believed not to be allergenic
    A systemic approach to recording adverse events (case studies)
    Definition of relative potency and thresholds for sensitization and the elicitation of allergic reactions
    Development, refinement, standardization, and validation of test protocols
Basic mechanistic
    Development of animal models of allergic disease
    Studies of the qualitative and quantitative relationships between antigen-specific IgE and overt disease
    Investigation of the influence of route, duration, timing, and nature of exposure on the development of sensitization
    Studies of the factors that contribute to susceptibility to food allergy
    Investigation of the mechanisms underlying food allergy
    Investigation of potential windows of vulnerability during development
    Identification of unique situations that cause children or other individuals to be at greater risk
    Epidemiology to establish the incidence of food allergy and whether it is changing
    Studies of the potential role of non–IgE-mediated reactions in food allergy

screening proteins of unknown allergenicity. Development of proteomic approaches to screen potential allergens (specific IgE on a chip) was also suggested as a research need. Characterization of allergens and development of serum banks require a systematic process for recording adverse events and obtaining informed consent for use of serum obtained in epidemiologic and experimental studies. Once developed, all tests for hazard identification will require standardization and validation—no small task. These research needs are summarized in Table 1.

Basic Mechanistic Research

Appropriate animal models (not necessarily the same as those used for hazard identification) and human clinical and epidemiologic studies are needed to assess the correlation between antigen-specific IgE and clinical disease and to investigate the influence of the route, duration, and nature of exposure on the development of sensitization. An important research need is to investigate the mechanisms underlying food allergy, including the development of and failure to develop oral tolerance, and identification of possible windows of vulnerability during immune development (including *in utero* and during lactation) or unique exposure conditions that might place children at greater risk. The mechanisms underly-

ing the development of tolerance to ingested antigens, whether by passive (anergy) or active (suppressor cells) processes, are poorly understood and may be crucial to understanding what makes a protein allergenic and what makes an individual susceptible. The contributions of *in utero* exposure, gut immaturity, and exposure via breast milk to children's risk of sensitization also need to be determined. Studies (possibly using tansgenic mice) are needed to assess the heritable factors that contribute to susceptibility to food allergy. Epidemiology is needed to determine whether the incidence of food allergy in the industrialized world, like the incidence of other types of allergic disease, is increasing.

The natural history of non–IgE-mediated food allergies (although somewhat beyond the scope of this current workshop) was also considered an important long-term research need. Questions were raised as to whether certain foods were associated with this type of allergy and whether IgE is a reasonable surrogate marker in this instance or if other biomarkers would be more appropriate. The context in which food is presented, including the matrix, concomitant infections, and other sources of gut inflammation, also deserves further attention with respect to both IgE- and non–IgE-mediated food allergies. Basic mechanistic research needs are summarized in Table 1.

Recommendations

In summary, there was consensus that research should progress quickly in the area of hazard identification to improve or replace the FAO/WHO decision tree. Support was particularly strong for the development, standardization, and validation of appropriate animal model(s) for this purpose. It was also generally agreed that there is much we do not know about the development of food allergies, and that more basic research in this area would help us to control the risks more effectively and efficiently. More work is needed than any one funding organization is likely to be able to support. Therefore, it is recommended that there be significant coordination between these organizations and an integrated approach to tackling this problem. Open and free exchange of information as it becomes available is needed to facilitate these research endeavors

[1]National Health and Environmental Effects Research Laboratory, Office of Research and Development, U.S. Environmental Protection Agency, Research Triangle Park, North Carolina, USA; [2]Syngenta Central Toxicology Laboratory, Alderley Park, Macclesfield, Cheshire, United Kingdom; [3]Johns Hopkins University Bloomberg School of Public Health, Baltimore, Maryland, USA; [4]Laboratory of Molecular Toxicology, National Institute of Environmental Health Sciences, Research Triangle Park, North Carolina, USA

References

FAO/WHO. 2001. Evaluation of Allergenicity of Genetically Modified Foods. Report of a Joint FAO/WHO Expert Consultation of Allergenicity of Foods Derived from Biotechnology, 22–25 January 2001, Rome, Italy. Available: http://www.fao.org/es/esn/gm/allergygm.pdf [accessed 11 September 2002)

Germolec DR, Kimber J, Goldman L, Selgrade MJK. 2003. Key issues for the assessment of the allergenic potential of genetically modified foods: breakout group reports. Environ Health Perspect 111: 1131–1139.

From *Environmental Health Perspectives*, Vol. 111, No. 8, June 2003, pp. 1140–1141. Printed by the National Institute of Environmental Health Sciences.

Glossary

Absorption   The process by which digestive products pass from the gastrointestinal tract into the blood.

Acid/base balance   The relationship between acidity and alkalinity in the body fluids.

Amino acids   The structural units that make up proteins.

Amylase   An enzyme that breaks down starches; a component of saliva.

Amylopectin   A component of starch, consisting of many glucose units joined in branching patterns.

Amylose   A component of starch, consisting of many glucose units joined in a straight chain, without branching.

Anabolism   The synthesis of new materials for cellular growth, maintenance, or repair in the body.

Anemia   A deficiency of oxygen-carrying material in the blood.

Anorexia nervosa   A disorder in which a person refuses food and loses weight to the point of emaciation and even death.

Antioxidant   A substance that prevents or delays the breakdown of other substances by oxygen; often added to food to retard deterioration and rancidity.

Arachidonic acid   An essential polyunsaturated fatty acid.

Arteriosclerosis   Condition characterized by a thickening and hardening of the walls of the arteries and a resultant loss of elasticity.

Ascorbic acid   Vitamin C.

Atherosclerosis   A type of arteriosclerosis in which lipids, especially cholesterol, accumulate in the arteries and obstruct blood flow.

Avidin   A substance in raw egg white that acts as an antagonist of biotin, one of the B vitamins.

Basal metabolic rate (BMR)   The rate at which the body uses energy for maintaining involuntary functions such as cellular activity, respiration, and heartbeat when at rest.

Basic four   The food plan outlining the milk, meat, fruits and vegetables, and breads and cereals needed in the daily diet to provide the necessary nutrients.

Beriberi   A disease resulting from inadequate thiamin in the diet.

Beta-carotene   Yellow pigment that is converted to vitamin A in the body.

Biotin   One of the B vitamins.

Bomb calorimeter   An instrument that oxidizes food samples to measure their energy content.

Buffer   A substance that can neutralize both acids and bases to minimize change in the pH of a solution.

Calorie   The energy required to raise the temperature of one gram of water one degree Celsius.

Carbohydrate   An organic compound composed of carbon, hydrogen, and oxygen in a ratio of 1:2:1.

Carcinogen   A cancer-causing substance.

Catabolism   The breakdown of complex substances into simpler ones.

Celiac disease   A syndrome resulting from intestinal sensitivity to gluten, a protein substance of wheat flour especially and of other grains.

Cellulose   An indigestible polysaccharide made of many glucose molecules.

Cheilosis   Cracks at the corners of the mouth, due primarily to a deficiency of riboflavin in the diet.

Cholesterol   A fat-like substance found only in animal products; important in many body functions but also implicated in heart disease.

Choline   A substance that prevents the development of a fatty liver; frequently considered one of the B-complex vitamins.

Chylomicron   A very small emulsified lipoprotein that transports fat in the blood.

Cobalamin   One of the B vitamins (B_{12}).

Coenzyme   A component of an enzyme system that facilitates the working of the enzyme.

Collagen   Principal protein of connective tissue.

Colostrum   The yellowish fluid that precedes breast milk, produced in the first few days of lactation.

Cretinism   The physical and mental retardation of a child resulting from severe iodine or thyroid deficiency in the mother during pregnancy.

Dehydration   Excessive loss of water from the body.

Dextrin   Any of various small soluble polysaccharides found in the leaves of starch-forming plants and in the human alimentary canal as a product of starch digestion.

Diabetes (diabetes mellitus)   A metabolic disorder characterized by excess blood sugar and urine sugar.

Digestion   The breakdown of ingested foods into particles of a size and chemical composition that can be absorbed by the body.

Diglyceride   A lipid containing glycerol and two fatty acids.

Disaccharide   A sugar made up of two chemically combined monosaccharides, or simple sugars.

Diuretics   Substances that stimulate urination.

Diverticulosis   A condition in which the wall of the large intestine weakens and balloons out, forming pouches where fecal matter can be entrapped.

Edema   The presence of an abnormally high amount of fluid in the tissues.

Emulsifier   A substance that promotes the mixing of foods, such as oil and water in a salad dressing.

Enrichment   The addition of nutrients to foods, often to restore what has been lost in processing.

Enzyme   A protein that speeds up chemical reactions in the cell.

Epidemiology   The study of the factors that contribute to the occurrence of a disease in a population.

Essential amino acid   Any of the nine amino acids that the human body cannot manufacture and that must be supplied by the diet, as they are necessary for growth and maintenance.

Essential fatty acid   A fatty acid that the human body cannot manufacture and that must be supplied by the diet, as it is necessary for growth and maintenance.

Fat   An organic compound whose molecules contain glycerol and fatty acids; fat insulates the body, protects organs, carries fat-soluble vitamins, is a constituent of cell membranes, and makes food taste good.

Fatty acid   A simple lipid—containing only carbon, hydrogen, and oxygen—that is a constituent of fat.

Ferritin   A substance in which iron, in combination with protein, is stored in the liver, spleen, and bone marrow.

Fiber   Indigestible carbohydrate found primarily in plant foods; high fiber intake is useful in regulating bowel movements, and may lower the incidence of certain types of cancer and other diseases.

Flavoprotein   Protein containing riboflavin.

Folic acid (folacin)   One of the B vitamins.

Fortification   The addition of nutrients to foods to enhance their nutritional values.

Fructose   A six-carbon monosaccharide found in many fruits as well as honey and plant saps; one of two monosaccharides forming sucrose, or table sugar.

Galactose   A six-carbon monosaccharide, one of the two that make up lactose, or milk sugar.

Gallstones   An abnormal formation of gravel or stones, composed of cholesterol and bile salts and sometimes bile pigments, in the gall-

213

Glossary

bladder; they result when substances that normally dissolve in bile precipitate out.

Gastritis Inflammation of the stomach.

Glucagon A hormone produced by the pancreas that works to increase blood glucose concentration.

Glucose A six-carbon monosaccharide found in sucrose, honey, and many fruits and vegetables; the major carbohydrate found in the body.

Glucose tolerance factor (GTF) A hormone-like substance containing chromium, niacin, and protein that helps the body to use glucose.

Glyceride A simple lipid composed of fatty acids and glycerol.

Glycogen The storage form of carbohydrates in the body; composed of glucose molecules.

Goiter Enlargement of the thyroid gland as a result of iodine deficiency.

Goitrogens Substances that induce goiter, often by interfering with the body's utilization of iodine.

Heme A complex iron–containing compound that is a component of hemoglobin.

Hemicellulose Any of various indigestible plant polysaccharides.

Hemochromatosis A disorder of iron metabolism.

Hemoglobin The iron-containing protein in red blood cells that carries oxygen to the tissues.

High-density lipoprotein (HDL) A lipoprotein that acts as a cholesterol carrier in the blood; referred to as "good" cholesterol because relatively high levels of it appear to protect against atherosclerosis.

Hormones Compounds secreted by the endocrine glands that influence the functioning of various organs.

Humectants Substances added to foods to help them maintain moistness.

Hydrogenation The chemical process by which hydrogen is added to unsaturated fatty acids, which saturates them and converts them from a liquid to a solid form.

Hydrolyze To split a chemical compound into smaller molecules by adding water.

Hydroxyapatite The hard mineral portion (the major constituent) of bone, composed of calcium and phosphate.

Hypercalcemia A high level of calcium in the blood.

Hyperglycemia A high level of "sugar" (glucose) in the blood.

Hypocalcemia A low level of calcium in the blood.

Hypoglycemia A low level of "sugar" (glucose) in the blood.

Incomplete protein A protein lacking or deficient in one or more of the essential amino acids.

Inorganic Describes a substance not containing carbon.

Insensible loss Fluid loss, through the skin and from the lungs, that an individual is unaware of.

Insulin A hormone produced by the pancreas that regulates the body's use of glucose.

Intrinsic factor A protein produced by the stomach that makes absorption of B_{12} possible; lack of this protein results in pernicious anemia.

Joule A unit of energypreferred bysome professionals instead of the heat energy measurements of the calorie system for calculating food energy; sometimes referred to as "kilojoule."

Keratinization Formation of a protein called keratin, which, in vitamin A deficiency, occurs instead of mucus formation; leads to a drying and hardening of epithelial tissue.

Ketogenic Describes substances that can be converted to ketone bodies during metabolism, such as fatty acids and some amino acids.

Ketone bodies The three chemicals—acetone, acetoacetic acid, and betahydroxybutyrie—that are normally involved in lipid metabolism and accumulate in blood and urine in abnormal amounts in conditions of impaired metabolism (such as diabetes).

Ketosis A condition resulting when fats are the major source of energy and are incompletely oxidized, causing ketone bodies to build up in the bloodstream.

Kilocalorie One thousand calories, or the energy required to raise the temperature of one kilogram of water one degree Celsius; the preferred unit of measurement for food energy.

Kilojoule *See* Joule.

Kwashiorkor A form of malnutrition resulting from a diet severely deficient in protein but high in carbohydrates.

Lactase A digestive enzyme produced by the small intestine that breaks down lactose.

Lactation Milk production/secretion.

Lacto-ovo-vegetarian A person who does not eat meat, poultry, or fish but does eat milk products and eggs.

Lactose A disaccharide composed of glucose and galactose and found in milk.

Lactose intolerance The inability to digest lactose due to a lack of the enzyme lactase in the intestine.

Lacto-vegetarian A person who does not eat meat, poultry, fish, or eggs but does drink milk and eat milk products.

Laxatives Food or drugs that stimulate bowel movements. Lignins Certain forms of indigestible carbohydrate in plant foods.

Linoleic acid An essential polyunsaturated fatty acid.Lipase An enzyme that digests fats.

Lipid Any of various substances in the body or in food that are insoluble in water; a fat or fat-like substance.

Lipoprotein Compound composed of a lipid (fat) and a protein that transports both in the bloodstream.

Low-density lipoprotein (LDL) A lipoprotein that acts as a cholesterol carrier in the blood; referred to as "bad" cholesterol be-cause relatively high levels of it appear to enhance atherosclerosis.

Macrocytic anemia A form of anemia characterized by the presence of abnormally large blood cells.

Macroelements (also macronutrient elements) Those elements present in the body in amounts exceeding 0.005 percent of body weight and required in the diet in amounts exceeding 100 mg/day; include sodium, potassium, calcium, and phosphorus.

Malnutrition A poor state of health resulting from a lack, excess, or imbalance of the nutrients needed by the body.

Maltose A disaccharide whose units are each composed of two glucose molecules, produced by the digestion of starch.

Marasmus Condition resulting from a deficiency of calories and nearly all essential nutrients.

Melanin A dark pigment in the skin, hair, and eyes.

Metabolism The sum of all chemical reactions that take place within the body.

Microelements (also micronutrient elements; trace elements) Those elements present in the body in amounts under 0.005 percent of body weight and required in the diet in amounts under 100 mg/day.

Monoglyceride A lipid containing glycerol and only one fatty acid.

Monosaccharide A single sugar molecule, the simplest form of carbohydrate; examples are glucose, fructose, and galactose.

Monosodium glutamate (MSG) An amino acid used in flavoring foods, which causes allergic reactions in some people.

Monounsaturated fatty acid A fatty acid containing one double bond.

Mutagen A mutation-causing agent.

Negative nitrogen balance Nitrogen output exceeds nitrogen intake.

Niacin (nicotinic acid) One of the B vitamins.

Nitrogen equilibrium (zero nitrogen balance) Nitrogen output equals nitrogen intake.

Nonessential amino acid Any of the 13 amino acids that body can manufacture in adequate amounts, but which are nonetheless required in the diet in an amount relative to the amount of essential amino acids.

Nutrients Nourishing substances in food that can be digested, absorbed, and metabolized by the body; needed for growth, maintenance, and reproduction.

Nutrition (1) The sum of the processes by which an organism obtains, assimilates, and utilizes food. (2) The scientific study of these processes.

Obesity Condition of being 30 percent above one's ideal body weight.

Oleic acid A monounsaturated fatty acid.

214

Organic foods   Those foods, especially fruits and vegetables, grown without the use of pesticides, synthetic fertilizers, etc.

Osmosis   Passage of a solvent through a semipermeable membrane from an area of higher concentration to an area of lower concentration until the concentration is equal on both sides of the membrane.

Osteomalacia   Condition in which a loss of bone mineral leads to a softening of the bones; adult counterpart of rickets.

Osteoporosis   Disorder in which the bones degenerate due to a loss of bone mineral, producing porosity and fragility; normally found in older women.

Overweight   Body weight exceeding an accepted norm by 10 or 15 percent.

Ovo-vegetarian   A person who does not eat meat, poultry, fish, milk, or milk products but does eat eggs.

Oxidation   The process by which a substrate takes up oxygen or loses hydrogen; the loss of electrons.

Palmitic acid   A saturated fatty acid.

Pantothenic acid   One of the B vitamins.

Pellagra   Niacin deficiency syndrome, characterized by dementia, diarrhea, and dermatitis.

Pepsin   A protein-digesting enzyme produced by the stomach.

Peptic ulcer   An open sore or erosion in the lining of the digestive tract, especially in the stomach and duodenum.

Peptide   A compound composed of amino acids that are joined together.

Peristalsis   Motions of the digestive tract that propel food through the tract.

Pernicious anemia   One form of anemia caused by an inability to absorb vitamin B12, owing to the absence of intrinsic factor.

pH   A measure of the acidity of a solution, based on a scale from 0 to 14: a pH of 7 is neutral; greater than 7 is alkaline; less than 7 is acidic.

Phenylketonuria (PKU)   A genetic disease in which phenylalanine, an essential amino acid, is not properly metabolized, thus accumulating in the blood and causing early brain damage.

Phospholipid   A fat containing phosphorus, glycerol, two fatty acids, and any of several other chemical substances.

Polypeptide   A molecular chain of amino acids.

Polysaccharide   A carbohydrate containing many monosaccharide subunits.

Polyunsaturated fatty acids   A fatty acid in which two or more carbon atoms have formed double bonds, with each holding only one hydrogen atom.

Positive nitrogen balance   Condition in which nitrogen intake exceeds nitrogen output in the body.

Protein   Any of the organic compounds composed of amino acids and containing nitrogen; found in the cells of all living organisms.

Provitamins   Precursors of vitamins that can be converted to vitamins in the body (e.g., beta-carotene, from which the body can make the vitamin A).

Pyridoxine   One of the B vitamins (B_6).

Pull date   Date after which food should no longer be sold but still may be edible for several days.

Recommended Daily Allowances (RDAs)   Standards for daily intake of specific nutrients established by the Food and Nutrition Board of the National Academy of Sciences; they are the levels thought to be adequate to maintain the good health of most people.

Rhodopsin   The visual pigment in the retinal rods of the eyes which allows one to see at night; its formation requires vitamin A.

Riboflavin   One of the B vitamins (B_2).

Ribosome   The cellular structure in which protein synthesis occurs.

Rickets   The vitamin D deficiency disease in children characterized by bone softening and deformities.

Saliva   Fluid produced in the mouth that helps food digestion.

Salmonella   A bacterium that can cause food poisoning.

Saturated fatty acid   A fatty acid in which carbon is joined with four other atoms; i.e., all carbon atoms are bound to the maximum possible number of hydrogen atoms.

Scurvy   A disease characterized by bleeding gums, pain in joints, lethargy, and other problems; caused by a deficiency of vitamin C (ascorbic acid).

Standard of identity   A list of specifications for the manufacture of certain foods that stipulates their required contents.

Starch   A polysaccharide composed of glucose molecules; the major form in which energy is stored in plants.

Stearic acid   A saturated fatty acid.

Sucrose   A disaccharide composed of glucose and fructose, often called "table sugar."

Sulfites   Agents used as preservatives in foods to eliminate bacteria, preserve freshness, prevent browning, and increase storage life; can cause acute asthma attacks, and even death, in people who are sensitive to them.

Teratogen   An agent with the potential of causing birth defects.

Thiamin   One of the B vitamins (B_1).

Thyroxine   Hormone containing iodine that is secreted by the thyroid gland.

Toxemia   A complication of pregnancy characterized by high blood pressure, edema, vomiting, presence of protein in the urine, and other symptoms.

Transferrin   A protein compound, the form in which iron is transported in the blood.

Triglyceride   A lipid containing glycerol and three fatty acids.

Trypsin   A digestive enzyme, produced in the pancreas, that breaks down protein.

Underweight   Body weight below an accepted norm by more than 10 percent.

United States Recommended Daily Allowance (USRDA)   The highest level of recommended intakes for population groups (except pregnant and lactating women); derived from the RDAs and used in food labeling.

Urea   The main nitrogenous component of urine, resulting from the breakdown of amino acids.

Uremia   A disease in which urea accumulates in the blood.

Vegan   A person who eats nothing derived from an animal; the strictest type of vegetarian.

Vitamin   Organic substance required by the body in small amounts to perform numerous functions.

Vitamin B complex   All known water-soluble vitamins except C; includes thiamin (B_1), riboflavin (B_2), pyridoxine (B_6), niacin, folic acid, cobalamin (B_{12}), pantothenic acid, and biotin.

Xerophthalmia   A disease of the eye resulting from vitamin A deficiency.

Index

Index

Test Your Knowledge Form

We encourage you to photocopy and use this page as a tool to assess how the articles in *Annual Editions* expand on the information in your textbook. By reflecting on the articles you will gain enhanced text information. You can also access this useful form on a product's book support Web site at *http://www.mhcls.com/online/*.

NAME: _____   DATE: _____

TITLE AND NUMBER OF ARTICLE: _____

BRIEFLY STATE THE MAIN IDEA OF THIS ARTICLE: _____

_____

LIST THREE IMPORTANT FACTS THAT THE AUTHOR USES TO SUPPORT THE MAIN IDEA:

_____

WHAT INFORMATION OR IDEAS DISCUSSED IN THIS ARTICLE ARE ALSO DISCUSSED IN YOUR TEXTBOOK OR OTHER READINGS THAT YOU HAVE DONE? LIST THE TEXTBOOK CHAPTERS AND PAGE NUMBERS:

_____

LIST ANY EXAMPLES OF BIAS OR FAULTY REASONING THAT YOU FOUND IN THE ARTICLE:

_____

LIST ANY NEW TERMS/CONCEPTS THAT WERE DISCUSSED IN THE ARTICLE, AND WRITE A SHORT DEFINITION:

We Want Your Advice

ANNUAL EDITIONS revisions depend on two major opinion sources: one is our Advisory Board, listed in the front of this volume, which works with us in scanning the thousands of articles published in the public press each year; the other is you—the person actually using the book. Please help us and the users of the next edition by completing the prepaid article rating form on this page and returning it to us. Thank you for your help!

ANNUAL EDITIONS: Nutrition 06/07

ARTICLE RATING FORM

Here is an opportunity for you to have direct input into the next revision of this volume.
We would like you to rate each of the articles listed below, using the following scale:

1. **Excellent: should definitely be retained**
2. **Above average: should probably be retained**
3. **Below average: should probably be deleted**
4. **Poor: should definitely be deleted**

Your ratings will play a vital part in the next revision.
Please mail this prepaid form to us as soon as possible.
Thanks for your help!

RATING	ARTICLE
	1. The Changing American Diet: A Report Card
	2. Pyramid Power
	3. Dietary Guidelines for Americans 2005: Executive Summary
	4. Healthier Eating
	5. 10 Megatrends in the Supermarket
	6. 51 Healthy Foods You Can Say "Yes" To
	7. Getting Personal with Nutrition
	8. The Slow Food Movement Picks Up Speed
	9. Who's Filling Your Grocery Bag?
	10. Moving Towards Healthful Sustainable Diets
	11. Omega-3 Choices: Fish or Flax?
	12. Revealing Trans Fats
	13. Good Carbs, Bad Carbs
	14. Are You Getting Enough of This Vitamin?
	15. Feast For Your Eyes: Nutrients That May Help Save Your Sight
	16. Get the Lead Out, What You Don't Know *Can* Hurt You
	17. Fortifying with Fiber
	18. Diet and Genes
	19. Metabolic Syndrome: Time for Action
	20. The Magnesium-Diabetes Connection
	21. Coffee, Spices, Wine: New Dietary Ammo Against Diabetes?
	22. Allergen Control
	23. Meeting Children's Nutritional Needs
	24. No One to Blame
	25. The Role of the School Nutrition Environment for Promoting the Health of Young Adolescents
	26. Still Hungry? Fattening Revelations—and New Mysteries—About the Hunger Hormone
	27. Eat More Weigh Less
	28. A Call to Action: Seeking Answers to Childhood Weight Issues

RATING	ARTICLE
	29. Social Change and Obesity Prevention
	30. Using Nutrition-Related Claims to Build a Healthful Diet
	31. Nutraceuticals & Functional Foods
	32. Herbal Foods: Are They Efficacious and Safe?
	33. Herbal Lottery
	34. The Latest Scoop on Soy
	35. Q & A on Functional Foods
	36. Are Your Supplements Safe?
	37. Food Colorings: Pigments Make Fruits and Veggies Extra Healthful
	38. Certified Organic
	39. Send in the Clones
	40. Seafood Safety: Is Something Fishy Going On?
	41. Suspect Produce: How To Be Safe From Contaminated Fruits, Vegetables
	42. Ensuring the Safety of Dietary Supplements
	43. Hunger and Mortality
	44. The Scourge of "Hidden Hunger:" Global Dimensions of Micronutrient Deficiencies
	45. Pushing Beyond the Earth's Limits
	46. Food Security, Overweight, and Agricultural Research—A View From 2003
	47. Confronting the Causes of Malnutrition: The Hidden Challenge of Micronutrient Deficiencies
	48. Contribution of Indigenous Knowledge and Practices in Food Technology to the Attainment of Food Security in Africa
	49. Taking Steps Toward Adequate Supermarket Access
	50. Helping Solve Hunger in America
	51. Assessment of Allergenic Potential of Genetically Modified Foods: An Agenda for Future Research

(Continued on next page)

BUSINESS REPLY MAIL
FIRST CLASS MAIL PERMIT NO. 551 DUBUQUE IA

POSTAGE WILL BE PAID BY ADDRESEE

McGraw-Hill Contemporary Learning Series
2460 KERPER BLVD
DUBUQUE, IA 52001-9902

NO POSTAGE
NECESSARY
IF MAILED
IN THE
UNITED STATES

llıllıııılıllllıııllllıııııllllılılılılllıııılılılıll

ABOUT YOU

Name

Date

Are you a teacher? ❑ A student? ❑
Your school's name

Department

Address City State Zip

School telephone #

YOUR COMMENTS ARE IMPORTANT TO US!

Please fill in the following information:
For which course did you use this book?

Did you use a text with this ANNUAL EDITION? ❑ yes ❑ no
What was the title of the text?

What are your general reactions to the *Annual Editions* concept?

Have you read any pertinent articles recently that you think should be included in the next edition? Explain.

Are there any articles that you feel should be replaced in the next edition? Why?

Are there any World Wide Web sites that you feel should be included in the next edition? Please annotate.

May we contact you for editorial input? ❑ yes ❑ no
May we quote your comments? ❑ yes ❑ no